Penny Meakin is originally from the East End of London and now lives and works on the edge of the Peak District in Staffordshire, where she has a passion for gardening, writing, running, philately and dabbles in art; making pictures out of English postage stamps.

She is married with a large family and currently teaches a variety of subjects at a local University, where she has spent twenty happy years entertaining and teaching teenagers.

Dedication

This book is dedicated to the brave young men of the Sheffield City Battalion

Where so ever they now lie

A Soldier's Cemetery

Written by 12/525 John William Streets who was killed and missing in action on 1st July 1916. He was aged 31.

Behind that long and lonely trenched line
To which men come and go, where brave men die,
There is a yet unmarked and unknown shrine,
A broken plot, a soldier's cemetery.

There lie the flower of youth, the men who scorn'd
To live (so died) when languished Liberty:
Across their graves flowerless and unadorned
Still scream the shells of each artillery.

When war shall cease this lonely unknown spot
Of many a pilgrimage will be the end,
And flowers will shine in this now barren plot
And fame upon it through the years descend:
But many a heart upon each simple cross
Will hang the grief, the memory of its loss.

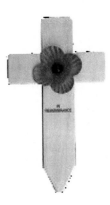

Foreword

"The Meakin Diaries are an honest, unpretentious account of one young, Sheffield man's journey to the Battle of the Somme, and the lovely Penny Meakin, with whom I spent a fascinating afternoon filming, has done a tremendous job bringing them to life for the general reader.
I heartily recommend this book to anyone interested in the First World War and those who fought in it."

Sir Tony Robinson

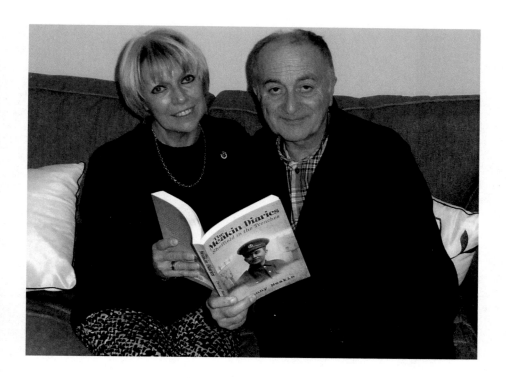

Penny Meakin

WORLD WAR ONE

THE MEAKIN DIARIES

SHEFFIELD IN THE TRENCHES

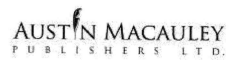
AUSTIN MACAULEY
PUBLISHERS LTD.

ISBN 9781849638883 (Paperback)
ISBN 9781849638890 (E-Book)
ISBN 9781849638890 (Hardback)

www.austinmacauley.com

First Published (2014)
Second Edition Published (2016)

Austin Macauley Publishers Ltd.
25 Canada Square
Canary Wharf
London
E14 5LB

Acknowledgments

To Frank, for writing his diary each and every day during the most atrocious and terrifying conditions.

To my wonderful husband Nick, for his help, support and patience during the long hours of typing and research, and for accompanying me on many occasions when visiting the Battlefields and for proof reading the many versions of this book ... and the cooking of wonderful meals when I was 'in my trench'.

To Dr Tony Price for his help and guidance in the early stages of reading the diaries, and for lending me his copy of Major and Mrs Holt's 'Battlefield Guide to the Somme', which I managed to get covered in mud and, of course, replaced.

To Ralph Gibson for his help and support in the early stages of development and allowing me to use his wonderful book 'The Sheffield City Battalion' as a source of invaluable reference.

To the York and Lancaster Museum in Rotherham, who put me in touch with Ralph Gibson and who passed my name on to the BBC as an 'expert' on the Battalion in order to feature them in the programme 'Time Flyers', with producer Sandy Raffan.

To my dear friend Roz Chimes at BBC Radio Stoke for allowing me on air on many occasions to discuss this book and to BBC Radio Sheffield for featuring this book on air.

To Hayley Knight and her team at Austin Macauley Publishers for their invaluable support in the final publication of the book and subsequent additions.

To Colonel I.G. Norton for checking my work for military accuracy and for inviting me to the Somme for the York and Lancaster Regiment Centenary Tour in 2016.

To the wonderful Jeremy Freeston of Dragonshead Productions, who brought Frank Meakin to 'life' by featuring him on a Discovery Channel programme 'The Somme the First 24 Hours' – what a life changing phone call that was!

To the amazing Sir Tony Robinson who visited our house one wet and windy November night, with a film crew, to record an interview with me for 'The Somme, the First 24 Hours' featured on the Discovery Channel and for taking the time from his very busy schedule to write a Foreword for this book.

Finally and most importantly, to the brave young men of the Sheffield City Battalion, to whom this book is dedicated.

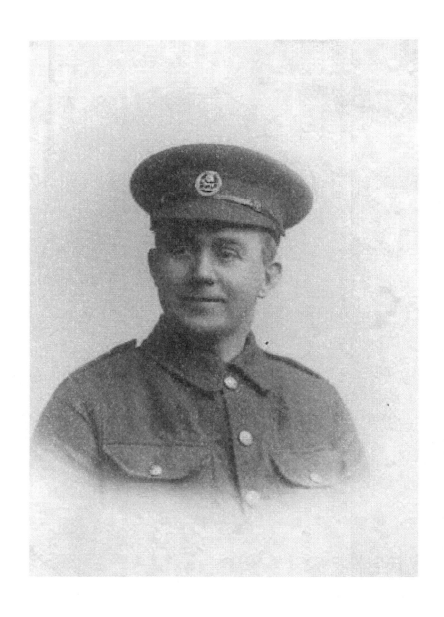

The Diaries of Frank Meakin
A Tribute to the 12th York and Lancaster Sheffield City
Battalion

Contents

Preface

Following a career change in 1995, I found myself with the luxury of having several weeks free in the summer of 1996. My husband Nick had always spoken of his Grandfather's diaries, which had been passed on to him from his Father. I had looked at them on several occasions and as a former diarist myself, they seemed absolutely fascinating. They consisted of two rather battered volumes, one for the 1915 leading up to March 1916 and one for the whole of 1917 with 'notes' for the beginning of 1918. I began to read them and found that I could, with practice, decipher the beautiful, tiny writing. It was obvious that the writer had been in action somewhere in France and on one occasion had actually killed a German in self-defence. Exciting stuff!

My knowledge of the First World War was pretty scant. Having been brought up in Hatfield in Hertfordshire, history lessons at school always focussed on the Romans and the Elizabethans because of the proximity to Verulamium and Hatfield House and the First World War was far too recent for the nuns at my convent to even consider. I always had an interest in both World Wars, mainly because of my maternal Grandmother with whom I stayed each school holiday in East Ham in London. I was very aware of the Battle of the Somme and like most people, knew that it took place on 1st July 1916. I was bitterly disappointed that the diaries did not include that date.

During a family visit to Nick's parents in September 1996, I asked about Frank and was given the standard response, that he was in the Battle of the Somme but he went to sleep. I had always known that this could not be true, as he would have been shot if he had slept. Upon leaving, Nick's father gave me another small diary, explaining that although it was for 1916, it did not include the 1st July. That night I began to read the new diary. Yes it was true that the 1st July was not in there but the 18th July 1916 certainly was. Frank had retrieved his diary on that day, having put away his personal effects prior to the Battle of the Somme. He then recounted the events of the previous three weeks.

History was jumping out of the pages and what I was reading was quite simply incredible - my quest had begun. Who was he? Which Battalion was he in? Why? Where? Nobody knew. My life changed dramatically that night, I was 'in my trench' and my obsession had started.

The next few weeks consisted of reading, taking notes, circling places on Michelin maps of France and buying any books that Nick and I could find on the First World War. One place kept cropping up - a small town in northern France called Serre...

We purchased a copy of 'War Walks' by Richard Holmes. Ironically we had watched the accompanying T.V. series, little knowing the importance of the episode relating to the Somme. Part of that episode had actually featured the town of Serre and there it was written in black and white – the 12th York and Lancaster, Sheffield City Battalion. My research had begun.

I concentrated in these early stages on what was written about the 1st July and we booked our first of many trips to the Somme the following month. In the intervening weeks we read as much as we could and then we set off, armed with a copy of 'Major and Mrs Holt's Guide to the Somme Battlefields'.

We visited Sheffield Memorial Park and the trio of Cemeteries that lie in No Man's Land. We visited the only piece of preserved British Front Line on the Somme, which was exactly where the Battalion had fought from on the 1st July 1916. We found many of Frank's 'pals' that are mentioned in the diary, the majority of whom lie in Queen's Military Cemetery in Serre or are listed on the Thiepval Memorial. It was an amazing and life changing trip.

My quest over the last fifteen years has been to get these amazing diaries into print. It is so important, not only for Frank's grandchildren and great grandchildren, but for the relatives of anyone mentioned therein. There has been a great deal of research involved. I have attempted to explain the 'language' that I did not understand but most importantly, I wanted to impart as much information about the individuals that are mentioned in those precious volumes - the unsung heroes of the Sheffield City Battalion to whom this book is dedicated.

Introduction

Frank Meakin was born on 16th March 1881 in Duffield, Derbyshire, the son of William Francis Meakin, a Railway Accountant Clerk born in Chellaston Derbyshire and Henrietta Meakin, born in Salford Lancashire. Frank was the eldest of the family, having a sister, Margaret, who was two years his junior and a brother, Arthur, who was seven years his junior. Arthur later served in the Army Cyclists Corp which was active during the First World War, controlling the Army's bicycle infantry.

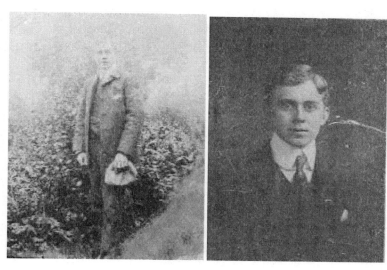

Frank was well educated and attended The Masters School in London where he studied architecture. His first job was working for the Midland Railway Company in the Engineer's Office located in Crewe and then Derby. He then progressed and was employed as an Architect and Surveyor at Sheffield City Council based in the Town Hall. It was whilst working in Derby that he met Dorothy Jane Smith, affectionately known as Doll.

Dorothy was the daughter of Sophia Jane Smith and Herbert Dagley Smith and lived with her three sisters, Maud Ethel, Lucy and Sophia Gladys in a large Victorian house called the Poplars in Elvaston Lane in Alvaston, Derbyshire.

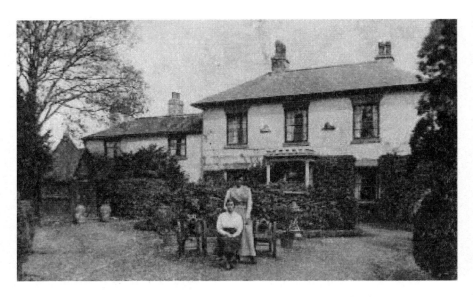

Poplars, the Family home in Alvaston. Doll can be see standing behind her sister.

On the 3rd April 1915, only seven months after joining the Sheffield City Battalion, Frank and Doll were married in Alvaston. They had been married for only six short months when Frank left for active service in Egypt and France. Sadly, for the duration of those six months Frank was stationed at the Redmires Training Camp situated on the moors above Sheffield. It for that reason that when he eventually returned to Sheffield in 1918, he was so excited as their married life together 'was about to begin'.

12/729 Lance Corporal Francis Meakin was a member of the Sheffield City Battalion for almost the whole duration of its existence, joining up with his colleagues from the Town Hall on the first day. He was discharged on the grounds of ill health twenty two days before the Battalion was disbanded forever. Frank kept his diaries throughout his entire campaign. Orders were given that banned the keeping of diaries during 'active' service. It is perhaps no coincidence that Frank, who was somewhat of a rebel, began his diaries on his first day of 'active' service and kept them until the day that he was discharged.

The 'Meakin Diaries' are virtually unique. There were many diarists from the Battalion who kept diaries prior to the Battle of the Somme but very few survived to recount the activities from July 1st onwards. Frank's diaries are well written and include vivid descriptions of the Battle of the Somme and consequent aftermath, the Battle of Arras and 2nd Battle of Vimy Ridge. There are also a variety of accounts including: a member of the Battalion who was shot for desertion; members of the Battalion being gassed; their squalid living conditions; being covered in lice and rats; aeroplane activity; accounts of one to one combats with the German Army and the shooting of Germans in self-defence. The diaries also depict that what began as a wonderful 'adventure' for King and Country, but quickly fell into despair and disillusionment. The diaries

14

also include entries every day about food and what became, because of his non-declared diabetic condition, Frank's obsession.

Frank's story, which begins in December 1915 as he departs on his 'adventure' to Egypt, is an inevitably sad one, with a tragic and unexpected ending.

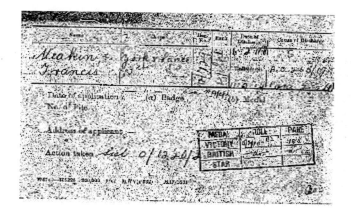

The war record of 12/729 Francis Meakin

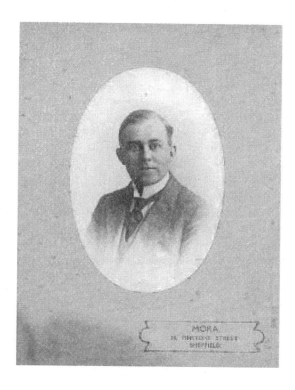

1

The 'Coffee and Bun Boys' – A Battalion is Born

It is the 3rd September 1914 and there is an air of great excitement in the Main Reception Room of the Town Hall in Sheffield. Frank Meakin, an architect working for Sheffield Council at the Town Hall, has arrived, with some of his friends and colleagues, to enrol as a volunteer for a new Battalion that would be for the men of Sheffield. Standing with him in the queue are **Percy Richards,**[1] **Edward Rogers,**[2] **Gilbert Unwin,**[3] **Harry Todd,**[4] **Horace Dowty,**[5] **Alf Thorne, Harry Hale, George Saddler**[6] and **Mr F. E. Pearce Edwards,**[7] the City Architect who has come along for morale support.

The room is packed with hundreds of men from Sheffield. Men of all ages and shapes and sizes - professional men: teachers, bank managers, business men, clerks and of course architects. They all had one common aim, to help their country in its hour of need.

Six weeks earlier, Europe had been plunged into war.

The 'Pals' Battalions were formed following a recruiting drive by the War Office in 1914. Across the country tens of thousands of men rushed to recruiting offices to join up as enthusiastic volunteers to help with the war effort. Men from similar working trades, professions, and sports or social clubs were encouraged to enlist together. The tragic consequences of this idea would be only too apparent when they all fought together. Volunteers for the Sheffield City Battalion were sought from the professional classes and specifically from Sheffield University, ex public school men, lawyers, clerks, journalists and architects. They became known by the Barnsley Pals, who were predominantly miners, as the 'Coffee and Buns Boys', as they were middle class and the 'cream' of Sheffield.

---

[1] **12/757 Private Percy Charles Richards** – was killed in action on 3rd May 1916. He is buried in the Sucrerie Military Cemetery, Serre.
[2] **12/767 Private Edward Gordon Rogers** – was killed in action on 3rd May 1916. He is buried in the Sucrerie Military Cemetery, Serre.
[3] **12/807 Private Gilbert Unwin** - was killed in action on 3rd May 1916. He is buried in the Sucrerie Military Cemetery, Serre.
[4] **12/802 Private Harold Todd** - was killed in action on 3rd May 1916. He is buried in the Sucrerie Military Cemetery, Serre.
[5] **12/638 Private Horace Bradley Dowty** – was killed in action on 15th May 1916. He is buried in the Sucrerie Military Cemetery, Serre.
[6] **12/663 Private Harry Thomas Hale, 12/799 Private Alfred James (Alf) Thorne, 12/771 Private George Henry Saddler** – were all killed in action on 1st July 1916. All three are buried in Queens Military Cemetery, within a few feet of each other.
[7] **Mr F. E. Pearce Edwards** was the City Architect at Sheffield Town Hall. He became a lifelong friend of Franks and also assisted in the design of the City Battalion Camp at Redmires.

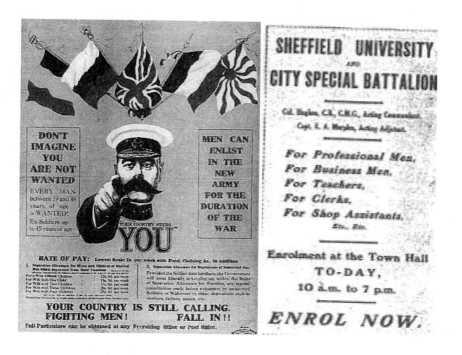

Within the first few days 1,400 forms had been completed and handed in to the Lord Mayor and his helpers. Enrolment included a cross examination and the completion of documentation by over forty volunteer clerks, followed by a medical examination by a small army of volunteer Doctors. Rejections were numerous and over the course of the first few days only 1,000 men were actually recruited. Frank knew that he was diabetic and did not declare the fact when enlisting. Had he done so, he would not have been passed fit for the service of his Country and this amazing story would not be told.

The Sheffield City Battalion was one of twelve Battalions in the 31st Division. All but two of the 'Pals' Battalions were recruited from Yorkshire, the others being from Durham and Lancashire. In the county of Yorkshire alone, within a matter of days, several Battalions had been formed at their maximum strength of 800-900 men each. These Battalions were attached to existing regiments and given a new Battalion number followed by the word 'Service', so the 12th Service Battalion, York & Lancaster Regiment became known firstly, as the Sheffield University and City Special Battalion, York and Lancaster Regiment, later to be officially titled 'Sheffield City Battalion, 12th (Service) Battalion, York and Lancaster Regiment. There was some criticism that Sheffield had only produced one Battalion when smaller towns such as Barnsley had produced two, but this was put down to the fact that Sheffield had already fully recruited two battalions of the Territorial Force; the 1st and 2nd / 4th (Hallamshire) Battalions of the York and Lancaster Regiment, as well as Regiments of Royal Artillery and Royal Engineers and others.

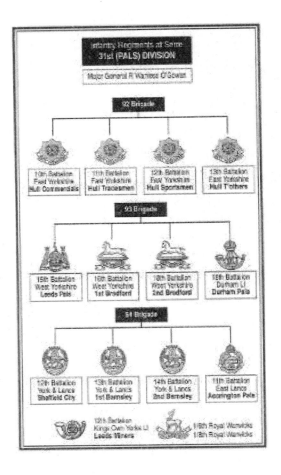

The Battalion was made up of four Companies:

A Company consisted of men from the University, some teachers, bankers and local business men, some of whom were earning £500 a year.

B Company consisted of men from the districts outside of Sheffield including Penistone and Chesterfield who were bankers, teachers, students, railway men and tradesmen.

C Company was a contingent of teachers, bankers, students, teachers, accountants and employees from the Town Hall. Frank belonged to this Company.

D Company comprised of mainly teachers, bankers, students and reporters from the Sheffield Daily Telegraph.

The first home of the Battalion was the Norfolk Barracks in Edmund Road, Sheffield. Training began on 15th September and men were marched to Bramall Lane Football Ground which the Directors of the football ground had kindly offered as a parade ground, an offer that they would later regret when the turf did not wear well. Other grounds were also used at Norfolk Road, Queens Road and Norfolk Park.

This strange mix of men who ranged in age from 19 to 35 (Frank was 34), dressed in their own clothes, some in bow ties, were described by their Commanding Officer, Colonel H. Hughes, as 'a crowd, a good looking crowd but a CROWD'. The first performance of the recruits was quite a shambles but they were a highly intelligent 'crowd' and learned very quickly.

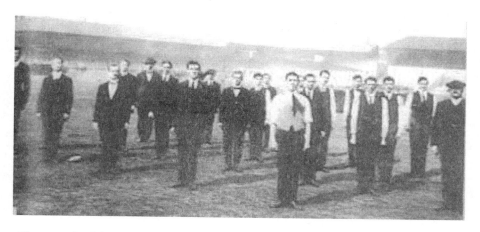

Photograph of the men parading at Bramall Lane Football Ground (please note the bow ties!)

For nearly three months the men lived in their own homes and those that lived outside of the area were provided with lodgings within the City. They received their first uniform but the sudden demand for khaki on the textile industry meant that the Battalion was issued with a temporary uniform which was blue/grey in colour. Some of the men were concerned that they would be mistaken for postmen. It was not until 1915 that they received their khaki uniforms, the delay being put down to the lack of khaki dye that was obtained from, of all countries, Germany.

On 10th October 1914 a new Commanding Officer, **Lieutenant Colonel C.V. Mainwaring**[8] took over from Colonel Hughes. He had vast military experience and was an ideal candidate to train the Battalion.

Once the men had reached a basic level of fitness they began a series of route marches one of which took them to Redmires, where the construction of their future camp was taking place on the site of an old racecourse. Frank's colleague and superior at the Town Hall; Mr F. E. Pearce Edwards had helped with the design of camp and local traders supplied furniture and other fittings.

---

[8] **Commanding Officer, Lieutenant Colonel C. V. Mainwaring** – was Commander of the battalion for a short time but was forced to stand down in September 1915 due to ill health as a result of his previous action in the Far East. He kept an interest in the Battalion throughout their campaign and later became President of the '12th Club' the survivors association.

Redmires was 1000 feet above sea level and was situated in a rather bleak location. Huts were raised off of the ground and were constructed of wood and measured 60 feet long by 20 feet wide, with a single door at one end. Lighting was by gas and there was a coal burning stove in the centre of each hut.

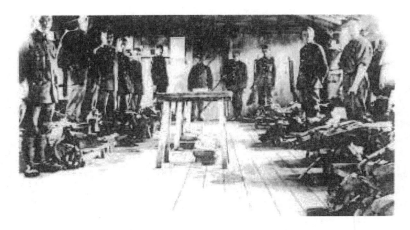

A photo of one of the interior of one of the wooden huts at Redmires.
Frank can be seen standing second on the left. In the centre is CSM Ellis.

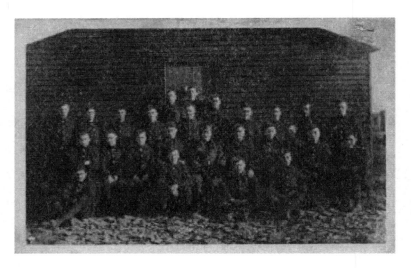

A photo of 'C' Company outside of their hut at Redmires
Frank can be seen standing in the centre behind Capt Colley

The Battalion marched here on 5th December 1914 and were joined by 13th and 14th Yorks and Lancaster Regiments, Barnsley Pals and the 10th Lincolnshire Regiment and were formed into 115th Infantry Brigade. In addition to the huts, a YMCA was built, which was successfully used as a Concert Hall, canteen and Post Office and there were also quiet areas where the men could write letters. Over the Christmas period, the men were allowed to return home for a short period of leave but the rota was staggered so that routine duties could continue.

The following months saw the men taking part in musket training and simulated attacks, digging trenches and a variety of physical training, which included quarrying and road making. It was not for the faint hearted. The weather conditions were atrocious and some of the men fell ill with pneumonia and as a result two members of the Battalion **died.**[9] Training on the moors and in such dreadful conditions stood the men in good stead and as a result they could outmarch other regiments and could triumph over them in athletic events.

On 9th May 1915 the men were given orders to move to Cannock Chase and were also told that due to a re-organisation, they were now part of 115 Infantry Brigade in 38th Division along with both Barnsley Battalions and 10th (Service) Battalion, Lincolnshire Regiment. This did not last long as by May 1915 they had been transferred to 94 Brigade in 31st Division (all part of the new fourth Army) and the Lincolns had been replaced by 11th (Service) Battalion, East Lancashire Regiment known as the Accrington Pals. The 'Coffee and Bun Boys' regarded the Barnsley Pals as a rough and ready lot and the Barnsleys were equally unimpressed by this 'white collar bunch from Sheffield' but over the coming months a mutual respect developed between them and they soon had a reputation as the best brigade in the Division. That mutual respect would become increasingly important when they were in action together on 1st July 1916.

Leaving Redmires was a big event both for the men and for the City of Sheffield. It was unfortunate that the timing of the train leaving for Stafford was extremely early, so they paraded at 5am and as a result of this and lack of notice, some people missed the departure of 'Sheffield's Own'. Many did turn out to see them off and the Hallamshires and **R.E.**[10] Bands played them through the City. The Lord Mayor addressed them outside the Town Hall and they then marched off to the station, through crowds of relatives and friends. There were emotional scenes at the station, as relatives thought that this would be the last time that they would see them – and it many cases it was. For miles after leaving the City they were cheered by people who were standing by the railway line.

Home was now Penkridge Bank Camp, on a high part of Cannock Chase, close to Rugeley. Cannock Chase looked very different in 1915 to the Area of Outstanding Natural Beauty that it is today; it was treeless, bleak moorland covered in deer. The men were now completing 'advanced training' which included attacks, tactical movements and night attacks. Route marches became more frequent and longer and those hard months at Redmires began to pay off. On 13th July 1915, there was a full parade of the Sheffield City Battalion and they were formally taken over by the War Office.

---

[9] **12/133 Private Charles Haydn Handforth** died on 8th February 1915 in the 3rd Northern General Hospital and **12/741 Private John Charles Ortton** died on 20th February 1915. He was buried with full military honours on 23rd February at the City Road Cemetery.

[10] **R.E.** – Royal Engineers.

The Battalion was turning into a well-equipped and well trained force. During the hot summer of 1915, the men were often called upon to deal with the many fires that broke out on the Chase. This resulted in a specific fire piquet of over 100 men being established. There were many route marches and on one occasion in July, the men, in full kit, embarked on a sixteen mile route march across Cannock Chase in blazing sunshine. It took over six hours and over 80 fell out with heat exhaustion.

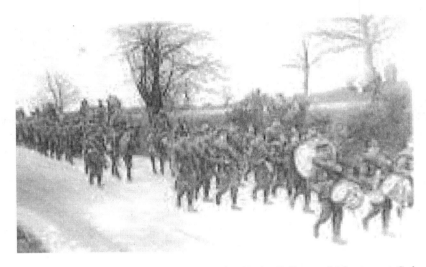

The City Battalion on a route march. Captain W. A. Colley and Lieutenant Colonel Mainwaring are the officers who are mounted.
Frank can be seen as the third man on the right in the group of marching men.

Orders had been given to move to Ripon and on the 31st July they caught the train from Rugeley to Ripon where they were based in the Fourth Army Training Centre. The camp was a large complex of camps located to the south of Ripon. The main emphasis of training here was 'musketry'[11] which included all aspects of weapon training, handling and shooting. At this point the new Commander of 31st Division, **Major General R. Wanless O'Gowan** [12] made his first visit to the Battalion. He was very impressed with the Battalion's turnout, physique and their handling of weapons.

Aside from their training, there was little else for the men to do at Ripon. Many spent their time in the town and many made visits to Ripon Cathedral and nearby Fountains Abbey. All members of the Battalion were allocated leave and on 10th September 1915 they celebrated the first year of their formation. A

---

[11] **Musketry** – a term which had survived from the days when the infantry had been armed with muskets.
[12] **Major General R. Wanless O'Gowan** – commanded, apart from a few short absences, the Division throughout the whole of their campaign until they were disbanded in February 1918.

celebration concert was arranged by the **Padre**[13] and many members of the Battalion took part. **Sergeant Roberts**[14] was the pianist and he was accompanied by **Captain Woolhouse**[15] and **Sergeant Crozier**[16] as the singers.

The Battalion left Ripon on the night of 25th September and began the journey to Sailsbury Plain, which was to be their base to complete their training prior to going abroad. Here they were based at Hurdcott Camp which was built in the grounds of Hurdcott House, close to the town of Wilton. During this time Lieutenant Colonel Mainwaring left because of ill health and was replaced by **Lieutenant Colonel J. A. Crossthwaite**.[17]

At this time there was a 'Munitions Scandal' which began to have an impact on the Battalion. Since the beginning of the war there had been a shortage of shells which manifested itself at the Battle of Loos, when attacks by the British infantry had failed because of a shortage of high explosive shells. The shortage was due mainly to the lack of a trained labour force in the munitions industry as many of the skilled workers required to run the factories had volunteered in 1914 to join the war effort. Many articles about the situation were written in 'The Times' but Lord Kitchener refused to accept that there was a problem, demonstrating how out of touch he was with the situation.

A Ministry of Munitions was set up under Lloyd George and one of their first tasks was to re-engage the workforce where they were needed. This meant that all men were interviewed by members of the Ministry and if they were considered to be essential to industry, they were forced to return to their jobs and were released from the Army. There were fifty men from the Battalion that returned to their pre-war jobs and a total of 40,000 throughout the Army as a whole.

On 16th November the Battalion, along with the rest of the 31st Division, moved to Larkhill Camp, which was located about ten miles north of Sailsbury and one mile from Stonehenge. Here they stayed in very basic accommodation. The reason for the move was to complete the musketry course which required the men to complete training of a more practical nature, which also required them to fire from trenches. There were good facilities for the machine gunners to practice at the Larkhill ranges. Here the men were finally issued with their **SMLE**[18] rifles.

It was while the Battalion was training at Larkhill, that orders were received for the 31st Division to go to France, which caused great excitement and

---

[13] **Captain J. F. Colquhoun** – became the Divisional Padre and won a Military Cross in 1918.

[14] **12/761 Sergeant A. W. Roberts** – took part in the attack on 1st July and was wounded in action.

[15] **Captain E. G. G. Woolhouse** – commissioned 18th September 1914 and served as Adjutant from 10th October 1914 to 16th January 1915 when he resigned. He was left out of the attack on 1st July 1916 when he arrived the next day with 80 reinforcements.

[16] **12/628 Sergeant Henry Cecil Crozier** - won a Military Medal (MM) on the night of 15th / 16th May 1916, a few weeks before being killed on 1st July 1916. He died helping eight men who had been wounded by the same shell and he had won the MM in similar circumstances. His body was never found and he is commemorated on the Thiepval Memorial.

[17] **Lieutenant Colonel J. A. Crossthwaite** – Regular Officer previously with the Durham Light Infantry. He fell ill on 30th June 1916 as a result of wounds that he received in Ypres in 1915.

[18] **SMLE** - Short Magazine Lee Enfield, sometimes referred to as a 'smelly' rather than S.M.L.E.

apprehension. **Captain A. N. Cousins**[19] was selected as the Battalion's representative on the Divisional Advance Party and became the **Adjutant**[20] in 1917.

The Battalion marched back to Hurdcott, having completed their musketry training and in the intervening days all members of the Battalion were able to take a few days precious leave.

The final orders came through and there was some disappointment when the destination was announced as Egypt. Final preparations were made and all the men were issued with sola topees (sun helmets) in preparation.

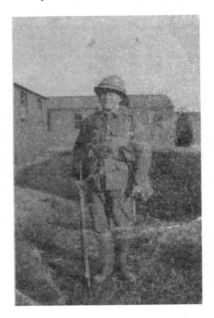

Frank at Hurdcott Camp having been issued with his new sola topee or sun helmet, in preparation for Egypt.

Kit bags were packed and the canteen stayed open all night as the men were due to leave early the next morning. On their final day they received many farewell messages, most notably from the King who wrote:

'Officers, NCOs and men of the 31st Division, on the eve of your departure for active service I send you my heartfelt good wishes. It is a bitter disappointment to me that owing to an unfortunate accident I am unable to see the Division on parade before it leaves England, but I can assure you that my

---

[19] **Captain A. N. Cousins** – a Sheffield University student. He was killed in action on 7th December 1917 and is buried in Rolincourt Military Cemetery.

[20] **Adjutant** – a staff officer in the army, air force, or marine corps who assists the commanding officer and is responsible especially for correspondence.

thoughts are with you all. Your period of training has been long and arduous but the time has now come for you to prove on the field of battle the results of your instruction. From the good accounts that I have received of the Division I am confident that the high tradition of the British Army is safe in your hands and that with your comrades now in the field you will maintain the unceasing efforts necessary to bring this war to a victorious end. Goodbye and God Speed. George V.'

On 20th December the Battalion then travelled by train to Keyham Dockyard at Devonport to board the **SS Nestor**.[21] This is where Frank's story begins, as they embark on their 'adventure' to Egypt.

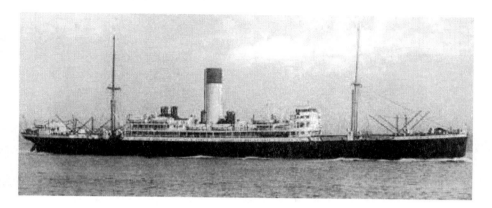

The SS Nestor owned by Blue Funnel Lines

---

[21] **SS Nestor / Holt Line** – The SS Nestor was owned by John Holt (Blue Funnel Lines) based in India Buildings, Liverpool. Prior to the war she had carried passengers and cargo to Australia. The cargo decks had been converted into a series of troop messes. Blue Funnel Lines lost 30 ships during the First World War.

2
Egypt – The 'Adventure' Begins

1915

December 20 Monday
We embarked on the SS Nestor of Liverpool, which belongs to the John Holt Line but is now called 'T71', at about 2 o'clock at Keyham Dockyard, Devonport. We were No.9 Platoon of course, bagged for fatigue, rolling bales of blankets from the wharf to the deck. We were said to be sailing at 5pm but didn't. There was very nice cold mutton served at 4pm which was tea with bread and cheese at 5pm. We then drew blankets and hammocks but there were not enough hooks to hang them on, so the result was tight packing and head and feet like sardines. I rolled out of mine in an approved manner and then had a most comfortable night.

December 21 Tuesday
We had coffee, stew, bread and butter for breakfast, which was very nice. We paraded at 10am for a roll call and were then were inoculated against cholera which was almost painless. The hypodermic needle slipped in with scarcely a twinge, much different to the typhus inoculation in the breast. We all then had to parade in our life belts to make sure that everyone had one. The voyage started about 11.40 am, the weather was fine but rather dull, the Sound (Plymouth Sound) was very pretty and interesting, dotted with islands and branching creeks as it is. There was much cheering from other boats and garrisons on nearby forts. Our band performed very creditably playing the Regimental March, 'Keep the Home Fires Burning' and 'God Save the King'. Dinner: soup and rabbit, beautifully cooked and very much enjoyed. We passed a British submarine in the sound and were escorted by two destroyers which rolled fearfully giving us an idea that the sea is fairly rough, though our boat is 14,000 tonnes and should hold steady. Many evidently don't find it so though, for only about half eventually turn up for tea. Lots are drawn among us for two permanent orderlies to our mess of 18. The blow falls on **Hale**[22] and myself.

I take over from the present day's orderlies before tea, as they are knocked out. Bread and butter with apple and pineapple jam, very good which made a good meal, then washed up and cleaned away. Bending must have brought on my first spell of sickness, for I went out and lost my days rations immediately after. I heaved again later on and then went into a slung hammock. It is reported off Ushant light, the destroyers have left us and we were now in the Bay of Biscay. I turned in at about 7 o'clock and had a good night. The canteen was

---

[22] **12/663 Private Harry Thomas Hale** – was killed in action 1st July 1916, he is buried in Queen's Military Cemetery, Serre.

opened in afternoon and I bought 50 Capstan cigs, no duty paid, so Capstan tobacco 2/- per 1/4 lb tin.

December 22 Wednesday

I am feeling a bit rocky but packed a ripping breakfast and felt much more stable; coffee, porridge and mackerel, the latter said to have been caught from the boat that morning. I was grieved to see loads of food being thrown overboard, as so few were in a state to eat them. I managed a couple of cigs but with no great relish. The cold headwind was enough to blow one over. We had soup, boiled salt beef (very hard), potatoes & parsnips, prunes and rice for dinner. We passed a big three-mast sailing boat, tacking in our direction and dead ahead. Later we didn't seem to be moving very quickly. We had bully beef and pickle, the usual lovely rolls and butter and I had a mouthful or two of tea and then had to rush to 'unload'. I came back and made very creditable repast, which I lost again.

I turned into my hammock about 7 o'clock again and it seemed a very rough night, there was a fearful seething of spray and hammering of spares on the deck overhead, I was rather disturbed but on the whole I had a good night's rest. I wondered however folks can take sea voyages for pleasure.

December 23 Thursday

I felt very groggy before breakfast but packed it down with porridge and liver and bacon. I managed to get through washing up and inspection before unloading again. I feel much better now and started on the diary. Our stern gun has just been fired, it is only a small quick fire but quite a jar – what must a 17 inch be like? We were supposed to have crossed the Bay of Biscay early in the morning so we must have passed Cap Finistere and be somewhere in the open Atlantic off Portugal now. Anyway, the chopiness of the bay seems to have given way to usual big Atlantic rollers. The weather is dull but fine and much warmer, and I am sitting without an overcoat. We had suet raisin pudding, soup, roast beef, peas and potatoes for dinner. It is a great feat for mess orderlies to toboggan down about 15 feet of steps with the mess dinner - yesterday I saw a man repeat the performance with the second lot that he fetched. The waves are occasionally sweeping the decks now. I was waiting outside the Galley and one came over the forecastle decks onto Galley roof and gracefully cascaded, dowsing my back. We are expected to arrive at Gibraltar tomorrow but here we are considerably off our course to avoid submarines, so we may not get there until Sunday. We only have bread and butter for our tea. The boat rolls fearfully but I feel that I have my sea legs at last and am out of danger from being ill again. Sling hammock at 6pm and read until lights out at 9.30, very comfortable indeed.

December 24 Friday (Christmas Eve)

Breakfast; coffee, Irish stew and porridge

I went for hot water after serving as last time and I wasted three quarters of my cold breakfast - not again! I had to hand scrub the mess deck this morning which was too much work. The day was mild and breezy with a good sea and a very fine sunrise. Dinner: soup, roast mutton, potatoes, cabbage, apple rings and rice. We waited for one hour after dinner for hot water. Hale turned sickly, and it looks as though he might be starting when the rest of us are better. We are due off Cape St Vincent at 3pm. Bread, butter and cheese for tea. There is a report that all letters are to be posted by 7pm, so I sent 7 or 8 sheets off to Doll and then read in hammock till lights out.

December 25 Saturday (Christmas Day)

The boat is now sailing northeast, so I judge that we must be turning up towards Gibraltar from North African coast. There is another fine sunrise and the weather getting quite warm. Breakfast: porridge, liver and bacon. There was no hot water till 9.30am. Drizzle sets in, the first rain since sailing. We also passed two steamers homeward bound. Dinner: Beef, potatoes, soup and 'ship' plum pudding. Like it better than the real thing. I notice that our letters have not yet been cleared. Stew for tea – what an insult – no Xmas Dinner! Our boat is making complete turns and going dead slow, evidently waiting for the right to pass Gibraltar. **Colley**[23] left cigs on all C Company tables except ours, being among D Company we got missed. We passed the rock of Gibraltar at about 8.30pm and the weather cleared. The straight seemed narrower that I imagined. The black mass of the **Costa**[24] on starboard side was looming large. The lights of town opposite Gibraltar seem very close – probably Tangiers. Searchlights were playing all round from Gibraltar and signals flashing about, the Rock was quite discernible with lights along both coasts. Today is the rottenest Xmas I have ever spent, absolutely no remembrance to celebrate the day.

December 26 Sunday (Boxing Day)

The most glorious sunrise I've ever seen, the colours were indescribable; deep orange predominantly and a beautiful balcony breeze. We are in the Mediterranean at last, with the North African coast just discernible. Orders - men orderlies only on for two days – Hooray! I draw breakfast; porridge then tripe and onions ad lib. I then went back and drew second allowance – the best meal for ages. I am enjoying my first morning of freedom. Dinner: Soup, mutton and rice pudding. I played solo this afternoon and evening and lost 3/6d. We are sailing quite close to the Algerian coast – only 8 to 10 miles away, one chain of the most rugged mountains, with sandy tracks discernible over passes between and also what look like houses. We had buns for tea.

December 27 Monday

I am on submarine guard

Breakfast: porridge & currie and rice. We are a bit nearer still to the coast, the wild ruggedness is more pronounced than ever. The coast disappeared about

---

[23] **Captain W. A. Colley** - killed in action 1st July 1916. He had a premonition of his death just before going over the top but despite this, was first out of the trench. Soon after he was hit by a shell and killed. This gallant gentleman had been a leading business man in Sheffield and was a member of the Council. He should not really have been at the front and certainly should not have been leading a company into action at the age of 47. His remains were never found and he commemorated on the Thiepval Memorial.

[24] **Costa** – probably the Costa de la Luz.

11am, probably where it dips away southwards. Dinner: rabbit, soup, prunes and rice. While writing to Mother, I looked up to see a mountainous land close to port. I thought at first it must be one of the European islands. I then saw we had turned completely around and were going back on our tracks, we must have been warned of a **submarine**.[25] I was late for tea, so only the smallest bit of bread was left, the cook acknowledged the shortage but said only one oven was available, the other was probably monopolised by his 1000 buns sold by him to cooks and retailed to troops at ½d, I wonder if our flour goes astray too. I couldn't get near to any of those 2d sandwiches either, which are made of meat which the cooks sneak into the galley. The cook gives me ripping big lump of cake though. We turned back east again about 9pm.

December 28 Tuesday
I am on ship guard. Breakfast: steak. We seemed to be about where we turned back yesterday. I was posted on top of the pre gangway boat deck, I was only there for 45 minutes though, then taken off for my 2nd cholera inoculation. Dinner: boiled mutton and broth, apple rings and rice. At 1pm we were off a small island shaped like a volcano crater, off the coast of Tunis. There is an alarming notice that letters were to be destroyed and cancelled with no censoring after all. My guard was 10 to 12 midnight and we passed the lights of each end of an apparent island on the starboard side, which was probably Pantelleria. I tried to visualise Doll all night but couldn't do it, I managed everyone I know but she.

December 29 Wednesday
Breakfast: porridge and had scaled fish, maybe mullet, very nice. We were quite close to Malta when I came off guard at 10am on the starboard side. There was a lovely panoramic view of the coast, as we sailed along till 12 noon. A beautiful day, at last the sea is a real Mediterranean blue. Dinner: salt beef, soup & rice and we were in the harbour when we had finished. There were many small boats and boys naked but for shorts like little brown monkeys, diving for money and getting it before a yard or so under. They refused pennies however. The fellows on board were very generous with 6d and shillings, two or three squabbling in water at once, they also picked up our meat refuse to eat. There were some boys with fair hair, alas! British subjects? Gondola-like boats were waiting for passengers with silver and exhausted boys who seemed designed to catch any pennies in nets.

Diagram of a gondola-like boat

---

[25] **Submarine** – The Nestor had turned back as the Suffolk had been torpedoed and sunk nearby.

It was a splendid rock harbour with flat roofed buildings rising in tiers, matching the rock to which they cling, partly classic Gothic and Moorish. The entrance to the harbour reminds one vividly of pictures of the Acropolis and the buildings are the same in keeping. The lack of vegetation is marked. A big hospital ship follows us in – the Don Mongolia, painted with white ensign, very spick and span, also a Greek troop ship has just came in, the Hermeverles. I would love to land but didn't for a minute expect that we should be allowed to. The letterbox has been pasted over and marked closed, I am glad I got mine off. I hear that boatmen started selling cigs 50 for 4d but were stopped. The boatmen quarrel and gesticulate murderously then quietly subside. The officers go off to shore in native boats, great resentment is felt. The men are allowed on forecastle deck as quid pro quo. The French Mail steamer leaves, I hope and trust our mails are going with it. My thoughts to those at home do anyway. There are many wounded soldiers rowed about the harbour, I wonder if we shall see Malta again in like cries. The boat leaves, during a tea of marmalade, and we are followed out by small British cruiser. I get a marvellously beautiful view of the town and the island backed by a gorgeous sunset. I read in a Maltese paper that five ships were sunk this week by submarines.

December 30 Thursday
We had sausages for breakfast. It is another glorious day, with clear blue seas. There are sports on deck but I hike up to canteen to buy one bottle of ink to continue this diary. There is boiled shoulder of mutton and raisin plum duff for dinner. I was trying to get a bath. I had it; boiling hot and salty. I soaped my head contrary to advice and the result was too sticky to wipe and it dried like a twisted rope and I had to wash it in the lavs. We had cheese for tea. The orders tonight - men are not to smoke on the deck etc. and it now applies to officers and about time too. That night I was on guard on boat deck, they were smoking all over the place, cigar ends or pipe plugs were sailing down from the bridge every ½ hour. I am on canteen fatigue tomorrow, which means actually carrying up stuff from the thief who runs the show making about 300% profit on cigs.

December 31 Friday
We had currie for breakfast. I carried two cases of tinned fruit and one empty case of lemonade. These ship fatigues usually consist of about half an hour mild exercise in the morning and I am glad I did it. We are supposed to arrive in Alexandria tomorrow. I played three games of chess with **Bart**[26] in the morning and won two. Dinner: mutton, soup, prunes and rice. We had sports in the afternoon – **Gus Platts**[27] took on four in succession, each round was 2½ minutes. Tea: Bread and butter. A petty thief on board, washed out my towel yesterday and tied it to a rope today. I bought a tin of peaches for tea and put them in the corner end of the rifle rack and by 2.15pm they were gone. This sort of thing creates a spirit of comradeship in the Army, that the men fighting at your side are perhaps thieves – an inspiring thought. I played bridge for love

---

[26] **12/293 Sergeant H Bartholomew** – commissioned to 6th York and Lancaster on 29th August 1917.

[27] **Lance Corporal Gus Platts** – Boxer and Physical Training Instructor.

and won two rubbers. The fellows kept up silly singing till late because it was New Years Eve. The officers, I hear were singing on deck till later. They should have more sense, if only for example and their orders. I slept in my shirt and pants as it was warm enough without a blanket.

1916

January 1 Saturday (New Year's Day)

We had porridge and herrings for breakfast. I have sight of low lying coast with groups of palm trees and flat roofed houses. Alexandria itself was soon in sight, the docks and buildings cover an immense stretch of front. We were berthed in the harbour at 9.30am, a truly wonderful sight with a breakwater composed of loose stones, which looked about three miles long. The amount of shipping here is enormous and I've never seen such a busy port. Numerous local boats put out to us with fruit but the native police drove them off. A thief of a newspaperman was allowed on board and sold ½d papers for 2½d, his fortune is made. We had rabbit for dinner and orders were given that we were to pack up immediately after, to be ready for 2pm. We docked at 2.20pm and saw crowds of beggars scrambling for pennies with the native police beating their bums as they stooped down. The pandemonium of unloading commences by native dockers. They make a game of it, swinging up and down with the load on a hoist.

We had cheese for tea and we paraded at 7.30pm on the quay. There were crowds of natives in the station throughout the night selling fruit, bread and eggs. The oranges were really luscious, finer than any in England. There was no need to but I bought bread and about 5lbs of biscuits. It was confirmed by Mr Ward, the story of the boatswain who had a very narrow escape from a submarine yesterday. The enemy sighted after us at 11am and chased us for three hours, which accounted for the zigzag course as we always showed him our stern as he manoeuvred to get us broadside. It seems he gave up chasing us and went for the **Ionic**,[28] the **East Lancs**[29] boat only five miles from us and actually fired a torpedo and missed. Our carriages jolt like thunder and we are tightly packed on wooden latched seats, too uncomfortable for us to sleep, so we played solo most of the night and I lost 1½d. I succeeded in the afternoon in getting a letter off to Doll and there was a soldier on the quay picking them up as we threw them to him.

January 2 Sunday

The railway is crossing a sandy waste with occasional green patches of cultivation though predominately trees which are palms, acacias and a soft feathering sort of pine, very effective in the distance. We are passing Arab camps all the way across with natives walking along tracks in picturesque garbs

---

[28] **SS Ionic** – was attacked by U-boat in broad daylight with 11th East Lancs on board. The submarine fired a torpedo from 500 feet off Ionic's port side missing its stern by 100 feet. The Ionic then proceeded at full speed and outran the German boat.

[29] **11th Battalion East Lancs** – Accrington Pals.

of various hues with some very handsome fellows among them. The sudden change of environment was very strange, more like a dream. I seemed to have been in England only yesterday, now I saw Egypt undiluted. We seemed to strike the canal about halfway down its length, which was rather desolate. I did not view the prospect of seeing the war out here with much enthusiasm. Soon the sea was almost up to the railway metals on our side and just over the banks of the canal on the other. We ran by the side of the canal to Port Said with a small freshwater canal between us, passing through Tel el Heber and Ismalar where the bells of English church were ringing. I was covered with mosquitoes as I stood on coach platform. We arrived at Port Said at 9.30 am and then tramp through the sand for a mug of tea. We were told to go off to tents and then had bully beef and biscuits for dinner.

We had a lecture by Colley on the temptations of the East. The flies are a big nuisance, what will they be like in the summer as this is an exceptionally severe winter for Egypt? We were allowed out between 2 – 8pm and we went into the English quarters where all natives are barred. I was most agreeably surprised as there was a fine bathing beach and first rate shopping streets, as gay as Paris. I shall be able to pass a very pleasant quiet holiday here.

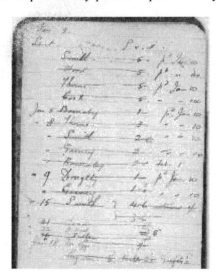

Page from diary showing Frank lending
money to the younger members of the Battalion

January 3 Monday
The morning was very cold but the tap water quite warm. We had bacon for breakfast. I bought some rush matting for the floor of the tent, 6 feet by 4 feet, for 2d. A lot of instructions were read out today, many completely disappeared in the native town. Only one third of us were only allowed out from 4.30 to 8pm. Our letters are to be censored. We had bully beef, cheese and jam for dinner followed by 1¼ hours march this afternoon. We had jam for tea and

butter seems to be off now. I also bought some tomatoes for my dinner. An Arab held out a lush specimen, I spat on it wiped it on his sleeve. I chose two smaller specimens from under the pile and washed them well. I Wrote to Doll asking her to tell me when she receives the letter, also a **PC**[30] to Mother.

January 4 Tuesday

The Army's latest enthusiasm for work suddenly awakens. We have an early morning parade from 6.45 to 7.45; a parade 9 to 12 and 2 to 3. It is one whirl of packing and unpacking, washing and shaving till 9am and all kit was packed before 9 and the valise of the tent rolled up. We had a square inch of bacon and one hard biscuit like a round tile and got no tea until after 9am.

We then marched round town at morning parade and I cleaned my rifle in the afternoon. We had stew for dinner.

Jam and cheese for tea, we bought our own bread, I haven't had a bit of army bread since I came, barring yesterday. It is my night out but it has been raining hard for an hour now. I found some postcards of Port Said and they are allowed to be sent all night. I send cards to Mother, Maggie, Mrs Brachern and Mrs Parker. I beat down an Arab for tangerines from 9c to 5c per dozen. My watch has stopped and I broke the hair spring messing with it.

January 5 Wednesday

We had bacon for breakfast and I bought two fried eggs. We then went on a march to the other side of the creek as far as Railway Bridge and stew for dinner. I have written PCs to Aunties Annie & Clara, Mrs Snead, Mrs Headland, Frank Twinn and the Architects Office in Sheffield. We had jam and cheese for tea and I then went into town and posted my cards. It was a very severe night and too cold to sleep.

January 6 Thursday

We had breakfast, dinner and tea as above. Grant stops all passes today because Cook leaves his service hat in tent. We had an early morning physical drill:

9.30 – 11.00 Company drill
11.30 – 12.00   Extended order
2.00 – 3.00   Physical and bayonet

January 7 Friday

Greek Xmas Day – many shops closed. Meals ditto. I was on transport fatigue all day. Orders then went out that anyone going out must have parade buttons bright and boots clean. It was a ruse to make us replace them for ourselves, button sticks and brushes were taken from us. No 10 Platoon went away on outpost, **Wood,**[31] **Cook**[32] and **Sadler**[33] were all with them. I hear that all letters

---

[30] **PC – Private Concerns** — censored private letters.

[31] **12/1803 Private F. Wood** – wounded in action 1st July 1916.

[32] **12/1469 Private Gilbert George Cook** – killed in action 16th May 1916, buried in Sucrerie Military Camp, Colincamps.

reaching London from the Mediterranean etc. between 15th and 24th December went down on a ship called the Persia. I went to the Music Hall on the quay, mediocre entertainment but the man lying on a spiky board was interesting. I then had a cup of tea and cake at Weslyn Soldier's Institute. Blankets were served out tonight.

January 8 Saturday
Meals: ditto. We re-pitched our tents 100 yards to the east and drew 120 rounds of ammunition in the afternoon. I went to the Cinema d'Art in the evening 5.30 – 7.45 then left before anything like over, very good indeed

January 9 Sunday
Meals ditto but small round of biscuits extra. We had Church parade at 9.30 and voluntary bathing parade at 2pm. it was splendid and not at all cold and we had fun in the breakers. I went to Café Splendid in the evening for grenadine picor to remind one of Paris. The constant boom of the big guns could be heard distinctly this evening.

January 10 Monday
Meals ditto but bacon – hot. The imaginary guns heard this morning, were only sides of beef thrown on hollow wood floor. I helped to move A's field kitchen to the station so missed early morning parade. The morning parade march was around the Arab quarter, a filthy hole the stinks absolutely like a pig-sty drainage, not at all inviting, we also passed old fashioned Arab school. We broke the march for a bathe which was very enjoyable again. Were paid when we returned – fellows without dependants £1, I got 4/-. We were then putting up tents for the Barnsleys in the afternoon. Five of us erected three and packed up one of A Company's. I was put in charge of the stable piquet tonight 6 – 6am and was one of one of 9. I hear that our mail arrived at Said yesterday but has gone to Alexandria to be sorted. We are eagerly awaiting its arrival.

January 11 Tuesday
Meals ditto but no cheese, we are supposed to forego this to get milk in tea but there is no milk today.

We are made to go on morning parade at first then **Cousins**[34] told us to report to SM for light jobs, and we cleared up camp lines. We went on a bathing parade in the afternoon and then to the Pathe Cinema in evening which was a good four-part drama but we had to come away as usual before end.

---

[33] **12/771 Private Gordon Henry Saddler** - killed in action 1st July 1916, buried in Queens Military Cemetery, Serre

[34] **Captain A. N. Cousins**- killed in action 7th December 1917, he is buried in Roclincourt Military Cemetery.

In our orders a new address is given, all as usual except Brigade is deleted and replaced with Egypt in lieu of **MEF**.[35] Today is the hottest day we have had and men must bathe in slips now.

January 12 Wednesday

Breakfast: cold bacon, bought tomatoes. Dinner: stew. Tea: cheese & dates, bought two eggs. The weather is cool and cloudy. I am put on **QM**[36] fatigue which is better than the parade. We have great skips of dates to break up which are tougher than rock and I eat to repletion. I have had slight diahorrea today, four times up to teatime. 12 letters are received for the Battalion today. A Company brought in a Turkish spy yesterday. I sent Doll a note with my latest address as per last night's orders.

January 13 Thursday

Meals - Breakfast: tinned meat. Dinner: stew. Tea: milk (at last), dates & bread – true decent fare. About twelve small letters arrive today for the Battalion. I find a chemist who sells chocolate at English prices. We had an early morning parade at 9am, 12 Company get drill and distance judging, followed by a one hour's march in the afternoon with the band.

January 14 Friday

Breakfast: cold boiled beef, milk in tea again. Dinner: stew. Tea: Hartley's Strawberry Jam. I bought a silver watch from **Coats**[37] for 7/-, it wants a glass which I bought for 10d. I also bought ¼lb butter which was 1/5d per lb, it was very creamy, a great treat. We hear that we are going to relieve A Company at **Salt Island**[38] on Monday. Tent and line orderly for No.12 and just a driblet of letters again.

January 15 Saturday

Breakfast: bully beef and No. 4 biscuits. Dinner: ditto with desiccated potatoes. Tea: Hartley's strawberry jam. We marched along the shore westward to the lighthouse which was about ten miles there and back, extremely hot and heavy going over sand and a fearful stench from animals beyond cemetery. We had a voluntary bathing parade in afternoon, with big breakers. Later I had tea in town at the **ASC**[39]Soldiers Rest. I bought three eggs and bacon, bread, butter & tea for 10d. Then I went to the Eldorado pictures in the evening, which was very good, a fresh Charlie Chaplin. There is a rumour that mails are in.

---

[35] **MEF** - The **Mediterranean Expeditionary Force** (MEF) was part of the British Army during World War I, that commanded all Allied forces at Gallipoli and Salonika. This included the initial naval operation to force the straits of the Dardanelles.

[36] **QM** – Quarter Master.

[37] **12/620 Private W. Coats** – wounded in action 1st July 1916.

[38] **Salt Island** – The Salt Island Redoubt were salt works that also contained the Vacuum Oil Company and The Shell Motor Spirit Company.

[39] **ASC** - Army Service Corps.

January 16 Sunday

Breakfast: bully beef. Dinner: roast mutton. Tea: bully beef and dates. I helped **Grant**[40] to fire N point by sun. A small jeweller actually gave me as second hand watchcase. I am on **piquet**[41] tonight, it was very cold and I am detailed to guard again tomorrow.

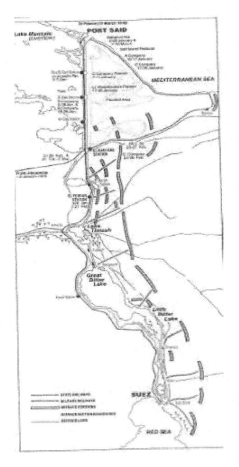

Map showing the position of the Battalion at Suez

January 17 Monday

Breakfast: corned beef. Dinner: stew. Tea: dates. The Company files in at 6.30am en route for the Salt Works. It is fifty minutes sail in a lighter on the canal, although it is only a short distance, and on the other side there are docks in a straight line and we passed a large American encampment on an island in the canal. In the distance there is what appears to be a chain of pyramids. I

---

[40] **Captain D. E. Grant** – served in Sheffield City Battalion until 11th May 1917 and later employed in the Ministry of Munitions.

[41] **Piquet** – Piquet duty.

surmised that it might be ancient burial places but they turn out on arrival to be nothing more than salt. One could think that it would be enough to savour the world forever. I am put on **Vacuum Oil**[42] guards meals fatigue, which only consisted of carrying them dinner and tea which was a quarter of an hour's walk away. Six of us and a corporal did it. We live in light shelter with a matting roof and boarded sides up to 3'6" and open. The fish are abound in the cut behind the tent. They are either shy of the hook or turn their nose up at the bait provided but can be caught in abundance by a net. I lost my igniter (cigarette lighter) somewhere near our quarters. No 10 Platoon with **Wood**[43] and party join us from El Tenah. They say that it's much nicer than here. The night is chilly and I have a skin irritation. I am on Vacuum Oil guard tomorrow. I left a letter for **Garvey**[44] to post.

January 18 Tuesday
Meals: ditto. I am on guard at Vacuum Oil. I weighed myself, without equipment and in my helmet - 70 kilos = 11 stone (1K = 2½lbs). The weight of the equipment and contents brought here is 58lbs. I then wrote to Mother. I bought eggs at 11/4d each, which I understand is a good price. I had quite an enjoyable guard.

January 19 Wednesday
Meals: ditto. We receive a very big mail at last and many fellows receive 10 letters or more. **Todd**[45] gets 8 from his girl alone. The only PC I received was from Doll, together with Maggie's belated letter of December 13th and one from Kniveton. The fisherman off Vacuum Oil gave me new fish which I cooked on a billy lid with suet, although not much flavour. Further special orders are given on saluting – RATS and chin straps must be over the chin - did you ever?

January 20 Thursday
Breakfast: ¼ loaf, ¼ of a 12oz tin corned beef but plenty of fish for No. 9 Platoon, very nice too, netted for us by natives at the Salt Works. Dinner: Stew. Tea: Stewed dates. I am on camp fatigue, chopping wood and cleaning pans. The order is given – our buttons are not to be cleaned, it seems that the General had been around the camp and had expressed indignation at seeing men cleaning buttons. It is a great relief to hear that there is evidently a real man somewhere at the top. A fellow posted my letter of 10th to Mother in Port Said.

---

[42] **The Vacuum Oil Company** - was situated in the position of the Salt Works, together with The Shell Motor Spirit Company.

[43] **12/1582 Private Harry Wood** – killed in action on 1st July 1916 and is commemorated on the Thiepval Memorial.

[44] **12/653 Private F. J. Garvey** – took part in the attack on 1st July 1916.

[45] **12/802 Private Harold Todd** - killed on 3rd May 1916 – he is buried at Sucrerie Military Cemetery, Serre.

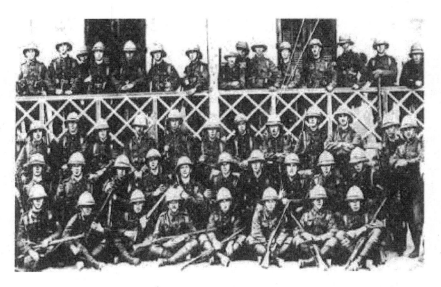

C Company at Ras El Esh. Frank can been seen standing on the right

January 21 Friday
Breakfast: 1/4 loaf, 1/4 small tin beef. Dinner: stew. Tea: stewed dates & rice. It is the first time I've had enough. **Tommy Hill,**[46] brought tin of milk. No.9 Platoon taken over the redoubt guard. We marched three miles along a neck of sand with 58lbs of kit and rifle, I envied the camels their comparatively light load. We are in tents here, last night the stormy sea covered all of the site. No. 11 Platoon were digging a trench and the embankment around, to keep the water back. Grant paraded us at 10.30am, we arrived 9.15am and it was announced that there was no work this morning. He then suggested battle but there was no eager response, so he gave us half an hour platoon drill, a bold bid for popularity at the start. We had 1½hrs filling sand bags in the afternoon. I had the most comfortable evening for some time. **Carter**[47] lets off his rifle on mounting guard and gets an extra 12 hours. The Redoubt is on a strip of sand, by the side of the sea, on the caravan route to Ras El Esh, the only route by which big guns could be brought. We had a cigarette and tobacco ration again.

January 22 Saturday
Breakfast: Bully beef. Dinner: Stew. Tea: Stewed figs and rice. I missed 11hrs day guard for being the first on parade, it was hard lines as I paraded at 7am for same, then a rifle inspection from 8.30am – 9am then sand bag revetting from 9.30am – 12noon and from 1.30pm to 3.15pm, then I had a bathe. A splendid

---

[46] **12/677 Corporal Tommy. W. Hill** – he was wounded in action 1st July 1916 and was commissioned to the machine Gun Corps on 25th May 1917.

[47] **12/1716 Private Arthur Carter** – Killed in action 1st July 1916, his body was never found and is commemorated on the Thiepval Memorial.

day, the weather is getting hot again and the sea is smooth again. Grant has been excelling himself in tiresomeness.

January 23 Sunday

Meals: ditto. We got a day ahead with our tea rations, so we trusted to something turning up. The fisherman with special permits to pass our shore, they extract fish as they return in accordance with old Turkish president, thus the Lord sends us fish for tea. I have been putting up sand bags and tents as targets 500 yards beyond the Redoubt as targets for sections 1 & 2 to shoot at this evening. I bathe in the afternoon - a bit chilly but perfect day again. I am on night guard which is very cold and windy, with continuous lightening all night. I sent a letter to Maggie.

January 24 Monday

Meals - Breakfast and Dinner: ditto. Tea: stewed figs. The rats are very tame early this morning when I am on guard. Three were in my bully can at once eating the tea leaves, I was only a few inches away. We are east of the Redoubt shooting with improvised targets and bottles, about six of us with Grant. I spent the afternoon, putting up targets again for sectional shooting. The General comes around later to inspect, so the shooting was put off. We have heavy rain storms in the evening.

January 25 Tuesday

Meals: ditto, tea about four figs. We had a tremendous storm of rain, hail, sleet and sand, quite blinding to face it and a very heavy sea which entirely swept over the strip of sand. It was a great fight to keep the waves out of our tent but by standing by frequently up to knees in wash of waves and furiously re-banking, we kept ours intact with scarcely a drop of water getting inside. Half of tents were down and the site was obliterated. The engineers went down in the night. We were relieved about mid day by the East Lancs 13th Division from the Dardenelles, a nice prospect for them to start with. We marched back nearly up to our knees in places. It was very cold waiting at the Salt Works to march to the ferry. We got back to Battalion camp about 3.30pm. Tea arrangements were very disorganised and I changed my clothes and had bacon, egg and tea at the ASC[48] in town. I wrote a letter to Doll and posted it there. We slept 14 in tent, very tight.

January 26 Wednesday

Breakfast: 2 hard-boiled eggs & bread. Dinner & Tea: a whole tin of beef. We had a Reveille 4.30pm and then we left Port Said in trucks at 8.30am, after stacking our tents and we travelled quite comfortably in 3rd class carriages. We arrived at El Ferdan about 12 o'clock but were shunting about till about 2pm, on unloading fatigue for about one hour, then fell out for dinner and hung about

---

[48] **ASC –Army Service Corps**, also known as 'Ally Sloper's Cavalry' after a children's comic character and as the Army Safety Corps, also known as Aunt Sally's Cavalry, so a ration truck became an Aunt Sally.

waiting for my turn on the inadequate ferry until 8.30. The East Lancs Band entertained us across the canal. We got tea about 9.30, and then had 14 sleeping in a tent. The day has been showery, very wet and uncomfortable. I felt pretty miserable waiting to be taken across. Sergeant Major starts to admonish me for bright buttons.

January 27 Thursday
Meals - Breakfast: ¼ tin of bully beef. Dinner: stew. Tea: figs, not quite half a loaf for the day. We had a little fatigue in the morning but we were mostly cleaning rifles which were very rusty. In the afternoon we were moving battalion stores, extra dates for tea sir! We moved two to four hundredweight (CWT) bags of sugar – which was a bit too stiff! from 1.45 - 5.30 pm. It was a very wet at night.

January 28 Friday
Meals: Breakfast: bacon. Dinner: stew. Tea: 1/4 loaf of bread and 3 biscuits for day and a taste of cheese. I was doing Engineer's fatigue at 6.40am - 5.30pm with only 20 minutes for dinner, moving rails and rolling stock during the morning. The afternoon felt very monotonous, moving wire. There was no time for a shave or a wash till night. The weather is still showery but night very cold.

January 29 Saturday
Meals - Breakfast: bacon. Dinner: stew. Tea: figs. Fatigue fell in at 7.45am and we were told we should finish at 11.45am. It was 8.45am before we got to work having to wait for the ferry as usual. I kept my hand in at work until 1 o'clock, moving packs of sandbags. Cousins is driving us like slaves, I have never been kept at it so. We had another half an hour wait for the ferry and a terrible crush. Dinner was about 2.15pm and we then had the afternoon off but were too done in for anything other than rest. It was a beautiful day and many bathed but said that the water was cold. Another big batch of letters came in but there was nothing for me, I am too dispirited to write myself. New orders - it is now a crime to eat the next day's rations in advance.

January 30 Sunday
Meals - Breakfast: bacon. Dinner: stew. Tea: very nice blackcurrant jam 5/8th of a loaf now allowed per day instead of 3/8th. We had fatigue from 10pm - 12noon which was not so hard as usual, loading revetting hurdles on trucks. I attempted a little washing this afternoon in the canal with soap and sand. There were 44 bags of mail for the battalion today with seven parcels in our tent and innumerable letters but none for me again.

January 31 Monday
Meals - Breakfast: bacon. Dinner: steak. Tea: stew and jam, regular ration of cheese for the last four days. We had another issue of tobacco today. The Pioneers paraded again. We go east about two miles to lay railway track with about 100 men, they carry spades and we don't. Grant gives me the usual bossing job without any authority as usual. We go forward about another two

miles with him marking out the direction for the extension, otherwise a pretty soft time. We paraded at 8pm arrived about 9.30pm, 12 - 2pm for dinner and finished by 4pm. I had a splendid surprise - a letter from Doll to raise my spirits. We go back to stay tomorrow.

February 1 Tuesday
Meals - Breakfast: bacon, plenty. Dinner: cold beef. Tea: blackcurrant jam. We marched out with full kit, blankets and groundsheet for a fatigue party carrying spades as well. We were paid before we set out, I received 12/-. Tents were set out and put up for us in the hollow of the second ridge of sand hills which has a few young date palms which about makes it almost an oasis. There are 15 in a tent now. A Turkish patrol sighted a few miles away, so we have a good proportion out on guard and listening patrols. I wrote to Doll and handed into Grant for censor.

February 2 Wednesday
Meals - Breakfast: bacon. Dinner: stew, very tough. Tea: blackcurrant jam. Water is now very restricted and only four mugs are allowed per day for washing and drinking. It is very clearly impregnated with chloride of lime and the stew and tea are also permeated with it. I was put in front of the fatigue party with about six fellows and we were allowed to go out without rifles or equipment. I am in high grace with Grant who takes me on one side and says he is going to have some rearrangement in the Pioneers. **L.C. Bradshaw**[49] is to go as he caught him slacking, I put in a good word for him but it is useless. We were working 7 -11.15am and 2.30 - 5pm. One man from each tent was allowed to go to the camp for purchases. I am the only pioneer excused guards. I can hear the jackals at night.

February 3 Thursday
Meals - Breakfast: 1/4 tin of beef. Dinner: stew. Tea: figs - 2 loaves between 15 and only three biscuits each were doled out. We have been relining and levelling the stretch over the sand hill near the camp. **Roberts**[50] kept with fatigue party. There are thirty more bags of mail in. I get parcel from the **A.A.**[51] which contained 2 slabs of chocolate, tin of peppermints, tin of tea, Gold Flake cigs and Royal magazine. Anecdotes I hear tonight:

---

[49] **12/602 Lance Corporal J. E. Bradshaw** – wounded in action 16th May 1916.

[50] **12/1029 Sergeant E. W. Roberts** – took part in attack on 1st July 1916.

[51] **A.A.** - Association of Architects.

- **Greaves**[52] at handing in **blue**[53] at **Redmires**.[54]

Major Plackett "Coat condemned, trousers good etc." Up came Graves slewed "Now Major how much for ragged frayed coat and this little lot?"

- **Captain Beley**[55] before we get uniform, treating fellows of battalion in town. "Now you chaps, it's all right being sociable here but I don't want you to come up to me on parade and say, Hello Beley, you old f---er"

- **Schofield**[56] without his puttees.
Colley "Where are your puttees?"
Schofield "They don't fit me"

- **Lieutenant Tyzack**[57] to slewed up private he meets out of his round about 11pm. "What are you doing here?"
"I saw a light sir, so came to investigate"

- Officer to Schofield in 'Thatched House'
"Why don't you get up when I come in?"
Schofield "I'll get up to you when you pay that £40 you owe me"

February 4 Friday

Meals - Breakfast: bacon. Dinner: stew. Tea: jam, apple jelly. We have been levelling and lining out all day. I wrote thanking Mrs Maurice Webb of A.A. for the parcel and thanks and appreciation for Winifred's card.

February 5 Saturday

Meals - Breakfast: bacon. Dinner: stew. Tea: marmalade, very nice lemon. 2/3 loaf each besides biscuits. Lining out and levelling again, we almost caught up early in the morning but got extra men and formed two parties and made very good progress. We should be about two days ahead now. There is a rumour about that the Baghdad Force is surrounded but we don't place much reliance on this now, about the Western Advance of 8 miles and the fall of Baghdad. Turkey are suing for peace and Austria are backing out. It was wet tonight.

Natural History related in tent:

---

[52] **12/1406 Private E. F. Greaves** – a member of C Company who took part in the attack on 1st July 1916.

[53] **Blue** – The textile industry could not keep up with the sudden demand for khaki , so the Sheffield City Battalion were issued with a temporary uniform which was blue/grey in colour. The men thought that they would be mistaken for postmen!

[54] **Redmires Camp** – a hutted camp on the moors on the outskirts of Sheffield where the Battalion trained from 10th December 1914 until it transferred to Penkridge Bank Camp, Cannock Chase on 13th May 1915.

[55] **Captain G. Beley** – was the officer in command of the reserves and was based in Sheffield Town Hall.

[56] **12/1185 Private H. Schofield** – wounded in action 1st July 1916.

[57] **12/1846 Lance Corporal W.H. Tyzack** – also served in the 13th York and Lancaster, Barnsley Pals.

-     The Great American brass billed bucking bullfinch, nests in the highest trees on highest mountains of the Andes. First finds his mate, then feels, fumbles and finally f---- her. He afterwards eats her to hide her shame and at the same time to get his own back

- The crocodile found in Egypt with square arse. He eats clay and s---- bricks, hence the pyramids

-     The Leopard - a spot for every day of the year.
Voice: "What about the leap year?"
"Hold up his tail and let the gentleman see"

February 6 Sunday

Meals - Breakfast: bacon. Dinner: stew. Tea: marmalade. We had parades from 7am - 11.30am and 3pm - 5pm and were then working as usual. We had a Church parade 12 - 12.45pm and then a rifle inspection at 2.45pm. The best four out of each tent were allowed to go to El Ferdan at 1.30pm. It was my turn but I was unable to make headway with the levelling, so decided to alter the line from the first diagram below to the second diagram below:

I received a letter from both Doll and Maggie each dated January 22nd.

February 7 Monday

Meals: Breakfast: bacon. Dinner: whole tin of bully beef but only one slice of bread & three biscuits for the day. Tea: jam. We are moving the camp about two miles ahead. We marched off 7.15am and piled across about 1½ miles ahead and fell out to word. I took six men to form two parties with me. **Atkinson**[58] was very annoyed and abusive, because I wouldn't take him. We got line altered as I decided and a little extra levelling was done by dinner time. The scrub in the desert is beginning to flower, some are rather pretty, one like a forget-me-not, only stiff. A variety of scrub smells just like the incense in a Roman Catholic Church when it is burnt. We had dinner around our rifles and dug holes in the sand for shade, the sun is so hot that it melted the jelly and fat in the tins of bully beef. There are infinite varieties of beetle which we encountered and several varieties of small lizards. The new camp is all nicely fixed and pitched or us with tea ready at 4.30pm and as it has been a very hot day, was exceedingly welcome. It was quite a welcome home. I must alter my line again in the morning – with a wider sweep near the main line. Tobacco rations were

---

[58] **12/1381 Private Cyril Atkinson** – killed in action 1st July 1916, his body was never found and is commemorated on the Thiepval Memorial.

missed again and I got three packets **BDV**[59] cigs and 2/3 of tobacco. I wrote to Mother and handed it in.

Anecdote:
- Lady in shop with little dog cocking his leg up against the sugar etc.
Grocer looks uneasy
Lady: "Carpenter, come here"
Grocer: "Funny name for a dog isn't it Madam?"
Lady: "Yes, I call him Carpenter because he is always doing little jobs about the house"
Grocer: "Do you think that if I kicked his arse he would make a bolt for the door?"

February 8 Tuesday

Meals - Breakfast: bacon. Dinner: stew. Tea: apple jelly jam, 1/8 of a loaf and about 4 small biscuits and a bit of cheese, as usual. We set our curves around the present camp. **Ratcliffe**[60] as he is levelling gets into trouble with Grant, so I have to level myself as well. I sent **Clarke**[61] ahead to line out which he does very well.

February 9 Wednesday

Meals - Breakfast: bacon and ¼ tin of bully beef. Dinner: whole tin of beef and 4 veg; potatoes, carrots, turnips, onions and gherkins. Tea: Robertson's 'Silver Shred' marmalade. Today **Roberts**[62] is levelling and I'm ahead lining out and putting in curves. Roberts gets chalked off for too much cutting and Ratcliffe yesterday for too little. I receive a parcel from Doll, postmarked January 15th which contains seed cake, pot of jam, tin of lobster, pack of cheese, plain biscuits and gingerbread, café au lait also letter. Anecdote told by night - contd.

Commercial traveller, hotel very full, Manager could only give him a double-bedded room, in one of which was a baby. He woke in night but could find nowhere to pee. So at last he transferred the baby to his bed and relieved himself in the baby's bed, only to find in the retransfer that baby had gone one better in his.

February 10 Thursday

Meals - Breakfast: bacon. Dinner: stew. Tea: ¼ tin of Robertson's 'Silver Shred' ¼ 'reputed' lbs of bread and a piece of cheese. I made café au lait at dinner. We finished lining out and levelling as far as the first trench at the foot of the hills

---

[59] **BDV** – Cigarette 'Silks' came about during WW1 due to the paper shortage making cigarette cards impossible or too expensive. By far the most prolific issuer in the UK was Godfrey Phillips, they issued more silks than all the other UK makers combined. Their B.D.V. brand was very popular.

[60] **12/1023 Lance Corporal F. Ratcliffe** – wounded in the attack on 1st July 1916 – he designed 12th York and Lancaster Memorial in Sheffield City Cathedral.

[61] **12/73 Private Arthur Clarke** - killed in action 1st July 1916, his body was never found and is commemorated on the Thiepval Memorial.

[62] **12/762 Corporal C. Roberts** – he was wounded during the attack on 1st July 1916 and was the last President of the 12th Club.

of the railhead, so got permission for myself, Ratcliffe and Clarke to go for a bathe at El Ferdan. We went down our own railway but I knocked my feet from time to time on the obstructions at the side of the trench when I was dangling my legs over the truck. I bought dates, tomatoes and butter at the **RFA**[63] canteen. The canal (i.e. Suez Canal) was open when we came back, so we had to come back by tea boat ferry. We had fine diving from a big barge about 10 feet away and swam across the canal. I wrote to Doll and handed in to Grant.

February 11 Friday
Meals - Breakfast: bacon. Dinner: whole tin of bully beef & three veg; cabbage, turnips, potatoes. Tea: ¼ tin jam, 1¼ reputed pounds of bread and cheese. Today I have been making a survey of line with a primitive compass, machine gun level and level staff. I made café au lait at dinner followed by a tent orderly.

February 12 Saturday
Meals - Breakfast: bacon. Dinner: stew. Tea: jam, bread and cheese as before. We are actually overdone with rations. The bully beef is in hand and as there is as much jam as we can eat and it is a problem to get in it all in the parcel tuck without neglecting rations. I am taken off the survey of line in the middle of the morning to complete the connection with transverse line at railhead and finished the same in the afternoon. Grant asked me for list of the men who had shown special efficiency or interest in the work that I had been in charge of. I gave him:

Clarke	A Battalion	Ratcliffe	D Battalion
Broomhead[64]	B Battalion	**Rideout**[65]	C Battalion

He insisted on crossing out Broomhead, saying he was all gas and wanted to boss everything, I gave him **Lockett**[66] instead. We are setting up tonight to unload the ration transport. There are rumours that we are going to India or **Mesopotamia**.[67] I shared **Lieutenant Corporal Smith's**[68] lobster which we upset in sand but carefully wiped same with the help of our trousers.

February 13 Sunday

---

[63] **RFA** – Royal Field Artillery

[64] **12/319 Private J. Broomhead** - took part in the attack on 1st July 1916 , Commissioned to York and Lancaster on 26 June 1917.

[65] **12/758 Private F.O. Rideout** – took part in the attack on 1st July 1916 and was commissioned to East Yorks on 28th May 1918.

[66] **12/717 Private G. Lockett** – took part in the attack on 1st July 1916.

[67] **Mesopotamia** - refers to the area between the Tigris-Euphrates Rivers in the Middle East. Today it includes Iraq and parts of Syria, Iran and Turkey.

[68] **12/1057 Lance Corporal Richard Elvidge Smith** – killed in action on 16th May 1916, he is buried in Sucrerie Military Cemetery.

Meals - Breakfast: bacon. Dinner: curry stew, figs and rice. Tea: jam. Bread and cheese as usual.

I continued with the survey as far as the canal and missed dinner so had three eggs and bread in the canteen and two cups of coffee. I had a bathe in canal and rode back on the main line and arrived at the camp at 3.30pm, most of men having had half day's holiday. I received two letters from Doll of January 26th and 30th and one from Mother of January 23th, also a postcard from Frank Twinn of January 27th who reports the birth of his son, 2 weeks and 3 days old weighing 8¾ lbs.

February 14 Monday

Meals - Breakfast: bacon. Dinner: tin of bully beef, potatoes, turnips and gherkins, figs and rice. Tea: jam (apple jelly). We had Reveille at 7am, with Grant as a favour without self. **Lieutenant Corporal Welsh**[69] and **Heslington**[70] are to visit the front line trenches, especially to study our strong point. We set off at 10.30am and arrived at 11.30am and set off back at 12noon and arrived for dinner at 12.45pm. We then left the camp for headquarters at 1.30pm in small advance guard. The fellows in camp seemed annoyed that we have had a good time. We were promised a holiday tomorrow and tobacco rations were issued.

February 15 Tuesday

Meals: Breakfast: bacon. Dinner: sea pie. Tea: jam, bread and cheese as usual - too much cheese. The engineering party turned out for two hours and a fatigue after all from 11.15am - 2.30pm. I was excused, to plot the railway with Grant. Lieutenant Grant, **Cowen**[71],**NCOs**[72] and the men were complemented by the Brigadier on the work done. It was a wet day so no working was done as intended. I wrote to Mother.

February 16 Wednesday

Meals - Breakfast: bacon and porridge. Dinner: stew and rice and dates. Tea: jam, bread and cheese as usual. We had a rifle inspection at 9.30am and a drill until 11am. We had a new Egyptian marching order 2pm and were then dismissed as there was a heavy rainstorm coming on. Then a fatigue from 9pm - 12 midnight, pushing water pipes up line on trollies, nearly for orderly room. **Windle**[73] and **Tagg**[74] dodged off on pushing the trolley back and the two men left with me refused to push any further and turned it off the line for others to pass. I made a protest in vain and the charge that should have been 'neglected

---

[69] **12/550 Lance Corporal W. A. Welsh** – wounded in action on 1st July 1916.

[70] **12/395 Private F. H. Heslington** – Took part in attack on 1st July 1916.

[71] **12/78 Private H. Cowen** – took part in the attack on 1st July 1916 and later transferred to the RAF.

[72] **NCO** – Non Commissioned Officer.

[73] **12/826 Private G. Windle** – also served in 6th and 13th York and Lancaster.

[74] **12/528 Private Reginald Tagg** – killed in action 1st July 1916 and is buried in the buried Australian Imperial Force Burial ground, Grass Lane , near Flers, which is some distance from the battlefield.

duty' was eventually overlooked by the Sergeant. I wrote to Doll and am feeling some indigestion.

February 17 Thursday
Meals - Breakfast: bacon. Dinner: stew. Tea: jam. I completely changed my underclothing. I handed in the letters that I had written to Mother and Doll and was on No 9 Platoon outpost from 6pm till 6am. We fell in at 3.30pm. I am in charge of the southern sentry post as I am the oldest soldier where I was disturbed about every half an hour by the patrol officer on changing sentry.

February 18 Friday
Meals: Breakfast: bacon. Dinner: stew. Tea: jam, poor quality again. I had the morning off followed by a rifle inspection. In the afternoon, we had a bit of aiming drill, then a bathing parade. We were turned out unexpectedly for fatigue 6 - 9pm, unloading 6lb pipes about 24 ft long out of barge which was very heavy dirty work. The bottom of the barge was full of grease, one man jumped down and was up to the waist in it. **Varley**[75] stepped back off the wharf into deep water. Grant, "Are you very wet?" We washed the rest of our clothes in the morning.

February 19 Saturday
Meals - Breakfast: bacon. Dinner: currie stew. Tea: poor jam. We manned the camp trenches 4.30am and then to the ASC Canteen for fatigue in the morning unloading carts. We were then putting in a few stakes to mark out a new camp in the afternoon which was an easy day. We strike camp tomorrow and go across the canal, then march to Kantara during the night or early morning. We were then packing up our kit bags to send away for good.

February 20 Sunday
Meals - Breakfast: bacon. Dinner: stew. Tea: jam (smooth blackcurrant or seedless raspberry). Test orderly, thereby prepared baggage fatigue and had a fairly restful day. We struck camp at 2.30pm and pitched again on the west-side of the canal and were then on fatigue, removing the officer's mess furniture etc.

February 21 Monday
We had Reveille at 4am and then struck camp for Kantara, loaded field kitchens, then breakfast which was bully beef and tea. We marched off 7.50am, did 45 minute stretches, then a rest for ¼ to ½ an hour. 1¾ hours for dinner which was bully beef, cheese and biscuits! We bathed feet in canal. I have a nasty blister through the hole in my sock and have been wearing my overseas boots for the first time for a long march. I would very much have liked to bathe but was not allowed. We arrived at our new camping ground at 4.15pm after about a 13 mile march. I was very done up. The tents on the baggage had not arrived. We had tea and jam about 5pm. The evening was very chilly and I was making up my mind to sleep with or without overcoat and blanket. The tents

---

[75] **12/808 Corporal J. S. Varley** – Wounded June 1916.

arrived at 8 o'clock and we were all up and settled by 8.30pm and had another ration of tea.

February 22 Tuesday
Meals - Breakfast: bacon. Dinner: stew. Tea: jam and lots of biscuits & cheese in addition. I have had the finest night's rest since arriving in Egypt, it was actually broad daylight when I awoke, which reminded me forcibly of a good old fashioned Sunday morning. I arose at 7.50am, it was a beautiful morning and I felt really happy. I then went to the canal in the morning about one mile away for a swim. We had fatigue after dinner, consisting of a 1½ mile walk to canal, loading a few articles and then back again. Tea was then ditto and we then had to carry up again ubiquitous kit bags. I received a letter from Mother dated February 3rd with an account of a **Zeppelin raid over Derby.**[76] We received tobacco rations but BDV are better. The blister on left foot is very sore. We prepare full marching order for a march off to first line trenches followed by a Reveille at 2am.

February 23 Wednesday
I was up at 2am, struck tents, had a mug of tea and bully beef and set off at 4.15am. My foot is very sore and my pack is the limit. We have frequent rests and arrived at 7am. We had complete rest all day but for a start at Officer's mess dugout which was just started and then abandoned past 10am but I was only superintending. Bully beef for dinner, bacon for tea, I am very thirsty, there was no water until the evening than only less than a quart, which is to last until tomorrow evening. I made half a cup of café au lait though.

February 24 Thursday
Breakfast: bacon. Dinner and tea: stew again. Up for Reveille at 5.30am, then breakfast at 6am, fell in 6.40am and arrived at work at 7.30am. We fell out 11.30 - 1pm for lunch and then worked till 5pm. We were wiring hurdles in revetments to piquets with the Pioneer party. We had dinner at 6pm and one and a half pints of water were drawn again and I handed in letter to Doll.

February 25 Friday
Breakfast: bacon. Dinner: bully beef. Tea: stewed figs and raisins and jam. Our working hours today are as before but we went out in ordinary way with No 9 Platoon to the strong point. I drew water twice today and had tobacco rations also. We started working ½ hour on then ½ hour off with an alteration after dinner with ten minutes rest per hour only.

February 26 Saturday
Breakfast: bacon. Dinner and tea: stew and jam. We marched off to the strong point for work this morning with all our belongings on our back, including a

---

[76] **Zeppelin raid over Derby** - Derby was hit by a Zeppelin raid in February 1916. Through bad weather and perhaps the force of nature they hit the Derby area thinking that it was Manchester. Instead the bombs hit many little towns around Derby, killing up to 15 people. Burton on Trent was also hit as it was mistaken for Liverpool.

shovel. We finished at 4pm but only had one hour for lunch and ten minute breaks. I had the supervising job again, marking out internal trenches and the camp moved for us further north. Splendid mail for me on arrival: two letters from Doll, January 9th and February 8th, one letter from Mother, February 10th, one letter from Maggie, February 7th and papers, one PC from Auntie Maggie, February 8th and papers, one parcel from Maggie, January 25th, one parcel from A.A. which contained chocolate, book, cigs and sweets. Maggie's parcel contained Heinz Baked Beans, apricots, cream, sweets, tea rations and seed cake. 'John Bull' in some paper says that the 31st Division consist of the **'Cream of the North'** [77] and are not intended for active service. We now call ourselves the 'Never Guards'. We have been promised holiday tomorrow afternoon.

February 27 Sunday
We were roused at midnight (Saturday) and given the particulars of the difference in clothing required at once. The move back to Kantara was announced. I went back to bed but was again disturbed as signallers out of our tent wanted. It was not Colley's fault as we had to get up. Message said details wanted immediately. He replied "The men all asleep, will tomorrow do?" The reply was crushing "Immediately, means at once!" The tents were struck at 7am, then a bit of loading up and not doing much besides. I went back to strong hold to look for my cardigan but the same had been lost. The march off was announced for 10.15am. There was plenty of water, so I decided on taking a waterproof sheet and having a bath and shave but we suddenly paraded in midst of it. I was the later to hand in the rum rations. Mine of course was at bottom of my valise. Biscuits were thrown indiscriminately into the tent bag and of course were utterly wasted. I had a quick wash but not a shave. We left **Hill 80**[78] at 11.15am, with Maggie's and A.A. parcels in addition to the back breaking loads that we came with. We marched in ½ hour to 50 minute spells and had about ¾ hr for dinner at 12.30 and 10 to 15 minutes fall out otherwise. Colley was on horseback and picked out hardened sand for us on the desert but unfortunately we struck lakes, which we had to skirt around, so this lengthened the march by 2 miles. Our new camp is by the canal. We arrived about 3.30pm but tents were not put up till dark. I had a bathe in the canal, immediately upon arrival and more letters and many parcels had arrived. I received one letter from Auntie Clara dated February 14th and parcels of cigs and tobacco from Yeomans. I had apricots and cream at the mid day halt in desert - Ye Gods! What next in the desert, it was well worth the carrying. I was absolutely fed up with good things in the evening and everyone was sharing out cakes, sweets and chocolate. It is reported that Cousins has already sailed to arrange our disembarkation which is probably Marseilles.

---

[77] **Cream of the North -** The Sheffield City Battalion were the 'cream' of Sheffield, as they were mainly office workers and were known as 'The Coffee and Bun Boys'.

[78] **Hill 80** – is described as a desolate pinpoint on a map surrounded by a sea of desert to the east of El Kantara.

February 28 Monday
Breakfast: bacon. Dinner: stew. Tea: household jam C&B (Cross & Blackwell). Breakfast was not till 7am and there was no special Reveille. We had rifle cleaning only in the morning followed by an inspection 10.30am. The loss of service hats is being enquired into and there is a rumour that we shall have to pay for them. No water was drawn till about 11.30am, then for me a good shave. I wrote a short letter to Maggie after breakfast, thanking her for the parcel and for sending some tobacco. I had the afternoon off, settling down to entering up this diary and letter writing, so fear there will be no time for bathing. We had some weird vegetables in our stew today, calabash, the stem end out of which pipes are made. I received a letter from Doll dated February 5th.

February 29 Tuesday
Breakfast: bacon. Dinner: stew. Tea: jam. We had a Reveille at 6am and fatigue from 8am - 1pm, carrying heavy bundles of prickly matting – I was very thirsty. We were paid after dinner, I received 12/- and a fifty piasta note included for 10/3d. I got another cardigan out of the clothes heap. Most kit bags are emptied now and fellows had to scramble to get their own things back. We were then putting up tents for B Company, including a large marquee. We also have to give one out of our four per platoon and the result was 16 in a tent. I then wrote to Doll.

March 1 Wednesday
Meals: ditto. Today was a pretty easy day for some of us. The poorer shots had six mile walk to Hill 80 for rifle practice. They had an early breakfast and only got back for tea and were very dusty and thirsty. We cleaned rifles and oiled our equipment, had an inspection from 9.30am – 10am and then a bathing and washing parade and the bathing was ideal. In the afternoon we paraded at 3pm for half an hour, which was an aiming drill then a C Company parade. I handed in my letter to Doll.

March 2 Thursday
Meals: ditto. We had rifle inspection which was **Sweedish and Musketry**[79] in the morning. We had a skeleton order to be inspected first thing in the afternoon and then had the rest of the day off. I read most of 'Spanish Gold' and it was the warmest night that we've had.

March 3 Friday
Meals: ditto. We had Sweedish, bayonet drill and musketry in morning and then the afternoon off. There was a Quarter Master's orderly, retreat to retreat. We reported at 5.30am and were dismissed immediately till 8.30am. There are strong rumours of moving at last. I had a beautifully warm bathe this afternoon. Finest rumour so far is that the Battalion is to have six days leave immediately after arrival in France, then to be ready for action by April 1st.

---

[79] **Sweedish and Musketry** – Shooting practice and bayonet fighting.

March 4 Saturday

Meals: ditto. The Quartermaster's orderly was the easiest day's duty I've had. I fetched a bottle of beer from **14th Barnsleys**[80] for **Marsden**[81] and then held his horse for five minutes. I took the indent to Marsden for his signature then went on to the Divisional stores. I received two letters from Doll, February 16th and 19th, the first enclosing a letter from Mrs Headland.

March 5 Sunday

Meals: ditto. We had a compulsory church parade in orders, then announced optional watersports in canal this afternoon. We were entered in tests in the morning with No. 9 platoon and **Rodgers**,[82] **Lambert**[83] and me were selected. All were not on the church parade were paraded for fatigue while I was away (I got wind of it in time). Colley was very annoyed that only a few turned up for church, so he took names. Next time voluntary 'C' is to be compulsory. I was told by spectators that I was first in the diving but it turned out that I was an also ran and that Lambert was first. It seems that I was disqualified for not finishing the dive but swimming it out. I was not aware of the rules but will remember next time. I wrote to Doll and handed it in. D Company paraded this morning to fill up the draught on the SS Manitoba and then didn't go after all.

March 6 Monday

Meals ditto but dinner bully beef. I am still peacefully passing my time. We had half an hour Sweedish and half an hour Company drill in the morning and then a bathing parade. Today is probably hottest day that we've had and the bathing was delightful. We repatched our tents in afternoon then slept. A big parcel of mail arrived in the evening, as usual on eve of our departure. I received one from Mother with a letter of February 11th and one from A.A. dated February 10th. Mother's parcel contained seed cake, sardines, beans, steak and kidney pudding and a tin of café au lait which was much too large. The parcel from A.A. contained cigs, chocolate, peppermints and a book. I wrote and thanked A.A. for the parcel that I received on February 26th.

March 7 Tuesday (Shrove Tuesday)

Called Shrove 'Stewsday'. Meals were as usual. From 9am - 9.30am we had Sweedish and were then it was a holiday all day for C Company. Colley is a Toff. We bathed in the morning and our Battalion played the Barnsleys at cricket and also swim with them, beating them thoroughly. We had scarcely finished our tea when an order comes to down tents and pack up. We sleep in open until 2am and then have a Reveille. Tea is served and we march off with

---

[80] **14th Barnsleys** – 14th Battalion York and Lancaster, 2nd Barnsley Pals.

[81] **12/2 Company Sergeant Major William H. Marsden** - Killed in action 17th June 1916 he is commemorated on Thiepval Memorial.

[82] **12/767 Private Edward Gordon Rodgers** – Killed in action 4th May 1916 he is buried in Sucrerie Military Cemetery.

[83] **12/711 Private A. Lambert** – Runner. He took part in the attack of 1st July 1916.

everything we possess, including blankets and our kit bags stuffed with a full complement of second hand rubbish and also four cans of tinned stuff, and the remainder of our parcels. We had 2½ hours to wait at Kantara Station, it was an exhausting walk and I dropped my ration bag to add to my troubles.

March 8 Wednesday

We left Kantara and entrained in high sided trucks at about 6.30am, and had a good run to Port Said without a stop. We were put on fatigue immediately on arrival, moving ammunition and then paraded. We went to the Golf House for tea which was bread and butter and French pastry served by the Red Cross. The tea was served by the Battalion after but I had no appetite to cook. Four rashers of bacon were served raw to cook for breakfast from the previous night. I had a tin of Mother's Heinz beans with bully for dinner, which made a very enjoyable cold meal. I also had **C&B**[84] steak and kidney dumpling from the previous day with sardines for tea. We had no further work and 50% of C Company were allowed to go into town from 2pm - 8.30pm. I went in after tea, and met Thorne and saw Eldorado at the pictures and was able to stop for the finish. **Register**[85] had been chucking his weight about during our absence and was taking the names of all who had gone without a pass. The campground seems very filthy after the clean desert sand and we imagine that it is lousy. I finished a letter to Mother but the Sergeant wouldn't take it.

March 9 Thursday

We had physical before breakfast and then I fried four rashers of bacon and tomatoes in a tin over a patent mentholated war cooker. It took ten minutes to do it and it was a very nice breakfast too. We paraded at 9am for main onshore sea beach till 12.30 and it was an interesting march back through the main streets and the Arab quarters. I had stew and rice pudding for dinner. We had the afternoon off again and passes were granted till 8.45pm but we unexpectedly had to parade for clothing etc. I didn't get my service hat till about 4pm and then went to town after tea. I bought a scarab and wing brooch from **Simon Astill**[86] which was 8/- but it was too late to register same, so shall have to take it with me. I wrote a short letter to Doll and was unrestrained and posted it in the ordinary way. I gave in a letter to Mother at 4pm but received the same back at night as it was too late.

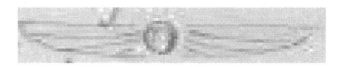

A drawing of the wing brooch

---

[84] **C&B** - Brand name - Cross and Blackwell.

[85] **12/755 Sergeant Bernard John Register** – Killed in action 16th May 1916, he is buried at Sucrerie Military Cemetery, Serre.

[86] **41080 Private A. Astill** – died of wounds on 19th September 1917 whilst serving with 8th York and Lancaster .

March 10 Friday

We had Reveille at 5am and breakfast 5.30am which was cold bacon. We packed up and had cleaned the camp by 7.30am and then paraded 8.10am. We marched off to the quay with all of our possessions as before at 8.30am. Only fiendish ingenuity devised rifles that slope with fixed bayonets to add to the pleasure of carrying kit bags. We embarked pretty quickly on the **SS Briton**,[87] a passenger boat but with our luck, we are on lower deck of the hold which is not even third class and smells very sour of the caked spew of countless troops. We hear that the lot before us were a very verminous lot. We were not allowed onto the deck at first and went up but **Elam**[88] drove us back like dogs. We were allowed above at about 11am. Some troops I hear had touched for 2nd class cabins. We were collared for storing ammunition at 12.30am, got off about 1.50am. In the meantime dinner had been served so I had it cold: mutton, potatoes and peas but no matter, as it was too hot to eat in the rancid hole. We gave out rifles in at 2.15pm to the armourer and were due for fatigue again at 3pm but dodged it by arresting ¼ hour stacking rifles. We had bread and butter for tea and weighed the anchor at about 5.15pm while at tea. We came below at about 7pm and I secured an early pitch for a hammock near to an electric light. The hold was very badly lit (electric) and ventilated. This accommodation is much inferior to the Nestor, poor as that was. The Officer accommodation is most spacious and palatial and the service appears princely and they have about two thirds of the boat. The boat is faster than the Nestor and does 22 knots but it is an old boat about 23 years old, I hear of the Union Line, who have amalgamated with Union Castle. It is the boat that Lord Roberts went to Africa on. I turned into my hammock to read before sleeping at 7.30pm and am told it was posted up in Port Said and that all parcels received in London from 17th to 23rd February went down on the **Maloja**.[89]

March 11 Saturday

I had a comfortable night in the hammock, although it was very rough and fellows in less fortunate positions than I got drenched by the seas pouring in from above. I was disturbed several times by fellows vomiting in buckets under me. I began to feel groggy very soon after getting up and soon brought up a little bile. I could have managed breakfast, so long as I was in the fresh air but it was impossible in the rancid hole we were in. There was no visible attempt at any ventilation and the few small port holes there were screwed up. I swallowed a little tea, which almost immediately came back and could eat nothing. At last I found a clean blank space on the poop deck and then set about comfortably

---

[87] **S.S. Briton** – a liner belonging to Union Castle Line that had seen service as a troop carrier during the Boer War.

[88] **Lieutenant C. Elam** – Sheffield University student. He was killed in action 1st July 1916, buried Australian Imperial Force Burial ground, Grass Lane, near Flers, which is some distance from the battlefield. Perhaps he was captured by the Germans.

[89] **S.S. Maloja** – the S.S. Maloja struck a mine laid by a German submarine, 2 ½ miles south west of Dover Pier. She sank in about 20 minutes with the loss of 155 lives.

dozing. Register comes to warn me for guard at 11.45am which was then about 10.30am. I had to go down to the 'Black Hole' again to get ready and was immediately bad again. I just pulled myself together for the parade and then collapsed again. I was on second relief. Dinner was brought to us at about 1pm but I didn't touch it but found half a small arrowroot biscuit lying beside me, which I managed to swallow and then ate an orange and kept it all down. I was on guard from 2pm – 6pm watching life belts on the officer's starboard deck and I got very peckish indeed towards the end. The machine gun section gave me the remainder of their tea, bread, butter and tinned salmon, which I stuffed down with gusto. The sea was very rough all day, which was completely washing the forecastle and often the front of the officer's deck and many men were frequently completely drenched. The sky was leaden with bright intervals and frequent sharp showers. I had eight hours off, which was very acceptable and got very comfortable on deck with a ground sheet, overcoat and a blanket. Coffee and biscuits were served to the guard at about 12.30, which was very acceptable. The guards were reduced on the 2am – 6am turn. I was one of three fortunates remaining and quickly got to sleep again.

March 12 Sunday
We had tea and stew for breakfast. I made a good one although it was in the stink pit. The sea is now calm and the weather bright, so there was nothing to do but make myself comfortable. I bask, write and read till the guard is dismissed at 12 noon. I am lucky to be on guard I consider, as I might have been on a nasty, dirty drudgery, swabbing up messes as I notice many of our chaps are doing. We have roast mutton, potatoes and peas for dinner. At about 2.15pm we describe complete spirals, I immediately look for a submarine but we slow down near a capsized lifeboat which is painted green, white and red, evidently the Captain wishes to identify it. We then proceed on our course again. I hear that our particulars are sent to Malta. There is the usual alarm and stand to from 5.30pm to 6pm. There is an announcement that letters may be given in at 8pm as we expect to put in at Malta tomorrow. I give in one that I wrote to Mother and write a letter to Doll as well. I then sleep on the deck which is very hot at first but rather chilly later. I have a fairly good night though although there is now more swell.

March 13 Monday
Breakfast: porridge, bread, butter and jam. Tea: bread, butter, rice and raisins. We have a mess orderly for the day. The weather is and the sea just crested. We arrived off Malta at about 4pm and expected to the enter harbour. The Captain expostulates forcibly with the harbour boat and then we proceed on our voyage. Some canvas air trunks were dropped into the hold. It is cooler so we sling hammocks below and I have a very good night. Our letters were not taken off after all.

March 14 Tuesday

Breakfast: porridge, bread and butter. Dinner: roast beef, potatoes and peas. Tea: bread and butter. I opened a tin of Heinz beans and bully beef. It has been a dull day with spells of sunshine in the afternoon. I sighted the coast of Sardinia in the afternoon and then slept in the hammock below and again had a very comfortable night.

3
France – The Adventure Continues

March 15 Wednesday

Breakfast: stew, bread and butter. Dinner: mutton, potatoes and carrots. Tea: bread butter and jam.

We passed what I took to be the Ile d'Hyeras about 11pm. It looks like a huge dark mountain mottled with grey the limestone showing through, the tops of which are lost in the clouds, numerous small isles on peaks in the foreground pure white by contrast, as if cleaned by the waves. It is by far the most coastal scenery I have seen since leaving England. We got the order to pack our kits at about 10am, which was a fearful scramble to sort out our belongings and not to pinch other peoples.

I was wrong! It was not an island at all but a promontory at the entrance to Marseilles harbour. I had no idea that Marseilles was so fine, what must the Riviera be like? The bay is very fine the mountains rise from the edge with taller ones behind, giving me the impression of the Swiss Lakes and the tops were veiled in mist. It was half inclined to rain but bursts of sunshine were frequent. The bay is enhanced by numerous islands, which appear well defended. Monte Cretos Island with the Chateau d'If is what one regards with the greatest intent. Furthest out is just a small arch with a lighthouse. Even the ordinary seafront type of town in front of us cannot mar the splendid background against which it rests and mingles. While on the right is a perfect picture, a study of orange and cream (Notre Dame) relived by vivid green, commanded by cream ground walls and tiled roofs. A most interesting looking railway runs round the foot of the mountain carried on viaducts for a great part of its length.

We docked in the afternoon and the West Yorks band played us in and they were a very fine band too. They have not been allowed to play the entire voyage, so we have missed some treats. At teatime an immense mail was brought on board and what a business it was getting it distributed, burrowing under those hanging equipments and baked to suffocation. As each letter or parcel was called out it was snatched up and hurried away into some quiet corner to be devoured, then return for more all to be digested later. There were no parcels for me as I expected, suppose they went down on the Maloja but I had five letters and a 'Passing Show' from Maud and Colin, two letters from Doll, Feb 27th and March 15th , two from Mother, Feb 20th and 27th and one from Maggie, March 5th. The West Yorks played most of the evening. I was nabbed for ammunition unloading but only for two cases apiece. We are told we are to entrain at 7pm. Mess utensils and hammocks are given in, then orders are amended and we are to disembark at 7am tomorrow. I had great difficulty to find a sleeping place, with the port side being the most sheltered but the orders are that the decks are to be kept clear. I try several dosses and settle down by the latrines and wake up very cold at 12.30 midnight. It looks like rain too, so I just find room at the bottom of the mess stairs and pass a very comfortable night. Of course, we were not allowed to go ashore but the officers go as usual.

March 16 Thursday (My 35th Birthday)

We had a Reveille at 5am. I got a wash and shave then had breakfast at 6am which was bread, butter and stew. Some boys came on board selling picture postcards. I buy one and give it to the boy to post to Doll, just to tell her of my safe arrival. We disembark at 7pm and the train goes at 11pm. We seem to be waiting for same in the dock hangar and are not even allowed to approach the door on the main street to look out. I have a thorough disgust with the Army. More mail was delivered while we waited but there is birthday cake for me though, sadly I am afraid that it has gone where all good cakes go, before it reached me, i.e. down but I did receive an Arabic grammar book. We then marched to goods depot station thro 1½ miles of dirty, dank streets in the pouring rain which reminded me of a wet market day in Derby. We halted opposite some second class carriages and our spirits rose, but no, we march on as they all seem thirds (third class). Hooray more seconds (second class), alas we pass them too, then - Oh horrors! Cattle trucks – '8 chevaux (en long) ou 40 hommes', and we are it - to hell with la Belle France and a grateful country. There is no room to move even a foot. A party of Bradfords (Bradford Pals) moves up and enquire 'are we defaulters?' as they are sent in cattle trucks for punishment. Alf Thorne has been out to investigate and calls for me. He has discovered an observation cabin at end of adjoining coach of which we take possession. He having been in it first has wiped thick soot off and looks like a sweep. We clean the windows, which transforms it.

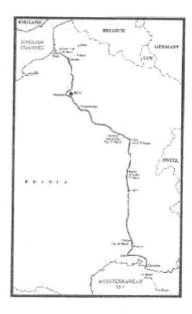

Map showing the train journey through France to the trenches

57

We started off at 11.30am and the weather clears up for commencement of journey. The scenery is beyond my description or imagination. I must bring Doll here when we can leave the children and there are beautiful hard smooth, winding roads for cycling. All colours are in the most delicate tints of cream, orange and green. Olive plantations are the principal culture with blossom abound; cherry apple and almond and conifer trees of conventional Italian shapes give dark relief. Vines are all cut down and resemble old gooseberry bushes and the vivid green of the grass gives the eye the greatest treat after the desert sand.

We travel along the coast for a long way crossing the viaducts that I noted yesterday. It licks Lucerne! Tunnels are numerous some are very long and go right through the mountains. From our observatory above the coaches we can see the glow of the engine fire and the smoke is very vivid and it is like looking into the pit of Hades or a cinema fire presentation. Turner might have designed the landscape. Presently it passes into the tunnels again, looking at the landscape through the wet panes is like trying to view a picture in a badly lit art gallery. We then have dinner of bully beef and biscuits and enjoy same. The sun comes out again with a fine cloud effect and we stop a little while in the ancient town of Arles, so closely associated with the Roman occupation. Here some of the fellows nearly get left behind, fortunately some of the officers are in the same boat so they could not say much. The country is flat about here and the train goes at a decent pace, stops at every station and shunts into sidings to let passengers pass. I wouldn't have it otherwise for every mile is a joy, feasting on the panorama from our glass cased observation tower. I wouldn't swop it for any first class carriage.

The next stop was Tarascon. There were crowds of quaint people, some in native attire who gave us a great welcome and were delighted with buttons thrown as souvenirs. A particularly chic piece of goods comes around corner and raises waves of ravenous delight from our fellows, which seems at first to render her shy but presently she is picking up buttons too and waving. There was also a fine castle at Tarascon. Presently we arrive in Avignon with the mountain background in outline of the blue evening shadows and tipped with pure white flakes of snow. There was a splendid medieval castle at Avignon which was probably the residence of the old Popes.

We received the most enthusiastic ovation here on the station and passing through the streets, past hospitals and barracks. We were all overwhelmed with kisses (transmitted by hand) 'par toutes les femmes tres jolies'. How they appreciate us here – 'les braves hommes Anglais'. In Marseilles no notice was taken of us at all, nor will there be any on our arrival I expect but by their fleeting glimpses their appreciation is aroused. Old men standing on bridges even took off their hats as we passed. I wondered how many have husbands or sweethearts at the front or had lost them, for many were in black. At Orange we stopped and had hot tea and had rum served. The people seem very honest. I asked two little boys if they could go and buy me a candle, they said they would so I gave them 2 centimes. In about ¼ hour they returned but reported that they were sold out and returned the money, which I told them to keep, for which they were very grateful. Wood gave me two carriage candles after. We started again at about 7.30pm and had tea which was bully beef and biscuits again. This makes a whole tea and a bit that I've eaten myself today.

At about 8.30pm we were swinging by the side of the Rhone with hills either side like the Rhine. The cliffs on our side were even, as if they were cut by a giant knife to form a cutting for the railway. I've been writing this off and on up on my perch all day, endeavouring to keep up with the interest as it occurred. Sleep is rather uncomfortable due to the tightness of our legs and fitful sleep. I roused frequently to note the magnificent Rhone and the mountain scenery that we were passing through.

March 17 Friday

We passed through Lyon at about 4am, which appears to be a huge manufacturing town. Presently all of the landscape is one great vineyard, evidently the Claret district and I note Beaujolis station. We stopped at Macon from 7 – 8am for hot tea and then more bully beef and biscuits for breakfast. I teach Thorne to say 'voulez vous ma donner d'eau bouillant?' He fires it at the engine driver, who fairly beams and mashes the tea tablets for him immediately. I got very cold this morning and my feet are cold for first time since leaving England. The day is opening very fine and bright and the country is losing its colour and looking more like English landscapes, except for the ubiquitous populous. The Rhone starts to be in flood above Macon and in some places is one and a half miles wide. There is a fine old Romanesque church at Tournus. We passed through Beaune at 11.20am, the country is getting very interesting and pretty again and a range of hills opposite us on left is full of colour and vineyards and the towns are very picturesque indeed. I have been writing to Doll but had to give it up, as it was shaking too much. I will post it at the next stop. *I think when I retire, shall come and settle down in the South here and tell my little French naturalised grandchildren how I came and saved the country for them in 1916.* We arrived in Dijon at 12.30 but we went into the sidings to change engines, where a big 12 wheeler was put on which was necessary considering that there are fifty coaches on this train carrying 2200 soldiers. It is the longest train that I've ever seen. We left Dijon at 1.45pm, meanwhile we had eternal bully beef and biscuits. After Dijon we hugged the side of most charming valley of the journey, a gigantic Dovedale and Derbyshire Peak with southern flashes of colour and a conical peak with a temple 'a la Tivoli' surmounted by a statue on summit. Malains has a regular fairybook castle with an ogre's stronghold.

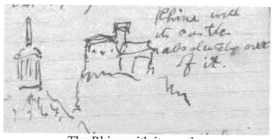

The Rhine with its castles

59

There was an extremely long tunnel from Malains to Blais Bus and I looked out for fellows sitting on our steps and noticed one that was that was on the roof has got onto the observation bus. Further on about Darcey, the countryside became rather tamer – absolutely Derbyshire, with hedgerows, brooks, cliffs and everything. We stopped at a small station for tea from 3.30 – 4.30pm. We had hot tea and rum served and also jam rations and I had a fine wash under the tap head as well. **Dowty**[90] has ridden with us most of the day, so it has not been quite as comfortable. The train rattles along at a fine pace now that we have a new engine. I gave the porter my letter to Doll to post. We then stopped at a regular picture of a town for a few minutes called Torinerre, which is 121 miles from 'Paris'. It struck me immensely. Thorne and I made toasted cheese over a candle for supper and I blew through the flame with a pipe to make a Bunsen burner. We were held up for long stops and after snatched some fitful sleep. We got in the environs of Paris at about midnight and were shunting about there till 4am. The engine put to the other end of train. I then slept better till 7am.

March 18 Saturday
We shunted into a siding at Epluges at about 7.30am and stopped for about an hour for breakfast. There was no tea but hot water was provided which gave out before I could get served. Anyway, I got water from the engine waste to melt Thorne's cocoa tablets. Pickles were served with bully beef which was a very good breakfast. We stopped just a little outside Amiens and I got a back view of the Cathedral which was very disappointing and the setting awful and viewed over a district one might compare with Attercliffe in Sheffield. Passing through a deep cutting and tunnels as we proceeded through town, there was no further chance of a better view. I just got a glimpse of the Southwest view but it was too far away to make much of it. After this country, it was pretty well incandented on the right and not very interesting and it came on to rain too. We disentrained at 3.15pm at Pont Remy, which was a very uninviting spot..... We immediately set out to march to our billets in the rain but after about two miles it cleared. The distance turned out to be about 9 miles and we were very weary and footsore and end of it with a full load and a blanket. We branched off the road to Abbeville, which we thought was our destination and arrived at Uppy. We were billeted at a deserted farm. No. 1 section are placed in a house, we are in barn – 25 of us. I had to settle down in the dark. I was soon feeling very wet on the seat and found that my bed was a heap of rotten turnips. I distributed the straw to better advantage and by aid of the ground sheet had the most comfortable bed I've had since leaving England. We made a fire in the yard and then prepared café au lait which was a most welcome refreshment.

March 19 Sunday
I had a splendid night. I helped to clear up the yard and unmade my bed by first throwing away the rottenest layer of turnips. I should now be very comfortable. We are pretty high up here and it was an uphill march nearly all the way. The

---

[90] **12/638 Private Horace Bradley Dowty** – Killed in action 16th May 1916 and is buried in the Sucrerie Military Cemetery, Serre.

country well wooded. We could hear what appeared to be big guns firing as we came. We got tinned butter for breakfast which was very good! The first dinner the Army has ever provided us was tinned stew, about one big tin per head and rice pudding with real milk. Afterwards I reclined in outstretched ease on a couch of straw or mattress of decaying vegetables, supping café au lait, as satisfied as any Sultan with that delightful fullness after a meal feeling. I only lack the presence of my Doll to make my happiness complete. I received a delightful letter from Doll of March 10th and another '**Passing Show**'[91] from Maud. I am writing my account of the journey to Doll in all my spare time.

I pulled the leg of the D Company fellows tremendously on journey about the brake box:

He – How did you touch for that job?

I - Oh, someone came along and just asked anyone to take it on.

He - Oh does the driver signal what you are to do then?

I - Not exactly I just apply brake if I think we are going too fast…

You notice we have been slowing down and stopping pretty frequently lately, well I just thought the scenery was worth stopping to admire so applied the brake.

He- But didn't the driver say anything?

I-   Oh no he seems a very decent chap.

Then he walked away quite satisfied. The liberties the fellows took on the journey were rather comical. They discovered the gas taps at the end of the carriage and when they wanted a light, they turned them on and then climbed on to the roof and lit the lamps, dropping numerous match ends into the bottom of the globes. When they wanted hot water they would go to any engine and turn the taps on indiscriminately until they found some. Tobacco and cigs were given out.

March 20 Monday

Breakfast: Splendid bacon. Dinner: Stew and rice pudding very good. Tea: Marmalade. Captain Colley evidentially missed the road for the Battalion rendezvous, for we marched at least three miles before meeting one mile away from happy **Captain Cousins**[92] who was barking "Cover off" all the way. Colley administers a splendid rebuke by passing up a message through the column to Captain Cousins "The Company are marching splendidly". Cousins then shuts up for a long time after that. We marched for nearly two hours without a rest and I am fearfully footsore as the roads are hard after the sand. However, the roads are very good and straight as a die. Our village reminds me more than anything of **Compton Chamberlaque**.[93] This afternoon, clothing was distributed and I received wool gloves, two pairs of fearfully knitted pants

---

[91] **The Passing Show** and John Bull was a paper issued in the post-WW1 period by Odhams Press in London - and it contained cartoons by some well-known artists and cartoonists in a similar vein to Private Eye today.

[92] **Captain A. N. Cousins** – Killed in action 17th Dec 1917 buried in Roclincourt Military Cemetery.

[93] **Compton Chamberlaque** is a small village in south Wiltshire, straddling the A30 road some 8 miles from Salisbury.

and a ditto vest. It has been a beautiful balmy spring day. We have had to give in our old clothing, boots and kit bag. How we shall carry our stuff now I don't know. I finished a letter to Doll and handed it in. I hear that green envelopes are to be distributed. There are persistent rumours of leave but Captain Grant dismisses the idea. I wrote to Arthur and handed it in and also sent Mrs Headland a field P.C. I received a green envelope. I have been sneezing frequently during the last two days – I do hope that it is only a chill. Water is very scarce in the village.

March 21 Tuesday

Breakfast: bacon. Dinner: stew. Tea: butter and jam. Today we have been digging practice trenches for bombers. I received a parcel from A.A. which contained cigs, tin of tongue and veal, chocolate, housewife writing pad and red magazine. I wrote thanks for same and for the one on leaving Egypt.

March 22 Wednesday

Breakfast: bacon. Dinner: stew. Tea: marmalade. We had a morning rifle inspection and ammunition cleaning. In the afternoon we had a firing farce, with five rounds deliberate and ten rounds rapid. I am too crushed to even get a decent firing position and it has been raining. *I received two letters from Mother announcing Doll's wonderful birthday gift and its quick withdrawal.* Doll is going on splendidly so what does anything else matter? I wrote to Mother and Doll and then spent a rather restless night, anxious to hear of any further news. Cutting for leave is one man per Company and two officers and eight days to start from 9th May to 22nd May.

March 23 Thursday

Breakfast: **Maconochies**[94] stew. Dinner: bully beef. Tea: marmalade and biscuits – no bread today. In the morning we had a physical drill and a short march. I spent the afternoon searching for lice and ironing my clothing. I seem entirely free but many fellows get a big haul and a few are entirely free. I handed in a letter to Mother and Doll in a green envelope and was then writing to Maggie. No. 9 cutting for one man to leave, 4 Section has it and **Waterfall**[95] wins.

March 24 Friday

Breakfast: bacon, which has always been splendid, have never had better in my life. Dinner: stew. Tea: stewed dates. I woke up to find about six inches of snow, the snow continued practically all day but in spite of that we went on a nine mile route march. The ways of the Army are very strange. Apparently we must never enjoy any comfort. We got back damp and cold and the only comfort was a chilly wet barn. We were given two gas helmets a piece and a

---

[94] **Maconochies** - suppliers of tinned food to the army rations, they consisted mainly of meat and vegetables .

[95] **12/1484 Private Nelson Waterfall** - Killed in Action 1st July 1916. His body was never found and he is commemorated on Thiepval Memorial.

pair of goggles were served. Independent parcels received and shared, I get 37 cigs, two ounces of tobacco and ten acid drops. More emergency rations served to Company.

March 25 Saturday
Breakfast: bacon. Dinner: stew. Tea: lemon marmalade. We spent the morning filling in trenches and had the afternoon off. No letters are being sent out at present and all leave is stopped. I hear an account of operations in the Channel. It has been a frosty morning with warm bright sunshine and the snow is fast disappearing and the afternoon was rather wet. I received a letter from Doll, March 20th. We have orders to move tomorrow. I chased all over the village to post a parcel of vest, pants and shirt but no go, so I shall have to carry part of them and leave the rest behind.

March 26 Sunday
We had Reveille at 5am and fell in at 7.30am. There was a delay waiting for our transport and the **East Lancs**[96] get in front and we really get going about 8.30am. The East Lancs were frequently halting so we had to continually stand to. We had very few fall outs and those that we had were short. The East Lancs had fallen out in groups which must have been 10% of them, there were none in C Company but many in 12th. We arrived in Longpre at about 1.30pm and were billeted in a ramshackle empty house, which was very uninviting but we touch for room with a hearth and a chimney, so make a wood fire and are soon at home. I make some café au lait and tea after a dinner of desiccated veg which was underdone. I also had butter and honey for tea and bought two eggs which were only 1½ centimes. I bathe my feet and have a wash in the brook where we obtain drinking water and then go for a walk around town in evening. Captain Cousins was in command of C Company, barking at all the waiters. I attempt to write to Doll again and have received a 'Passing Show' from Maud. It was dreadfully wet for half of the march, followed by rain and sleet.

March 27 Monday
Breakfast: bacon. Dinner: desiccated stew. We left Longpres at about 8am but hung about outside as usual till about 8.40am. We were told last night that the march would be seven or eight miles and it turned out to be fourteen. We arrived at Vignacourt at 2.15pm, absolutely done in and sore all over. This was not improved by spilling a scalding cup of tea down my back at breakfast. The town street is two miles long and it was heartbreaking work marching along wondering when we should fall out. We passed Amiens in the night about five or six miles away. We are billeted in a very clean barn with good straw, an inhabited farm with a café that is exceedingly clean with no muck heaps in the yard but no electric light. Rum was served out. I wrote to Doll with an enclosure to Maggie and handed them in. Valid reasons required now for leave this time.

---

[96] **East Lancs** – 11th Battalion East Lancs – Accrington Pals.

Ward places me first and **Driver**[97] second. I revel in pleasurable anticipation instead of going to sleep and I did not get into my billet until after 10pm. I was on mail fatigue which was seventeen bags of parcels, fortunately there were nine for me. I woke up in the night to hear hiccuping **Tommy Webster**[98] and the hiccuping gradually develops into the sound of vomiting. I light a candle to see if I can be of assistance and find him peacefully asleep as a babe in a drunken slumber, unconscious of the mess. He'd been begging rations of rum off fellows who didn't want it. I feel that I'm developing a cough and cold.

March 28 Tuesday
The Reveille was to be at 4.30am but everything was put ahead for one hour. I rise to find my shoulders are covered in blobs, because of my scald, which burst as soon as I rubbed them. Fortunately my pack clears the mess. We fell in at 7.45am and messed about as usual till 8.30am, probably waiting for the East Lancs to finish their breakfast. The 13th Barnsleys are ahead today, and they march better than the East Lancs. **Major Clough**[99] fell off section horse as he started to mount and all but landed on his back in pond. We arrived in Beauquesne at 2.45pm and had to wait ½ hour for our billets to be evacuated. I got into a billet at about 3.30pm which is a lot like a small army hutment with bare floors only. Longchamps is six kilometres to the right. We had only a little stew for dinner and butter and honey for tea and were drawing rations till after 6pm. I wrote to Doll and handed it in telling her about my leave. There is a strong south-west wind which has dried the roads and we had a slight shower about 2pm. There was plenty of rum served again. It was a cold hard night. We hear that the East Yorks lost 130 men by shellfire over the road that we are to march along tomorrow.

---

[97] **12/641 Private Horace Driver** – Killed in action 1st July 1916. He is buried in Luke Copse Military Cemetery, Serre.

[98] **Tommy Webster – 12/1165 Private Albert (Tommy) Webster** – Killed in action 1st July 1916. He is buried in Queens Military Cemetery, Serre.

[99] **Major T. C. Clough** – Ex Territorial Forces. Left 12 York and Lancaster in June 1916 - shortly before the Battle of the Somme.

4
The Trenches – Reality Strikes

Before reading the next chapter it is important to familiarise yourself with the layout of a British trench system and the terminology of a front line trench as there are many references made to these.

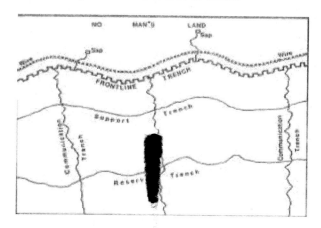

A typical British Trench System

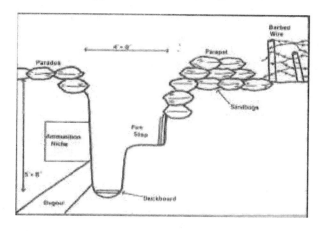

Cross section of a frontline trench

March 29 Wednesday

Breakfast: plenty of good bacon. We had Reveille at about 5.45am and fell in at 7.45am and got properly going at 8.30am. The guns could be heard as we marched along. We arrived in Bertrancourt at 12.15pm and saw an aeroplane being shelled some miles away. We are billeted in low corrugated iron and canvas huts. We had only done about eight miles, so this quiet fallout is the pleasantest surprise of the whole four days march, it was to be the longest of the longest. I had Maconochies for dinner and then drew for guard, I'm it - second relief. There is a heavy snowstorm for first spell and the tent was terribly wet and muddy, so it was as comfortable on guard as off. A little straw arrives about 9pm and we then hang out mainly around the field kitchen and keep fire in, brewing Oxo and tea all night.

March 30 Thursday

It starts freezing at about 4.30am, so the ground gets hardened over. I shaved at 6am and get a good wash in the snow and have a ruddy glow. We had Reveille at 7.30am but we all came up by 6am, this cold and discomfort had many running about throughout the night. It turns out to be a bright morning with a clear blue sky. Two hostile aeroplanes look just like gnats overhead and they are shelled violently by our guns but they miss by a mile. We have been firing pretty heavily throughout the night. We hear that the billets in the village three miles away were bombed yesterday with twelve casualties, two killed and two wounded in the 13th Yorks and Lancs. We had bacon for breakfast and I buy honey and butter from **QMS**[100] Doncaster. I am very disappointed at hearing nothing of my leave yet. One of our Sergeants was wounded by bomb from the aeroplanes this morning and we hear that one fellow was killed but there is no confirmation. I was not relieved from my guard till 11am. We have poor stew for dinner and honey for tea. We then had gas helmet drill in the afternoon and I feel better in it after 20 minutes than five. I received a letter from Doll, March 25th and one from Mother, March 26th. I was paid today – 10 francs, 100 francs between ten men and we had much difficulty in changing it.

I wrote to Doll, a short letter telling her nothing more has been heard of my leave yet. **Sergeant Charlesworth**[101] insists on me seeing the Doctor with my scald. The Doctor immediately says it will never heal and I must go to the hospital this afternoon. I tell him that I don't want to as I am down for the next leave, so he just resorts to an oil and borax dressing and says that my arm is to be regularly trussed up with bandages. How I would have welcomed the comfort of the hospital if it wasn't for my leave. We have one bale of straw between four men on wet ground and it is dreadfully cold. I was awakened at 10pm and told to go on leave the next morning and to report at 4.45am. I was delirious with excitement, rushing about through the mud and losing my boot and making preparations till 11pm.

March 31 Friday

I was up at 3.30am told that I must take my blanket and was then allowed to leave it. I started off at 5am for a three mile walk to Acheux Station and the train leaves at 6am. I go to Longpres and back out again, Amiens ditto and there

---

[100] **QMS** – Quarter Master's Stores.
[101] **12/561 Sergeant F. Charlesworth** – commissioned to the West Riding 31st July 1917.

was always an uncomfortable feeling that we might be recalled. The Worcesters give me tea and Maconochies and I mash tea tablets at the engine. Coffee and cognac was served at 4pm. The fellow opposite is at present picking lice off his shirt. It was a most tedious journey, the only window is in the door and it is very uncomfortable. Under the seats is an oil lamp that goes out immediately when lit. We were passing through Rouen at 7pm and I recognise the churches and the transport bridges, the scenery is rather more interesting around here. The tea I made gave me a thick headache. After about one hour getting through Le Harve docks, we go straight away on the **Canberra.**[102] We are underway at 12.30 midnight. It is a turbine boat with good accommodation but we are too late for a bank. The troops seem to have the run of the ship, there is a note 'Officers and troops' and for the first time in my ship experience I see officers dossing where they can like men (with a double meaning). I buy ½ a bottle of tea and three pieces of cake for 6d. I am not sleepy but I get down at about 1am after reading.

April 1 Saturday
We got up at 4.30am and the sea has been as smooth and as a calm as the Mediterranean. I got hot water in a billy can and had a wash and a shave then a cup of tea. Although I was the last to put my kit on and get on deck I was among the first thirty to leave. The train was waiting and only four were allowed per carriage which was very comfortable. We depart at 7.55am and arrive at Waterloo at about 10.30am. A free breakfast was provided which was sandwiches cake coffee etc. I go to catch 12 o'clock train (telegraphed home arriving Derby 2.30pm) then find it withdrawn as all the country is flooded and the telegraph poles down. I was very crowded and I was hot and very tired.

Leave April 2 Sunday - April 7 Friday (their first Wedding Anniversary was on April 3)

Frank now starts a brand new diary that he brings back from England

April 8 Saturday
Alas! My leave is up. I see the last of dear Doll and Mother as the train steams out of Derby. We arrive at St Pancras fifty minutes late and I am disappointed not to see Frank Turner. I try to find the Union Jack Club for dinner but get out of the wrong entrance, so fall back on the station restaurant and pay two shillings for a plate of ham and tongue and a bread roll, butter and tea. I travel to Southampton in the second part of the train. The London soldiers and the crowd are rather hysterical and very cheerful. I embark a rather larger boat than the one we came home in but it is more 'troopy' and not so comfortable. We start about 7.30pm and I sleep on the deck but get very cold about 1.30am and go below, only to arrive half an hour later.

---

[102] **S.S. Canberra** – cruise liner belonging to P&O Shipping Lines.

April 9 Sunday

I left Le Harve about 2.30 am and I seem to have been on the march or in a train every Sunday since we set out from Egypt. Sunday is truly a moving day with me. Coffee and rum is served out about 11am and the **FMCA**[103] refreshments are moderate and I bought a big roll and helped myself to butter for 4d. My own cake comes in very happily for consumption. We arrive at 2.30pm and I sent Doll a PC and then paid 5d for a mug of coffee. It was an extremely tedious journey and we didn't arrive in Acheux until 11pm. I marched to Bertrancourt to find that the Battalion had gone and had great difficulty in tracing its whereabouts by telephone. I found that they were in the trenches and had been there a week during which they had a very hot time with about **20 casualties**[104]. I arrived about 1.30 am and was finally accommodated in a Company command HQ dugout about 2.30am.

April 10 Monday

I got up soon after 8am to find the gruesome sight of **2 dead bodies**[105] in an adjourning ruined building wrapped up in blankets. One poor fellow was killed just after he had returned from leave and went into the trenches carrying sandbags to the front line and the other chap had been in a fierce bombardment. I was put on water tank guard at 3.30pm. The fellows gave me letters from Arthur dated March 29th, Doll March 29th and Maggie March 27th .They had opened parcels from Maggie and A.A. and eaten the perishables. We get food when and how we can now and the guards on rest time are sent on fatigues now. I get a five mile walk in the trenches, taking rifles for grenade firing which don't seem to be in demand, from 11.30am to 1.30pm. The whole place swarms with rats as big as rabbits. I had a comparatively quiet night.

April 11 Tuesday

Breakfast: boiled bacon. Dinner: Maconochies. Tea: marmalade. Brigadier Carter Campbell stops all our Battalion leave for one month because **Sergeant Loxley**[106] neglects to salute him - what news for a grateful country! The day was very wet and cold and I was fortunate to be on CHQ guard. If there is no sleep, we have a snug dry dug out. We are to carry on with guard another day and take barbed wire down to the trenches in the evening when there is a small bombardment. I get another letter from Doll, March 31st. The Brigadier orders the Battalion to work eighteen hours per day repairing the trenches. C Company went in firing line straight away and we were not relieved for three days and were not allowed to sleep. I had a bath at Colincamps, one tub per platoon.

---

[103] **FMCA** – Field Military Catering Arrangements.

[104] **12/991 Private Alexander McKenzie** was killed on 4th April 1916 and is buried in the Sucrerie Military Cemetery, Colincamps. He was the first fatality of the Battalion, which deeply shocked the men. Death was all too soon to become an everyday occurrence.

[105] **12/358 Private William Arthur Emerson and 12/388 Private Harry Handbury** – were the two men who died on 8th April 1916, they are both buried in Sucrerie Military Cemetery, Serre.

[106] **12/983 Sergeant C.W. Loxley** – wounded during the attack on 1st July 1916.

April 12 Wednesday

Breakfast: boiled ham. Dinner: Maconochies. Tea: marmalade & rice. We marched back to Bertrancourt which was five miles without halt and I am pretty jiggered with a full pack. It is not same camp as last but similar, with no straw on a mud floor but a brazier is provided. It is the first night's sleep I have had since leaving England; very warm and comfortable. Dowty gives me the residue of my A.A. parcel - a book and packet of toilet paper and I manage to get Margaret Gropier's parcel intact.

April 13 Thursday

Breakfast: boiled ham - 6.30. Dinner and Tea: Maconochies stew and marmalade. We marched back to near the **Sucrerie,**[107] and were trench digging for four hours. Why cannot they let us rest? I received another parcel from A.A. The day was just showery and there was a cold wind. I send Doll a Field PC and was then writing an unfinished letter to her. Rumours are rife that 31st Division are to be sent home for East Coast defence. The East Lancs have had orders about conduct when peace is declared. Our Colonel is said to have expressed indignation at the Battalion having to go trenching today. He said there were limits. I received a letter from Doll, April 9th.

April 14 Friday

Breakfast: fried bacon in plenty. Dinner: Maconochies. Tea: marmalade. We marched off trenching again at 7am and were back at 1.10pm. We were shelled most of the time but none came very near. I was then cleaning up in the afternoon, had my first wash and shave since Tuesday and gave in my letter for Doll.

April 15 Saturday

Dinner: Maconochies. Tea: honey. I was on day guard at the pond, mount 7am and was done out of breakfast, so I bought eggs and coffee at the billet. I have a thick head and a hard cough. I received a letter from Doll, April 12th. There was a terrific bombardment from our guns for half an hour during the night.

April 16 Sunday

Breakfast: bacon. Dinner: sea pie. Tea: marmalade. We are on church parade only today and have a hut orderly so we are kept on the go pretty well. We paraded at 6.35 pm for trenching again and then worked four hours up to midnight. I was raining all of the time so I was wet through but my cough got easier and marching back I felt absolutely fit, while most of the fellows were jiggered. There was tea for us when we got back. There is a nasty rumour that **Verdun**[108] has fallen with 180,000 prisoners.

---

[107] **Sucrerie** – the site of a sugar refinery, close to Euston Dump on the road to Mailley Maillet, now the site of the Sucrerie Military Cemetery.

[108] **Verdun** - The Battle of Verdun in 1916 was the longest single battle of World War 1. The casualties from Verdun and the impact the battle had on the French Army was a primary reason for the British starting the Battle of the Somme in July 1916 in an effort to take German pressure off of the French at

April 17 Monday

Breakfast: boiled bacon. Dinner: plum duff. Tea: stew & marmalade. I had a delightful nights rest and my cough is much looser. We are having absolutely slack days but I am detailed for the second party tonight. I got my mackintosh and handed in my letter to A.A. and Margaret Cooper and one to Arthur. I wrote to Doll, Mother and Maggie and will post them tomorrow. I am detailed at night for an induction in **flammenwerfer**[109] tomorrow morning and excused trenching tonight. I was fearfully wet and cold.

April 18 Tuesday

Breakfast: bacon. Dinner: stew. Tea: marmalade. I had a long and comfortable nights rest. We had flammenwerfer and **lachegrouse**[110] shell demonstration at other side of Bus at 10.30am, was back by 12.30am. We were required to capture portable liquid gas apparatus and fellows were positioned in a trench just in front of it, to show the harmless effect if they keep low. It was rather piffle. We had lachegrouse gas too and fellows were with and without goggles. I handed in green envelope to Doll with enclosures for Mother and Maggie. We paraded at 11pm for trenching again, as wet as ever.

April 19 Wednesday

Breakfast: bacon. Dinner: stew and rice. Tea: marmalade. There was a fine lunar rainbow right across lines this morning. I got to the trench at 12.45am and they are practically finished. The day is too wet and sticky to be at all workable. We had orders to stop till 4.30am which nevertheless must be adhered to. Colley makes us repair a sodden parapet – how long this fooling? We leave at 4am because it is daybreak, so Colley halts us in the road till 4.30am. We get back for breakfast about 6.30am. I slept until 1pm then had dinner and paraded in an adjoining hut for a lecture. Rain, Rain! Rain! I get my hair cut. We the parade again for the trenches, under **Wood**[111], thank goodness. I get to work about 9.45pm, very stiff and sticky, deepening the old fallen in and shallow trenches of the French. I should work till 12.30 midnight but Wood takes us off at 12.00 and we arrive back at 1.40am for tea and rum.

April 20 Thursday

Breakfast: bacon. Dinner: stew & rice. Tea: Golden Shred. I had another good night's rest and just sat up for breakfast and then slept till 11.30am. I had a good wash and shave in a billy and we had a short instruction in barbed wiring in the afternoon. I received a letter from Doll, April 17th with an enclosure from Mrs

---

Verdun. The Battle of Verdun started on February 21st 1916 and ended on December 16th in 1916 and made General Phillipe Petain a national hero in France.

[109] **Flammenwerfer** - a flame thrower first used by the Germans at Hooge on 30th July 1915. It was a steel cylinder filled with inflammable liquid and fitted with a long steel nozzle that projected a jet of flame approximately twenty yards long.

[110] **lachegrouse** –tear gas shells.

[111] **12/559 Lance Sergeant Thomas Harper Wood** – Killed in action on 2nd November 1916, he is buried in Sailly au Bois Military Cemetery.

Watson and also a letter from Mother. We are due for trenching again at 6.30pm but we started fast with only a reduced party so we went at 11pm with eleven others out of our platoon. I escaped to dinner and it rained again all day.

April 21 Good Friday

Breakfast: bacon. Dinner: stew & raisin duff. Tea: stewed dates. We were up at 8am for breakfast then had:

Parade	10am – 12 noon	Platoon drill
Parade	2pm – 3pm	Physical drill
Parade	3.30pm - 4.25pm	A few words from Colley

We were off trenching at 11pm tonight and it has been raining hard since 3pm. We lurched out in mud and inky blackness and marched to Courcelles, we then did an about turn again as we hear that the trenches are flooded. I was back in bed by 12.30 midnight.

April 22 Saturday

Breakfast: bacon. Dinner: boiled mutton & potatoes. Tea: marmalade. I had breakfast at 6.30am and the weather was drizzle and rain for most of the day. We had rifle exercises and a gas helmet drill from 10am – 12 noon, physical 2pm - 2.30pm and then paraded in the next hut till 4pm, just messing about. There was no working party tonight. P.S. I wrote to Doll somewhere about here.

April 23 Easter Sunday

Breakfast: bacon. Dinner: stew and plum duff. Tea: marmalade. We had a short church parade then were sent trenching 11am - 1.30pm. I was drawn for a night party but **Greaves**[112] swaps with me as his sleeping partner is going and Hale isn't. It is the first fine day since we came back to Bertrancourt – a splendid day. We had a tobacco allowance and pipes from the **Buffer Girls.**[113]

April 24 Monday

Breakfast: bacon. Dinner: stew & rice. Tea: marmalade - only half a loaf each. We were digging this morning and there was no parade in the afternoon. We hear that C Company are not trenching this evening, only D Company. I receive a letter from Doll April 21st and a parcel from Auntie Annie which contained chocolate and cigs. It has been a fine day again.

April 25 Tuesday

Breakfast: bacon. Dinner: cheese. Tea: Maconochies and marmalade. We paraded at 8am for a working party and marched off at 8.30am. I was a beautiful day so I am looking forward to trenching and taking a fair amount of rest. I was disappointed to pass the trenches and then proceeded to Colincamps for something vaguely described as wiring work. It was frustrating as the working hours were announced as being 10am till 12.30 noon and 1pm till

---

[112] **12/385 Private T. A. Greaves** – was wounded on 1st July 1916.

[113] **A buffer girl** was a worker in the Sheffield cutlery industry who used the polishing machinery on the steel tableware: a hot and dirty job which needed protective clothing.

3.30pm which was a very pleasant surprise, as we are able to nap after all. In the morning we thread tufts of grass into wire netting which the other half gathers up. This is to cover over our gun pits. It turned into a kindergarten game in the afternoon as we changed round. I managed to get some good naps. Meanwhile the Germans shelled heavily about 200 yards off, apparently trying to find our gun emplacements.

April 26 Wednesday
Breakfast: bacon. Dinner: day rations. Tea: stew and marmalade. We were grassing as yesterday but now piecework and we finished at 2.45pm and then marched back. Hale and I try to find a little joie de vivre in a bottle of Medoc for 1 franc 50 and 15 centimes on the bottle with no glass. We religiously consumed that bottle as though it were medicine and with as much enjoyment. We then retired to the church hut concert and consume gingerbread and nap in the half hour intervening. *The idea of wasting valuable years of one's short life at this game and being treated like beasts shows that we have truly sold our birthright.* Even green envelopes containing Private Concerns are opened at the orderly room now which is quite contrary to regulations. On waking up at concert time we were told that the East Lancs band had played half an hour ago and had gone.

April 27 Wednesday
Breakfast: Maconochies. Dinner: ditto. Tea: marmalade. We were charged for a trenching party today and fell in at 7.30am and marched off at 8am and were back at 2pm and were not overworked. It was an exceedingly hot day and I received a letter from Doll dated April 23rd.

April 28 Friday
Breakfast: cold bacon. Dinner: stew. Tea: Dates. We were allowed to go to Colincamps in the morning and are billeted in a farm two deep on sacking stretched over a frame. I have to repair Hale's and my portion. It is very hot which is stifling my cough and cold and I get no better and feel rather done in. We have only one hour's lecture in the afternoon on gas by **Jeremy Hill,**[114] then a good nap afterwards. G (Grant) is in charge of C Company, the Colonel and most of the officers are away for one month's instruction, when it comes to actual fighting it seems we can dispense with this expensive element! We fell in at 6.45om for a night working party. G claimed me as we marched out and I got Hale off as well. Some replicas of the German trenches wanted setting out next morning for rehearsal. I stopped with G in his billet until after 10pm and he treated me very well, giving me good coffee whisky and cigarettes. He told me he would have put me down for a stripe the other day but couldn't get at me. I mentioned a commission idea to him and he promised to do his best.

---

[114] **12/676 Corporal J Hill** – a member of C Company.

April 29 Saturday

Breakfast: bacon. Dinner: Maconochies. Tea: dates. One of the fellows in the working party that I missed last night, was wounded by machine gun fire. We were up at 5.30am, left at 6.30am and met G at 7.15am. We had work set out and were going well. G told us we could go back at 2pm. I had a fright during the morning and thought that I had lost ordinance map but G found that he had it. It was rather amusing as the owner of the land wanted to know what we were going to do. G told me to say just 'military business' and tell him to clear off. There was then much heated volubility on the part of the native. Eventually we had to threaten him with personal violence and arrest before he would clear himself and his cows off of his own domain. I received a letter from Doll of 26th and Mother 25th, and handed in a letter to Doll with an enclosure to Auntie Annie and sent a Field PC to Mother. It was a compulsory foot wash tonight. The Germans fiercely bombarded in the late hours of the night for 1½ hours. I managed to get to sleep before it was over though and the air was filled with the continuous roar of shells.

April 30 Saturday

Breakfast: bacon. Dinner: Maconochies. Tea: marmalade. My cough is now fearful and I feel quite jiggered up, but I had a restful day, so sleep off and on till teatime. There was a heavy shower in the afternoon. I am on trenching fatigue in the evening, parade at 6.50pm and didn't get back till 3.20am when we had to finish. We were swept by machine guns now and then and we heard the bullets whistling overhead. Tea and rum was served when we got back, which eased my cough and I got the most restful 2½ hours sleep for some time.

May 1 Monday

Breakfast: bacon. Dinner: Maconochies. Tea: marmalade. Bacon is in abundance lately. I was roused at 6.30am and am detailed for town common fatigue (burning rubbish in incinerators) but go sick with my cough. The Doctor hears my tale of woe at 9am but doesn't examine or ask me anything, just gives me two lozenges. I go back for duty but **Crozier**[115] puts me on a bath party. I have a good hot bath in the usual cream but get a rinse in a bucket of fresh water. I don't get on my incinerator till 11am. I was actually sent trenching again at 5.30pm and was back at midnight. It took two hours to march there where I was on top of the parapet all the time making bacon. I witnessed a lively skirmish in the front lines only one or two hundred yards away in a field adjoining which was screened by hedge. It looked as though we might be making a bombing attack. We had a rum ration and hot tea on our return. There was just a sprinkling of rain while we were out.

---

[115] **12/628 Sergeant Henry Cecil Crozier** - won a Military Medal (MM) on the night of 15th / 16th May 1916, a few weeks before being killed on 1st July 1916. He died helping eight men who had been wounded by the same shell and he had won the MM in similar circumstances. His body was never found and he is commemorated on the Thiepval Memorial.

May 2 Tuesday

● Breakfast: bacon - took rations lying about for the rest of the day - I easily scraped up a whole tin of butter. Dinner: Maconochies. We set off for the trenches 1.30am and there were severe thunderstorms on the way. The trenches were vacated when we arrived. It was a fairly quiet both day and night and there were no questions about standing with your head above the parapet at night. I am coughing and fearfully cold, this is the limit. No sleep is allowed and G says we must be working all the time, scraping mud out of the trenches. I have the greatest difficulty in keeping my eyes open even while on guard, possibly due to the cough lozenges.

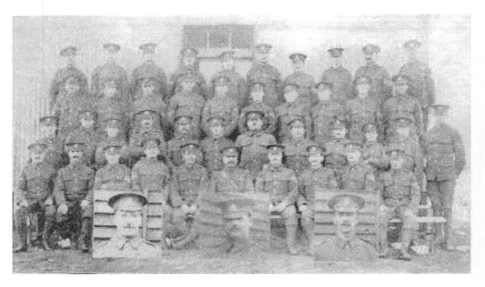

Top row left to right: Sergeants Jones, Faker, Buckley, Unwin, Furzey, Madin, Bardsley, Turner and R.G. Roberts
Second row: Sergeants Atkin, Bingham, Wells, Register, Crozier, E.W. Roberts, Wilkinson, Simpson and Horncastle
Third row: Sergeants Sleigh, Philbey, Chappell, Bevington, Powell, Heppinstall, Kirk, Nutt, Bridgwater, Atkinson, Connell and Everitt
Fourth row: Company Quartermaster-Sergeant Bilbey, Company Sergeant Majors Morley, Cavanagh and Marsden, Regimental Quartermaster Sergeant Doncaster, Regimental Sergeant Major Polden, Company Quartermaster Sergeants Charlesworth, Badger and Shepherdson, Company Sergeant Major Loxley
Inserts Sergeant Hutton (Regimental Cook, Company Sergeant Major Ellis, Sergeant Henderson

May 3 Wednesday

Breakfast: very indifferent cold bacon. Dinner: bully beef. Tea: jam. We were allowed from 6am - 12 noon for a sleep. I didn't get much as the Germans shelled us. In the afternoon they fired shells, rifle grenades and **pis cans**[116]in great profusion and the accuracy of their range is steadily improving. One dud rifle grenade hit the **parados**[117] above me. Two next seemed to fall in the trench near and covered me with dirt. **Atkinson**[118] got **shell shock**[119] and thinks that he has been badly hit but it was only a stone. Todd gets a slight wound in his leg and confesses disappointment at it not being good enough for **blighty**[120]. While having it dressed a shell does for seven of them - poor fellows. They were all instantly killed apart from Todd who lived nearly till they got him to hospital. The victims were: **Sergeant Major Ellis**[121], **Hardwick, Rogers, Richards, Frost, Unwin** and **Todd**[122], two of whom were casualties previously. A fellow next to **Gus Platts**[123] is wounded in the leg and tumbles back on him putting his shoulder out. G sends me to doctor at headquarters for my cough. He gives me lozenges and a gargle. Coming back I meet a stretcher party of three trying to carry **Richards**[124] so turn back and lend a hand and put him in a trench deeping. When I get back – there is no post! My cough frightens fellows. I received a letter from Doll April 29th. The weather today has been fine.

May 4 Thursday

Breakfast: cold bacon. Dinner: bully beef. Tea: jam. We had a stand to from 2.45am until 3.45am, Grant comes along and curses because I'm not smart enough and immediately a stand down is given. I'm to start my rest at 12 noon. Our communication trenches near where I'm working are heavily bombed apparently mostly pis cans but I get a good rest being asleep from 1.30pm to 4.30pm and I am then awakened for tea. We have to stand to in support at 5pm and then we go off on a wiring party. I'm not allowed over the parapet on account of my cough so I can only help behind. I return for further all night digging in the trenches that I have been in all day and I failed to realise this until

---

[116] **Pis cans** – German trench mortar bombs of about 10-inch diameter, also known as flying pigs and oil cans.

[117] **Parados** - an elevation of earth behind a fortified place as a protection against attack from the rear, especially a mound along the back of a trench. See diagram on page 65.

[118] **12/1381 Private Cyril Atkinson** – Killed in action on 1st July 1916. His body was never recovered and he is commemorated on the Theipval Memorial.

[119] **shell shock** – derangement of the nervous system resulting from exposure to shell explosions at close quarters.

[120]**Blighty** – soldiers slang for a wound that secured return to England.

[121] **12/560 Company Sergeant Major John William Ellis** – killed in action on 4th May 1916 when a minewerfen shell landed in his dugout. He had trained the Battalion from the very beginning. He is buried in Sucrerie Military Cemetery, Serre.

[122] **12/668 Lance Corporal Stafford Hardwick, 12/767 Private Edward Gordon Rogers, 12/1238 Private Arthur Douglas Frost, 12/807 Private Gilbert Unwin and 12/802 Private Harold Todd** - are all buried in the Sucrerie Military Cemetery, Serre.

[123] **Lance Corporal Gus Platts** – Boxer and Physical Training Instructor.

[124] **12/757 Private Percy Charles Richards** – worked with Frank Meakin at Sheffield Town Hall, hence the reason he stopped to carry him. He is buried in the Sucrerie Military Cemetery, Serre.

dawn. **West**[125] comes to support the trench for the farce of standing to at dawn and I found myself frequently dozing off. It was a fine day again.

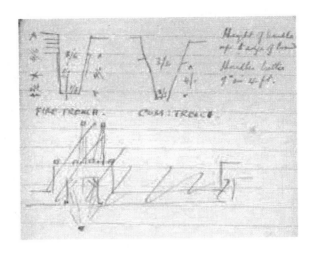

Frank's illustrations of the plan of the trenches

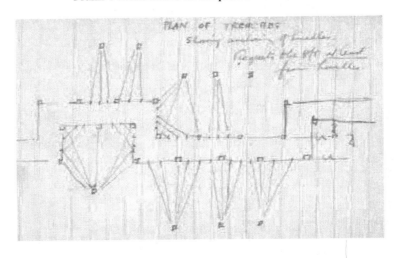

[125] **12/262 Private P. M. West** - a Sheffield University student. He was wounded in the attack on 1st July 1916 and killed in action on 12th May 1917. He is commemorated on the Arras Memorial

May 5 Friday

Breakfast: cold bacon. Dinner: cold beef. Tea: peaches, dates and jam

G says we are to dig all day today without a rest. I went soundly to sleep between each mouthful of my breakfast and the ration party misses us with tea. I go to the headquarters and fill a water bottle - water and cold tea at the same time and I had a delightful wash and clean my teeth and gargle. They had difficulty in waking me at dinner time and again at tea, in spite of being under very heavy shellfire. I am detailed for the ration party in the evening. I walked to **Charing Cross** [126] near **Euston**[127] and made two journeys carrying rations to the A Company headquarters. It was a wet night and chilly and I am glad that I took my overcoat in spite of the weight. I had an hour's rest in the dugout on the way back and a stand to 2.45 am.

May 6 Saturday

Breakfast: cold bacon. Dinner: bully beef. Tea: peach jam, bully beef and pickle. It is midday already, making this morning so far a well earned rest. I wash and shave, clean up and put some sandbags in the trench bottom and get some more decent sleep. I received a letter from Mother dated May 2nd. There are the prospects of a bright day again and it is rather more peaceful now, although there is still the usual spirited contest between our trench mortar and the guns on the left, the shells from both which pass over us. We have dinner and then we march out about 1.30pm, our party carrying suppliers stores with many bottles of rum, shame! Then back to Euston Dump. We get there about 3pm and then have to wait for Grant and C Company until about 6pm. We are then marched to camp three miles beyond Bus without a halt. I was absolutely done in and Jeremy Hill collapses. We are in a canvas hut in the wood as before, with a fine leaf mould floor and it is dry. We get tea immediately on arrival. It is very crowded but I manage to get to sleep immediately on getting down. I received a letter from Doll May 2nd and the weather has been occasional drizzle during the day.

May 7 Sunday

Breakfast: bacon. Dinner: stew. Tea: jam. I slept until breakfast at 8am and then again until 11.30am. I was then resting all day and wrote to Doll. The camp is beautifully situated on a hillside in fine woods which are carpeted with violets. The floors of the canvas huts are dry with leaf mould this time. The East Lancs band has been playing so peacefully that I might be in Hyde Park in Sheffield or the River Gardens. It has been a dull and wet day.

---

[126] **Charing Cross** –The trench railways ran from here to the front line, hence names such as Euston, Charing Cross, Waterloo, Railway Avenue and Blackfriars,

[127] **Euston also known as Euston Dump** – a large store dump, full of barbed wire, sandbags etc. close to Colincamps.

May 8 Monday

Breakfast: bacon. Dinner: mutton, mashed potatoes, currant duff. Tea: marmalade. I reported sick again but was given duty and three brown lozenges and one pink one. Our hut was detailed for bathing so I did orderly in morning instead. It was a wet afternoon so we only had helmet inspection and a bit of bayonet fighting. The dinner was the best that we have had for a long time. I received a parcel from A.A. which contained a rhubarb pudding, oxtail soup, chocolate, cigarettes, toilet paper and a novel. My green envelope to Doll has been opened, G called me to account for stating that we had only one hours official sleep whilst in the trenches, I proved the statement to him. I am told B Company have had about forty letters burnt, I wonder if mine has met the same fate but Doll's remains in suspense. I hear that the engineer who blew his hand off with a German rifle grenade at Colincamps has got 21 days field punishment for it. **Rush**[128] has shown me a stone chat's nest with three eggs. There were nine killed and thirteen wounded in our last spell in the trenches

May 9 Tuesday

Breakfast: bacon. Dinner: bully beef and stew. Tea: Marmalade. I reported sick again. The Doctor examines me a bit this time and he asks the reason for my black eye. I explain that it is bunged up with my cold and that also my ear and head are very thick. He looks for a rash but finds nothing. I expected light duties at least this time but no, he said I could carry on with my work. I asked if I could be excused any night work and he said it would not hurt me to go on with it. Anyway, I managed to dodge the parade for the rest of the morning and got an easy time on fatigues in the afternoon, I am feeling very done in though. Many fellows have just had their green envelopes returned as they wrote of wanting to come out of the trenches. Much to my surprise mine was not, although it contained what they consider 'forbidden matter'. I wonder if it was destroyed? **General Sir Douglas Haig**[129] is coming to inspect our camp tomorrow and the order is that all buttons and badges are to be cleaned but there is absolutely nothing to clean them with. We have even been picking the sticks and dead branches up out of the woods, putting them in heaps and cutting down the undergrowth. It was wet for most of the day. I received a parcel from Maggie with a letter dated March 5th.

May 10 Saturday

Breakfast: bacon. Dinner: stew. Tea: Marmalade. We had an early morning parade then again from 9am - 12 noon and 2pm – 4.15pm. We were at it all the time and it was probably arranged so that we will be looking busy when Sir Douglas Haig arrives! I report sick again at nine and was given the usual three lozenges and duty. I manage to dodge one hour of parade anyhow. Sir Douglas Haig and staff arrive on us about 11am. We see them just in time so get very

---

[128] **12/770 Private B. Rush** – a Sheffield University Laboratory Assistant and a bandsman. He took part in the attack of 1st July 1916.

[129] **Field Marshal Douglas Haig** – Commander-in-Chief of the British Expeditionary Forces (BEF) from December 1915.

busy, passing point and guard, which we do very effectively. I hear him remark "very good indeed". They stop at our platoon and ask several fellows what they did before the war. The 'Curios' are giving a concert this evening in the village but I fail in the draw for passes. I scarcely felt like going though, as I felt rather done in after tea. It has been a fine spring like day but it felt rather cold in the evening. I wrote to A.A.

May 11 Thursday
Breakfast: bacon. Dinner: stew. Tea: marmalade. I reported sick again and I feel all right but my voice is still missing. The Doctor gave me three white lozenges instead of brown ones, as I told him the latter gave me diarrhoea. I just missed the working party, digging trenches nearby so I was given light duties and had a soft day. I wrote to Doll and Maggie and received a letter from Doll dated May 7th. It has been a nice balmy, spring day.

May 12 Friday
Breakfast: bacon. Dinner: stew. Tea: marmalade. I reported sick again as my voice is still unregained. The Doctor tells me to persevere and gives me four more white lozenges. The Battalion marches, so I am put on camp fatigue and am digging by the sump holes and the exertion takes it out of me, with much perspiration. It is a nice, fine day. I hear that the Colonel on seeing many empty tins and boxes in a hut, enquired the reason. He was told that many parcels had been received. He said in that case they would have to be stopped.

May 13 Saturday
Breakfast: boiled bacon. Dinner: stew. Tea: marmalade. I reported sick again and was given three brown lozenges this time. The Doctor, I hope jokingly, remarked that I shouldn't recover my voice. It was a wet morning, so we only had rifle competence and about ¾ hour of physical. Grant tells me he has been seeing about a commission and advises that a special form of such, can be obtained from **RIBA**.[130] I then wrote to RIBA enquiring.

May 14 Sunday
Breakfast: boiled ham. Dinner: Stew and currant duff. Tea: marmalade. I reported sick again. The Doctor didn't think it was much good giving me any more medicine but instead gave me three different white lozenges to gargle with which seemed to do my voice good. I managed to dodge the digging party to Bus. I then went to Bus to have a bath and was given clean pants and socks but no shirt. The water was very scarce and I could not wash face or head. I received a letter from Doll dated March 10th. We are ordered into the trenches for 10 days from tomorrow. Our blankets were given in afterwards and all orders are cancelled and we must wait until tomorrow for our new orders. I took a walk to Authie and back, which is not much of a place.

---

[130] **RIBA** – Royal Institute of British Architects.

May 15 Monday
Breakfast: bacon. Dinner: stew and currant duff. Tea: marmalade. It has been a very wet day. The new orders for trenches were received in the morning after all, we had a few fatigues in morning, but it was fairly restful. We fall in 1.30pm and marched off at 2pm, with no fall out until 7.30pm. We were all posted in **Rob Roy**[131] and set to work at once. We had to walk two miles to collect our shovels and in the trenches we were half way up our legs in mud. The Germans gave us the most intense bombardment for over a year which lasted until 2.30am. Dowty was killed and 11 men out of 21 were casualties in No 9. I bound up one fellow's head and helped out a fellow with half his foot blown off and supported **Dowty**[132] until he died.

May 16 Tuesday
Our rations have been lost as they were burned in the general blowing up of the trenches, so we fended as we could on what we had. I found half of my bayonet rifle blown to blazes and my overcoat is lost and my gas helmet has been blown from the parados, opposite to where I was sheltering. The Colonel congratulates C Company on their stand as Berkshires abandoned part of their trenches and had 30 men captured. We had a lazy day and were then ordered to the front line in the evening. We were put in No 11 post which was absolutely blown to pieces the previous evening and where **Sgt Register**[133] and **five others**[134] were killed. I'm put in charge of the post. Grant congratulates us on the work done. My cold is getting better and I feel in fine spirits and worked hard all night repairing the parapet, never sleeping until stand to a quiet moonlit night.

May 17 Wednesday
There is an abundance of food, as many from the platoon are now missing. We have had cold bacon, mutton, butter, jam, Maconochies, cheese etc and we also find Officer's rations which have been buried, including sausages, jam, prunes, bacon etc. We carry on resetting the parapets and get a good sleep in the morning. **Cloud**[135] takes my name for my experience in road making and laying out. We get a lot of rifle grenades over in the afternoon and our trench mortar and guns are pretty active. I received a letter from Mrs Headland of April 1st and it has been a very hot afternoon. Our steel helmets are scarcely a summer

---

[131] **Rob Roy** – the support trench behind Railway Hollow and Campion.

[132] **12/638 Private Horace Bradley Dowty** - buried in the Sucrerie Military Cemetery, Serre.

[133] **12/755 Sergeant Bernard John Register** –was noted for the gallant way in which he helped to dig out his comrades without regard to his own safety and was killed during the action. He was not decorated for his bravery and is buried in Sucrerie Military Cemetery, Serre.

[134] **Five others** – there were actually 15 men killed during the two hour raid including Sgts Register & Dowty: **12/25 Private A. E. Arrowsmith, 12/291 Private Wilfred Barlow, 12/516 Private Alfred Slack, 12/1267 Private Percy Burch, 12/1057 Lance Corporal Richard Elvidge Smith, 12/1469 Private Gilbert George Cook, 12/1480 Private Joseph Strickland, 12/1145 Private Thomas William Stubley, 12/651 Private Edwin Furniss, 12/805 Private Wilfred Henry Cranstone Tucker, 12/700 Private Clement Johnson, 12/1268 Private Richard Henry Walker and 12/568 Private Robert Haly Bruce Matthews** and all are buried in the Sucrerie Military Cemetery, Serre.

[135] **Lieutenant C.C. Cloud** - Commissioned on 22nd July 1915 and served in 12th Y&L from 31 March 1916. He took part in the attack of 1st July 1916.

weight and fellows are burning their fingers touching them. Grant tells Colonel that my post No. 11 and No. 15 did most of the work.

May 18 Thursday

The night is quiet except for a few rifle grenades and we hear the Germans whistling and singing. It is a misty morning and we have orders to carry on as the night operations. I am pulled up by the Colonel because men were breakfasting with equipment off, due to Crozier's orders, against which I have protested. **Hollis**[136] also was not standing to his post, as he should have been. My explanation was apparently accepted though. I received a letter from Mother dated May 12th and cough lozenges from Doll. We are ordered by G to move out in the afternoon and to wash, clean and shave beforehand. It is my turn for a sleep at 10.30pm. I then have dinner with plenty of Maconochies, butter and blackcurrant jam and then sleep again from 11.30pm - 12.30 midnight and move out soon after 1pm. G seems very decent and in good humour. I am quite comfortable out in the dugout in afternoon and we only had to have equipment on ready to turn out during stand to, which was a decent concession of G's. We are carrying very heavy cases of rifle grenades from 10pm - 1am and I then got down for hours sleep before stand to at 2.45am and then waited ready in the dugout. It has been a very hot day again.

May 19 Friday

The morning was rather chilly. We had breakfast at 4.30am and we then were left to rest till dinner at midday. Rations included cold fried bacon, Maconochies, bully beef, dates (a few) and no jam or butter but we had that in reserve. We were then working from 12.30 noon - 5.15pm, carrying and then had tea. It was a very hot afternoon and a quiet day. I hear that the Battalion have lost 17 who were killed and have about 60 casualties that there were a 14 killed and about 40 casualties in the bombardment. We were trench digging from 9pm - 12 midnight. We should have gone on till stand to but G is very considerate lately and I am sorry to hear that he is leaving us for the Brigade.

May 20 Saturday

Breakfast: cold bacon. Dinner: Maconochies and bully beef and bags of biscuits which were left behind. I got two hours sleep before the stand to, then all we had to do was clean up dugouts and then wash, shave and clean ourselves. We stood to for relief at 11.30am then marched to the camp at Courcelles which was tents, with several good rests along the way. We had tea on arrival with plenty of jam and butter. I received a letter in morning served up with bacon from Doll of May 13th containing two photos of **'Poplars'**[137] with my dear wife in the foreground looking perfectly stunning. There was also a parcel of papers also from Maggie. I was entertained to fine ham supper by **Freddie Cork** who

---

[136] **12/687 Private Arthur James Hollis** – was killed in action on 1st July 1916 and is buried in Luke Copse Military Cemetery, Serre.

[137] **Poplars** – the Family home, one of an important group of Regency villas that still survive today at Alvaston near to Derby.

had received a fine parcel. I got down about midnight and had a perfect night's sleep, what a perfect treat after the trenches. I received a PC from Arthur, May 18th who is at Hardebot, resting for a few days by the sea.

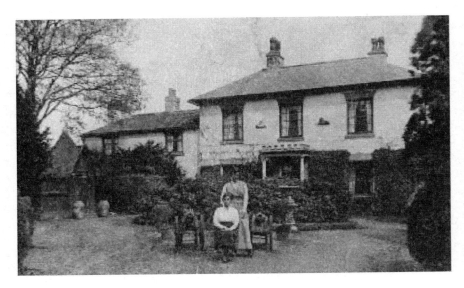

Poplars' the Family home in Alvaston. Doll can be see standing behind her sister

May 21 Sunday
Breakfast: bacon. Dinner: sea pie. Tea: jam and honey. We were only awakened at eight and had to turn out for a permanent working party at 8.20am. It was rather a blow and we had a big scramble for breakfast but it proved easy. We were trenching just outside the village itself from 9am – 12 noon and 2pm - 4.30pm. Parkin[138] was in charge, who expressed approval of my work and I made it show in my portion. I received a letter from Doll of May 17th, bless her, in spite of the scarcity in which I've written to her, she keeps up the correspondence finely. I have to report to G about some special work tomorrow. It has been perfect weather lately although a trifle hot. I have seen G about the alterations to the German trenches and I am to take the same in hand and have 15 men to do the work. I am then employed for the rest of the evening planning out the work.

---

[138] **12/1161 Lance Corporal Horace George Parkin** killed in action on 1st July 1916, his body was never found and he is commemorated on the Thiepval Memorial.

May 22 Monday

Breakfast: bacon. Dinner: Stew. Tea: peach and blackcurrant jam, plenty of butter too since we got to camp. There are lots of parcels for fellows in our tent, so I am living no end. I was pegging out trenches with Hale in morning and then take out a working party in afternoon. There was a little misunderstanding with Corporal Macement, who wouldn't take a shovel at first but he did in the end and has since worked as hard as any. Almost the whole camp was on the night working party to which we escape so long as the job lasts, long may it last but we are supposed to finish tomorrow. I was writing out my application for a commission in the evening. G approved the draft and suggests the addition of my taking charge of special details continuously. I wrote to Mother and put it in the letter bag in **Sergeant Philbey's**[139] tent.

May 23 Thursday

Meals ditto. I am with my party in the trenches from 8.30am till 12 noon and from 1.30pm to 5pm. We have all worked hard and still not finished part of our work, sandbagging a section of the trench. G came round this afternoon and gave me a bit of his old self re the portion of trench I had set out. I had done it in relation to one portion and he viewed it in its relation to another portion. I gave Captain Colley my application for a commission, which he said he would pass through at once.

May 24 Wednesday

Meals ditto. I expected to finish my trenching in the morning but it took until 4.30pm in the afternoon and it rained hard all day after dinner. An officer came round in the afternoon, who seems to be in charge of the proposed attack. He said he didn't expect us to get so far on the left as the big hole meant some alterations, which didn't work out with plan. The poor old working party; every available man goes out as usual in the pouring rain. I received a letter from Doll dated May 20th mentioning an accompanying parcel. I took **Garfitt, Cook** and **Kellington**[140] out for a fried eggs and coffee supper. The letter I that wrote to Mother was returned and described as 'too thick'. I obliterated such words as 'trenches' and rewrote the second page and posted again. We had a rum ration again tonight and we need it. Our ground sheets were wet through and our clothing and blankets are damp. I wrote to Doll about this date.

May 25 Thursday

Breakfast: bacon. Dinner: roast mutton and potatoes. Tea: apricot jam. I was resting practically all day. I was down for surveying in the afternoon, correcting trench plans, but one only chosen after all by **Roberts.**[141] I was on the working

---

[139] **12/1018 Sergeant George Philbey** – Died on 10th July 1916 from wounds received on 1st July 1916, buried in Couin Military Cemetery.
[140] **12/652 Private L. Garfitt, 12/622 Private F. Cook, 12/1193 Private F. W. Kellington,** a very lucky trio - all three were 'only' wounded on 1st July 1916.
[141] **12/765 Lance Corporal N. W. Roberts** – he took part in the attack on 1st July 1916.

party but we don't go out till 1am. We had **lice straffing**[142] after tea and I filled a big bag. I received letters from Doll and Mother dated May 21st. I find that Arthur was 21 miles away from me as the crow flies.

May 26 Friday
Breakfast: bacon. We welcome orders before midnight but the one o'clock party would not turn out until 9am as it was raining in torrents and they showed an example of consideration. It turned out fine and we were remaking a firing trench. I got congratulations from Cloud on my steps down to the traffic trench. I worked till 4.15pm and we were held up when we got to the road on account of the high explosive shells, which had been falling all afternoon, trying for our gun emplacements. I got out soon after 5pm and were back at the camp at 6 o'clock where they had fine cold mutton and mashed potatoes for us. I received a parcel from Doll, so made some extra good tea, with peaches, Hovis bread and butter, gingerbread, glass of lemonade and chocolate. I was then writing to Arthur.

May 27 Saturday
Breakfast: bacon. Dinner and tea: boiled meat and pickles, marmalade. We were working as yesterday but quicker and we got back at 5.30pm. My steps were further commended and I am given a general supervising job. There was a nasty mess in Colincamps as we marched home, there were dead horses and pools of blood and **eight men were killed**[143] and seven wounded by a few shells that I saw dropped as we were working. I try and get our tent tidied a bit as there have been frequent complaints made regarding the same. We are sleeping in boots and **puttees**[144] all the time that we are here, which is most uncomfortable.

May 28 Sunday
Breakfast: bacon. Dinner: hot meat and raisin duff. Tea: marmalade. In the morning we went to Bus for a bath and a clean change of underclothing and I found lice again in the same day. We were on holiday all day by order of Rickman, Colonel of the East Lancs, who is now acting as Brigadier. I received a letter from Doll dated May 24th and wrote to Doll and Mother. Our **9.2s** [145] were busy at night retaliating for Colincamps.

---

[142] **Lice straffing** – the picking of lice out of clothes, sometimes soldiers would 'burn them off' with cigarettes.

[143] **12/1084 Lance Corporal Frederick Walker** was one of those killed and is buried in Sucrerie MC. Before the war he was a fish and poultry dealer in Sheffield.

[144] **Puttees** – 4 inch wide pieces of cloth bound around the lower leg. They were very unpopular with the men as they were difficult to make presentable for parades.

[145] **9.2s** - A British heavy howitzer comprising of a segment shaped ground platform assembled from a steel section bolted the ground with a carriage that was mounted on the platform, it was pivoted at the front and traversed up to 30 degrees left and right. It was only used on the Western Front and initially batteries were in Heavy Artillery Groups, usually a single battery of 9.2-inch, the other four batteries being differently equipped.

May 29 Monday

Breakfast: bacon. Dinner: cooked meat, potatoes and cabbage mashed. We are on the working party again in trenches and were rather heavily shelled as we go in. I am given a supervising job again but I prefer to spend most of the time working revetting the parapet in the backward bay. I received a parcel from A.A. which contained tinned fruit, chocolate, acid drops, Eiffel Tower insect powder, magazine, writing pad and cigs. We were then clearing up for our departure to Bus tomorrow. It was a very wet night.

May 30 Tuesday

Breakfast and dinner: Maconochies. Tea: jam and marmalade. We left Courcelles at 9.30am for Bus Wood and then rested for the rest of the day. I felt rather done in with a full pack and slept through. My throat feels sore now when I swallow. I received a **'Public Opinion'**[146] from Colin and wrote to A.A.

May 31 Wednesday

Breakfast: bacon. Dinner: stewed beef. Tea: marmalade. Fine woods and a fine day, I could hear the owls and nightingales at night. We are back to parades all day, with more buttons and boot cleaning. Whilst scouring Bus Wood for wherewithals, I incidentally listen to the Leeds Band concert outside the YMCA. I received a letter from Doll who hasn't had one from me yet.

June 1 Thursday

Breakfast: bacon. Dinner: Maconochie's. Tea: marmalade. We paraded just for inspection and to present arms. General O'Gowan, Division General inspects us this afternoon and we were cleaning and burnishing in anticipation all afternoon. We fell in at 3.40pm and then messed about till 4.30pm and fell out till 4.45pm and were inspected at 5pm. He congratulated us on our stand and our fight under fire but suggested that we perhaps lacked experience; the 31st is the only new Division in the 4th Army. I received a parcel from Mother which contained cigs, salmon, Kampfire, cake, caramels, coffee squares and I wrote to Doll.

June 2 Friday

Breakfast: Maconochies. Dinner: stew. Tea: marmalade. We had a sharp shower early in the morning but it brightened up for a fine day. We fell in 8.30am for route march and were back by 12.30 noon. We only paraded in the afternoon for the usual few words from Colley and more instructions and light marching orders. Colley asked for a man who knew French and German for an observation job. I think I would have got it, had I come forward but somehow I felt that I should like to see things through in the fighting line. I have been playing Solo every evening and my losses and gains are pretty even.

---

[146] **Public Opinion** — A Magazine similar to 'Private Eye'.

June 3 Saturday

Breakfast: bacon. Dinner: bully beef and tea. Tea: apricot jam. We paraded at 7.30am for aeroplane signalling, which is just had a red flare to light in reply to an aeroplane's signal and to watch for the same. We were back at 11am and fell in at 12.20 noon for baths then ½ hour physical, then the day's work was done. I wrote to Mother and received a letter from Doll of May 30th. I won three frames at Solo and had ¼ of a pint of rum in my coffee which made me feel very rocky and I got out in the night between the roof and the side of the hut for a quick spew, no one suspected.

June 4 Sunday

Breakfast: bacon. Dinner: meat and cabbage. Tea: jam. We were to parade at 7am but waited until 7.30am and were supposed to go for a day's tree felling but it got turned on to stone breaking however **Flint**[147] was very industrious but wouldn't pay even for my keep. We finished at 12 noon but hung about napping and dining and arranged to get back to camp at 3.30pm, where we rested for the remainder of the day.

June 5 Monday

Breakfast: bacon. Dinner: Maconochies. Tea: jam. We had Reveille at 5am and marched off for Gazaincourt at 9am with the heaviest pack we have had consisting of steel helmets and Mackintoshes, in addition to anything we have carried before. We encountered the Corps Commander three times on the way and he remarked on our loaded appearance. We arrived at our billet at 2.30pm rather tired. We were not supposed to drink on the way and the particulars of the contents of our extra bottles were taken on arrival. I'd only had about ¼ of my bottle owing to sterilisation which made it like some foreign matter like creosote. I had a look round the village and found a decent café but it was terribly crowded. I then went to bed, too tired to write to Doll as my symptoms of diabetes are rather prevalent lately.

June 6 Tuesday

Breakfast: bacon. Dinner: sea pie. Tea: honey. We had a morning parade 7am till 8am. It was a wet morning and we just messed about experimenting with the equipment. Just as I had started a letter to Doll, we were unexpectedly fallen in at 1.30pm, digging grips to represent trenches and the whole countryside of corn is apparently to be sacrificed. We were working as hard and quickly as possible at each task set for us. I was thinking that when we were finished we should go but were kept hanging about till 7 o'clock after all. I fell off the end of the column with **Gunstone**[148] and another and we entered a café in Gezaincourt. Gunstone ordered three bottles (big ones) of Alsops Ale. I was so thirsty that at first I simply chucked down glass on glass and had quite enough though before

---

[147] **12/1375 Private W. Flint** – wounded on 16 May 1916 with 12th Y&L and wounded on 28 May 1918 with 7th Y&L.

[148] **12/661 Private William Walter Gunstone** brother of **12/660 Lance Corporal Frank Gunstone** who both signed up on the same day and who were both killed in action on the same day - 1st July 1916. They are buried in Luke Copse MC, Serre within a few feet of each other.

I'd finished. I got a little tea at the YMCA, then something more to eat at the billet. I received a 'Public Opinion' from Colin and it was time for bed then.

June 7 Wednesday
Breakfast: bacon. Dinner: stew. Tea: jam and marmalade. We had an early morning parade 7am - 7.45am and marched up to the Brigade parade ground after taking wrong direction for two miles. We had rifle and bayonet exercise and a trenching party in afternoon again and were at it till 6.30pm.

I had a letter from Arthur, June 1st his address is now: Cyclist A. Meakin, 'C' Company, Cyclist Battalion, 4th Corps Mounted Troops, BEF. I also received a letter from Maggie of June 3rd and then wrote to Doll and then it was bedtime again.

June 8 Thursday
Breakfast: bacon. Dinner: roast beef and mashed potatoes. Tea: watercress and marmalade. We had an early morning parade 7am - 7.40am, followed by a short brigade route march in the morning with a full pack. It was only six miles and we fell in at 8.45am and were back at 11.15am. The Colonel notes that C is the only Company with duty helmets. I was paid before dinner; 20 francs. We had a demonstration with a **Stokes gun**[149] and trench and wire, to which the whole brigade are marched at least 3 miles. It was rather disappointing in effect I thought. We got back at 5.15pm and I handed in a letter to Doll and received a letter from Doll, June 3rd with an enclosure from W Kenland of May 8th. We set off for Doullens at 6pm which is a quiet quaint town. It was quite a treat though to see some real shops again, although only those of a country town. The smell from the grocers was very homely. I found a café where I got three fried eggs, bread and butter ad lib, aperitif, café au lait and muscadet wine, all for 1.75 francs. We got rather wet coming home.

June 9 Friday
Breakfast: bacon, always very good, best smoked and liberal allowance. Dinner: stew and tea. Tea: watercress and jam. There was no early morning parade and we fall in 8.45 and have a new advance order. We marched to the training ground and rehearsed taking German lines. The field kitchen came up and we fell in from 12 noon - 1.45pm to dine, then resumed till 5pm. I bought three eggs and some butter for tea and received a letter from Mother, June 4th.

June 10 Saturday
Breakfast: bacon. Dinner: stew, rice pudding and tea. Tea: marmalade. We had a rehearsal as yesterday, with showers in morning but it set in pouring after dinner; for which we only had ¾ of an hour. It was the absolute limit - we practised entering trenches and then stood in the rain for over an hour, just rehearsing the time of waiting for the advance. We finished up by walking 100 yards through high corn and getting over our knees, making us thoroughly wet.

---

[149] **Stokes Guns** – a trench mortar of the type invented by Sir Frederick Stokes K.B.E.

I bought two eggs and butter for tea and got back about 6pm. After reading the Daily Mail and cleaning my rifle, there was no time to write to Doll again. I drew first for a pass for Doullens tomorrow.

June 11 Sunday
Breakfast: bacon. Dinner: stew and rice. Tea: marmalade. There was no parade in the morning but dinner at 11.45am. We fall in at 12.30pm for more rehearsals as before. I wrote to Doll and Mother in the morning. We were back again about 5.30pm and went to Doullens in the evening and had fried eggs as before. I received a letter from Doll.

June 12 Monday
Breakfast: Maconochies. Dinner: stew and rice pudding. Tea: jam. We had rehearsals again as before, both in the morning and afternoon with field kitchens out. It was pouring with rain most of the time but got back about 3.45pm. I just missed the working party, who didn't return until 5.30pm and have been enjoying eggs at both breakfast and tea lately. I had a good rest and an undisturbed night.

June 13 Tuesday
Breakfast: bacon. Dinner: cold beef and mashed potatoes. Tea: blackcurrant jam. We fell in at 7.30am and marched off at 8am, right through to the billets in Bus. We arrived at 1.30pm, in the pouring rain for the latter half of the march and I felt very damp. We had the YMCA, opposite our barn which was the Leeds Band concert. I wrote to Doll and sent a field PC to Kniveton.

June 14 Wednesday
Breakfast: bacon. Dinner: stew. Tea: blackcurrant jam. I sent a field PC to Mother. Captain Colley tells us the news of the great advance. We fell in at 1.30pm for the trenches and marched there in easy stages with plenty of fallouts. I thought that we were in for a softish time at first in support, with no details for work, till the next morning. We then turned out before 11am to fetch tools from Euston Dump but there were none of these when we arrived. Coming back we encountered some stray machine gun fire. A fellow a yard or two away utters a prolonged 'Oh ...' and stumbles forward, he has the luck of the evening, a bullet though the arse. We were back at 1.45pm and it has been raining off and on most of the day. There are twelve of us in a shelter and the roof leaks at my end and the floor is very slippy. The weather is cold, with nothing but ground sheets and no overcoats. The rations party had **one killed**[150] and three wounded right away.

June 15 Thursday
Breakfast: cold bacon. Dinner: Maconochies. Tea: jam. I was awakened at 4am for a salvage party, after a cold, wet, scratching night. Then later we were told

---

[150] **12/1354 Private Francis Gleave** – Killed in action 14th June 1916 and is buried in Bertrancourt Military Cemetery.

we are going to be left till after breakfast. I change into **Devey's**[151] place and use his overcoat and have two hours of most cosy sleep. We turn out 7.30am picking up stray picks and shovels all over the trenches. I take it easy through the morning and the afternoon. High explosives are very close in the morning which burst just over our parapet. The weather is dull and it is drizzling again. I wish we could get hold of the daily papers as we did at Doullens to verify the rumours we get in these stirring days. We were fetched out again about 9.30am to cart staff from Euston. I just missed a splendid Blighty, a bullet between the legs as I left the shelter and Hale picked the warm German bullet up afterwards. We turned onto rations when we got back to **Observation Wood**[152] and carried two bags right down to the front line. A hunt in the night was arranged for a 12.30am start so we were told to stay in Rob Roy. There was nothing doing however, so we come back. The bombardment started at 1.30am and we are turned into the German mine and it looks like a mess up with new time. We clear out while the bombardment is still on and return to the shelter for something to eat. I have had no sleep since last night.

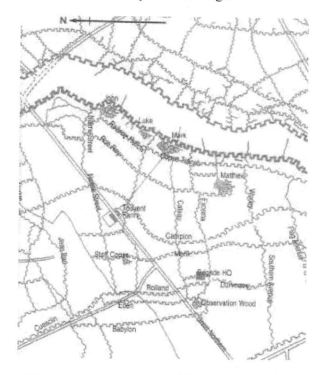

Map of the trenches showing the location of Brigade Headquarters and the four copses

---

[151] **12/1336 Private Rodney Frank Devey** - Killed in action 1st July 1916, his body was never recovered and he is commemorated on the Thiepval Memorial.
[152] **Observation Wood** – was the site of the Brigade Headquarters dugout.

June 16 Friday

There is no rest for the wicked! We were turned out 2.45am and went back to Euston carrying back shovels. Two hours allowance were given for breakfast which was cold bacon, bread and tea made with thick muddy water, as those damned engineers have not repaired the water main. We went back again to Euston carrying sandbags and then had six hours of sleep and a dinner of cold beef and bread and nothing to drink. We went back to Euston carrying trench boards and returned for tea at 6.30pm which was dry bread and jam and some better water, which had been fetched from the Sucrerie. We turned out at 9pm again to fetch water in pans and a thermos flask from the water cart at Euston. Saddler and I carry an empty flask, which was tremendously heavy on a pole. We waited for about two hours for the water cart and rations on a trolley which keeps coming off the line. We went to back to Observation Wood at about 1am.

June 17 Saturday

We find that we still have to take wine bottles to fill at **Sackville Street**[153] where the water is now back on and then go right down to the front line, to deliver them. I stagger under a load of fourteen quart bottles. We get back at 3.35pm and are turned out again at 5.30pm and are given a short time to eat a breakfast of cold bacon and tea which had just arrived. We are then carrying trench boards and bags down to **Matthew Copse**[154] which was one 9ft trench board and 100 sandbags for the two of us what a rotten load. We were back at 9.45am to finish breakfast and sleep. I received letters from Doll and Mother of 11th and 12th June. It has been a fine and bright day. Four men were buried in the sap during the night, by an explosion of a German land mine. We were supposed to have had a rest but were turned out again after four hours at 11.45am to carry mine props down to John Copse from Observation Wood. We were back for a dinner of cold beef at 1.45pm when we hoped to rest again. The enemy have levelled part of our front line this afternoon, killing three including **SM Marsden,**[155] **S Clay**[156] and **Thomas.**[157] I have had a good rest since dinner and a wash and shave after tea (of marmalade and butter) for first time since coming in. It has been a bright and fine day but cool. We were turned out 9.45am on a ration party and had to wait in Observation Wood till after midnight for the bodies of Clay and Thomas. We were to take them to Euston with us and helped carry them to the railhead. It was fearfully cold waiting and I had an attack of diarrhoea and sickness meanwhile. We got back at 2.30pm.

---

[153] **Sackville Street** – a long communication trench leading from La Signy Farm.

[154] **Matthew, Mark, Luke and John Copses** – group of four copses named after the evangelists, Matthew, Mark, Luke and John which are situated on the British Front Line opposite Serre. The Battalion headquarters were in a large dugout in John Copse .

[155] **12/2 Company Sergeant Major William Marsden** – was buried in his dugout despite many attempts his body was never recovered. He is commemorated on Thiepval Memorial. His remains probably still lie in the groups of copses opposite Serre, which mark the British Front Line.

[156] **12/1388 Sergeant Henry Charles Clay** – he was a policeman in Sheffield prior to the war and was killed in action on 17 June 1916. He is buried in Bertrancourt Military Cemetery.

[157] **12/249 Private Ernest Clifford Thomas** Born in Bengal India was killed in action on 17 June 1916 and is buried in Bertrancourt Military Cemetery.

90

June 18 Sunday

Breakfast: bacon. Dinner: cold beef. Tea: jam. I had a good rest in the morning and we were not turned out till after dinner at 12.45pm when we went to Euston and back with 100 sandbags and were back at 2.45pm. We were pretty heavily shelled with shrapnel in the open between the dump and the trenches and **one artillery man**[158] was knocked out as I walked across. I filled a good bag at louse straffing in the afternoon and then turned up at 6.30pm for carrying ammunition. Meanwhile our trench was shelled for first time and we were back at 8.30pm. We were turned out for rations at 9.30pm with no waiting or messing about, so we were back at 12.30pm. I was rather pleased as other available men on working parties are clearing trenches after shelling. It was a beautiful fine day and not hot. I received a letter from Doll of June 12th.

June 19 Monday

Breakfast: bacon. Dinner: cold mutton. Tea: jam and butter. Colley returns from a court martial and as is the usual course, the officers go in when we are in trenches. We are awakened at 2.20am for a formal stand to. I get to sleep again at 4am and rouse for breakfast and then sleep again till 9.30am. We are then called out on a **revetting**[159] party for a damaged trench. We are off at 12.30pm and then have dinner and are awaiting relief. **Varley**[160] is wounded in the front line. The Germans fire heavily all day and damage the front line again, we reply in turn with interest. Rumours of peace pour parlez, the Kaiser's terms are received and ours are given in return within three days for him to think it over. We are relieved by the East Lancs at about 7.30pm and arrive in Authie Wood at about 10pm and find a very good supper provided of tea, rice pudding and a very good stew. We have prepared a board announcing 500,000 Austrians have been captured to show to the Germans. I receive a fine parcel from A.A. which was awaiting me which contained tinned fruit cake, tea, tongue, turkey, tea, cigs, Eiffel Tower lemonade, chocolate, foot powder, two handkerchiefs and a novel. Our huts are filled with wire beds in two layers. The East Lancs had three fellows knocked out ten minutes after relieving us.

June 20 Tuesday

Breakfast: bacon. Dinner: stew. Tea: marmalade. The Battalion is practically given a day's rest but Colley has me correcting the plans of the German trenches. He tells me that he will give me something light tomorrow and instructs the Sergeant Major to leave me off the working party. There is a shortage of men, so he goes back on his promise and I am detailed last thing. I wrote to Doll and also sent a Field PC. It has been a very fine day.

---

[158] **2nd Lieutenant H. H. Lumb** was wounded on 17th June 1916. He was commissioned to 11th Y&L on 2nd April 1915 and served with 12th Y&L from 23rd April 1916.

[159] **Revetting** – strengthening of the walls of trenches or parapets with stakes or sandbags.

[160] **12/808 Corporal J. S. Varley** – was wounded on June 19th 1916.

June 21 Wednesday

Breakfast: bacon. Dinner: beautiful stew and tea. We fell in at 7.10am and marched to Colincamps which was about 4 miles and there we were given two cases of Stokes 3" shells to carry to John Copse, 3 miles away. The contents of each case was 42lbs, the two with the case was say 100lbs, besides the rifle bandoleer and gas helmets. We started about at 10.30am and I delivered my load by 5.30pm and I felt as though I had been pulled in the rack. I got back to camp about 9pm for dinner. It was the heaviest days work that I've ever had - the absolute limit. The Colonel threatens to stop parcels coming, if our huts are not kept perfectly tidy. We had **one killed**[161] and one wounded on our working party. I fill in my diary and have a short read and then go to sleep.

June 22 Thursday

Breakfast: bacon. Dinner: stew. Tea: jam. We do not have breakfast till 8am and only paraded from 10.45am – 12 noon for a rifle and ammunition inspection and a little drill. I made bath from a ground sheet and washed my feet and legs in the afternoon. I received a parcel and letter from Doll; cake, gingerbread, butterscotch and toothpaste dated June 14th and wrote to A.A. We are going carrying in the trenches this evening. We turned out at 9pm carrying gas cylinders from Euston to the front line on the right section, we had 4 men to one cylinder which were 140lbs in relays of two. It was fearfully rough on the shoulder and took about four hours. The other three men in party cracked up. The last hour I was carrying continuously and 11 fellows were registered I hear, in hospital.

June 23 Friday

Breakfast: bacon. Dinner: stew. Tea: jam. We were back for breakfast at 6.30am and I slept all day except for meals till 5pm when we turned out again. We had a heavy thunderstorm in the afternoon which has upset the weather and it was pouring all night. We were carrying 60lbs of Stokes mortars bombs from Euston to Matthew Copse the long way round. It took us four hours for first journey and back. It was a pitch dark night and many fellows fall and injure themselves. I attempted a second journey and carried them for about half a mile. We were held up for an hour by troops relieving. Daylight was breaking and the commencement of the bombardment was expected, so we cart them back again. My new uniform was soaked through in mud. I received a letter from Mother of 17th.

June 24 Saturday

Meals: ditto. We were back for breakfast at 5.30am and I slept till the middle of the afternoon, except for dinner. I am clothed in dirty a vest and pants and everything is wet through. We paraded at 5pm for a gas helmet inspection and I cleaned my rifle after. All letters are to be in tonight, so I wrote to Doll and Mother.

---

[161] **12/416 Private Cecil George Ibbotson** was the member of the working party who was killed, he is buried in Bertrancourt Military Cemetery.

June 25 Sunday

Meals: ditto. I bought a good feed of peaches, biscuits and chocolate for tea, and was eating sweets all day. I do hope that the diabetes doesn't suffer. We have a complete rest all day, after a beautiful night's rest too, although the bombardment started last evening and even here produced a continuous rumble. There was a German aeroplane over us this morning and our empty shell cases were dropping dangerously near. I received a letter from Auntie Annie dated June 21st and two from Doll, bless her of 20th and 21st. I cleaned up my uniform and puttees and there are rumours rife of a local success already. I made a big supper of toasted cheese and pickles.

June 26 Monday

Meals: ditto but rice at dinner. We paraded at 8.30am for an attack rehearsal but did nothing when we got to the ground. The General passed up message '9 German sausages[162] were brought down yesterday'. We got back from dinner at 1pm and paraded for an address by General O'Gowan at 5pm. His parting words before the attack were very optimistic. We turned out at 7.30pm for water carrying party in the trenches. We were shelled heavily with shrapnel near Euston with large fragments flying within a few feet of me. Coming back, I was over my knees in water and arrived back 5am drenched through.

June 27 Tuesday

Meals: ditto. We were awakened at 11.15am to pack my valise and private effects and to carry them to Bus at 2 o'clock. My boots socks and trousers are all ringing wet.

I am now putting this away with my private things.
My last thought as I close this - Oh Doll, my darling how dearly I love you and my Mother too.

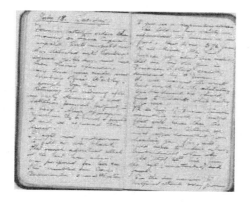

---

[162] **Sausages** – a 'sausage' shaped observation balloon more often referred to as a 'Maiden's prayer'.

5
The Battle of the Somme - Serre

July 18 Tuesday

I was down in battalion orders this morning as Lance Corporal unpaid, quite unexpected now. I was detailed with bombing squad yesterday and have been having exceedingly easy time since under new bombing officer **Westby**[163], who is quite simply barking. On returning this morning after an early dismissal, I saw the Battalion personal property in a heap with mine appearing conveniently to hand, so I pinched it and so have regained this diary. I will now endeavour to fill in the blanks.

The much advertised attack at the last hour almost was postponed for two days. This enabled our Corps Commander, General Weston to give us a preparatory address. He told us how vastly we outnumbered the Germans on out front and how to our 596 guns of all kinds, they had perhaps got about 200, including the big old gun at Gommecourt Wood, which was casually dismissed by O'Gowan. We were warned that the worst part would be the retaliatory bombardment we should have to endure while waiting to go over. The four lines of German trenches meanwhile would be levelled flat with lanes through the barbed wire. Certainly we might suffer somewhat from machine gun fire and would have to endure a heavy bombardment when we held that fourth line, from the left (unattacked) and front. On the day previous to the postponed attack and the day previous to the attack itself, we were extra well fed. We had a meat tea, as well as a dinner with rice pudding. Meanwhile the weather was very wet.

---

[163] **2nd Lieutenant F. H. Westby** – commissioned to 15th Battalion West Yorks (Leeds Pals) served with 12th Y & L from mid July 1916.

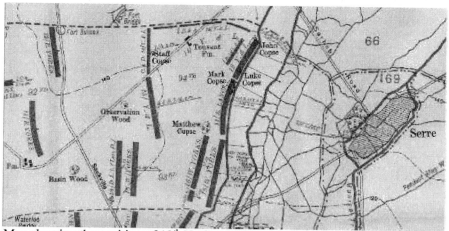

Map showing the position of 12th Yorks and Lancs in John Copse on 1st July 1916, opposite Serre

On *Friday 30 June* I was detailed with the **tape**[164] party under McCloud and left Bus Wood at 6.30 pm in advance of the Battalion. Thus, I missed the promised rest and tea at Courcelles. **Sergeant Thompson**[165] had a small flask of rum provided instead but the cork came out and the contents were lost. About midnight we went out into No Man's Land and pegged down the lengths of tape, 100 yards beyond our wire, this being the line at which our first wave were to get down, until the barrage on their front line lifted. I read afterwards that the Germans must have removed these again. I had finished between 1.30am and 2am and was then left to find my section, the Battalion now being in position. Copse Trench where we were to be, I found empty but just before daylight found my Company and section behind the front line parapet in shell holes and short shallow temporary trenches. Some of the fellows were digging themselves little **funk holes**[166]. I chanced to ask **Lieutenant Wardill**[167] what time zero was. He told me 7.30am much to my surprise, as we expected it to be just before dawn. Our bombardment started at 3.30am and the big guns were certainly off it, mostly dropping in our own wire. The Germans soon replied and gave us probably better than we received. They seemed to know precisely where we were, for that "old gun" or guns from Gommecourt searched for us in and behind that front line most methodically. They dropped them all round the

---

[164] **Tape** – tapes were laid down before the front line to mark the starting line for the attack and to mark routes across the ground which as a result of continual bombardment could have no recognisable features.

[165] **12/1069 Sergeant Walter Thompson** – killed in action 1st July 1916 his body was never found and he is commemorated on the Thiepval Memorial.

[166] **Funk hole** - a dug-out.

[167] **Lieutenant C. H. Wardill** - Killed in action 1st July 1916, his body was never recovered and he is commemorated on the Thiepval Memorial, brother of **12/ 816 Private Sidney George Wardill** also killed in action 1st July 1916, his body was also never recovered and is also commemorated on the Thiepval Memorial.

lip of our shell hole, but never got one in but the sections on each side of us suffered severely. I got the bacon and as I was making my breakfast it was smothered in muck. Fortunately I had enquired beforehand re zero as no one afterwards came along to give us any information.

At about 7.15am I looked over to see what the section on the right had done and saw the small trench filled up with Wardill standing up dead and partially burned. Then I saw the first wave going over, so we got into the front line and followed at 7.25am. I found **Captain Colley**[168] in the front bay and asked him the correct time, he pulled out his watch but could scarcely hold it, so shattered were his nerves. The poor fellow followed us all the same and was killed before he got very far. Our parapet was literally swept by machine guns and shrapnel fire and a large proportion only got a few yards.

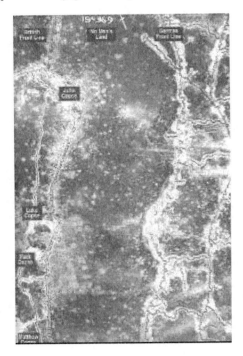

An aerial Photograph taken on the morning of the 1st July 1916 showing John Copse from which the Battalion fought

---

[168] **Captain W. A. Colley** - killed in action 1st July 1916. He had a premonition of his death just before going over the top but despite this, was first out of the trench. Soon after he was hit by a shell and killed. This gallant gentleman should not really have been at the front and certainly should not have been leading a company into action at the age of 47. His remains were never found and he commemorated on the Thiepval Memorial.

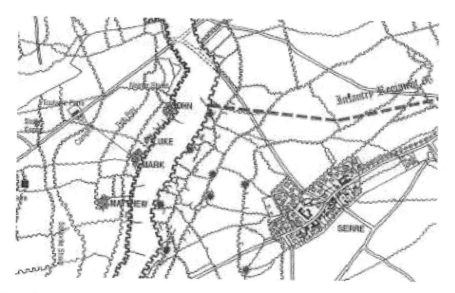

Trench map show the location of the trenches on 1st July 1916 showing John Copse

Previously the German bombardment of four hours had proved very deadly with sections being wiped out almost completely out. I was among the first of the wave to get over and I noticed **Devey**[169], thought now missing was ahead of me and apparently off his head, for with his rifle slung and thumbs in arm pits he was just shouting and swearing. Tommy Webster followed me. I stumbled several times in our barbed wire, and cursed freely, but probably these stumbles saved my life time after time.

Ahead I saw the first wave badly attenuated now but forming a well-dressed line lying down as near as they safely could to our barrage. So **Webster**[170] and I took cover in a shell hole about 20 yards behind. When the barrage lifted and the first wave went forward I closed up and joined them. I have a recollection of Webster grinning at me with his face covered with blood. The din of machine guns all round us was infernal but of the deadly missiles themselves I was quite unconscious and the idea of getting killed never struck me at all. In taking cover in that shell hole half way over I became aware of a terrible dry throat so resorted to my water bottle. On arriving at the German wire I found it quite untouched in front of me, but seeing what appeared to be an opening on the right about 40 yards away I made for that. There I found a series of shell holes had destroyed it half way across, but the other half was impenetrable. I found some A Company machine gunners here with their Lewis's and also a few bombers. There were eight of us in all.

---

[169] **12/1336 Private Rodney Frank Devey** - Killed in action and his body was never recovered and he is commemorated on the Thiepval Memorial.
[170] **Tommy Webster - 12/1165 Private Albert (Tommy) Webster** - Killed in action 1st July 1916. He is buried in Queens Military Cemetery, Serre.

The Germans were right on top of their parapets behind their wire, which was so thick it almost hid them. They even brought up a machine gun there to face us. We made good rifle practice for a time accounting for several of them till they took more careful cover. One of our group was killed. One shot through the face and he bolted straight back for our lines with blood streaming through a ghastly hole in his cheek. I don't think he ever got back. Another fellow was shot later through the hand and one in the afternoon wounded in the forearm. It was not long before the German machine gun was apparently knocked out by one of our shells for it never fired afterwards. We were subjected to showers of stick grenades but they got none actually in our hole. Soon after arriving here I had to have another swig at my water. Never have I experienced such a parched mouth and throat.

After we got over the Germans placed a fearful barrage of fire on our 1st and 2nd line preventing anyone else getting to us, only an odd man or two of the 3rd and 4th waves reached us. I looked back and saw our trench bridges flying hundreds of feet in the air. The enemy all afternoon were sweeping No Man's Land as near up to their own line as they dared with shrapnel getting our fellows lying out in the open and even some of us lying right in their wire. I dug a short trench of a few feet out of the crater we were in, into their wire, and this made nice cover for my head and body if I sat down. At first I kept a good look out for an attack from behind, but presently spent most of the afternoon dozing. The other fellows wanted to beat a retreat before dark and actually started out to do so in spite of my persuasion, for they feared being bombed out at dusk. They soon thought better of it however. A sniper only a few yards away but unseen actually called 'Sheffielder's, pass us some water' and he was shooting our wounded too. The **star shells**[171] had been going up for about quarter of an hour when I left and I was the last. I should have stopped longer still but I saw a form creeping through the wire towards me. It was in all probability a German. I might have shot him easily but refrained just on the chance it might be one of our fellows.

I made tracks darting from shell hole to shell hole. In the 180 yards back by a judicious use of craters I think I only did the odd eighty in the open. By waiting for a star shell to just go out and a burst of shrapnel to pass over then making another dart for cover I got back untouched. Our front lines were full of wounded fellows. I helped a couple into the sap in Mark Copse and bound up their wounds. I then made tracks for Staff Copse. There were some ghastly messes in **Cateau**[172], forms in the bottom of the trench and several times in feeling if they were alive, my hand would be plunged into a gory mess of flesh, once the neck of a headless trunk. I encountered loose limbs too. I could get no water that night except a few drops that I found in bottles lying about. I slept in the open in Staff Copse that night and had a good rest. The Doctor seemed hard at work all the time with a continuous stream of wounded coming in.

---

[171] **Star Shells** – incendiary shells.

[172] **Cateau** - a communication trench leading to Copse Trench.

6
The Aftermath

Out of the 650 of us who went over the top only 47 returned unwounded. Almost all the fellows considered my pals were either killed or wounded chiefly the former alas, **Hale, Thorne** and **Saddler**[173] are all missing. Only one of our officers viz. Cloud returned unwounded. **Colonel Crossthwaite**[174] returned sick a day or so before we went into action. **Major Clough**[175] also **Major Plackett**[176] left during engagement with broken nerves. We have now scarcely any officers and the Battalion such as it is composed mainly of new draught men. All of the Battalions of the Division seemed to have suffered as heavily. In some places the 1st line was broken through, about 50 yards on my right I saw a dozen of our fellows go over in file but they soon came back. Some got past the second line; even up to the fourth line I've heard but never came back. Some of the East Lancs were seen in Serre and throughout the morning reports from the Brigade said we had obtained our objective and were holding that village.

The next morning at daybreak I went to Observation Wood and was reluctantly supplied with a little water. I napped in the morning out, then fetched some water from **La Signy Farm**[177] and had a good shave and wash and also mashed tea.

That afternoon the remnant was paraded and we remained on duty in the trenches when we were relieved by the Gloucesters. We left the trenches at about 10 o'clock at night on *July 4 Tuesday*, the enemy were shelling **Railway Avenue**[178] pretty seriously and we passed some casualties. I think I felt more nervous then, than I had all the previous time including the attack. Safety was so near, and yet there was the idea of the chance of a shell. We were over our thighs in water going through that trench. We were promised a rest and tea at Bus but we were disappointed and marched straight to **Louvencourt**[179] ten or

---

[173] **12/663 Private Harry Thomas Hale, 12/799 Private Alfred James (Alf) Thorne, 12/771 Private George Henry Saddler** - all killed in action 1st July 1916. All three are buried in Queens Military Cemetery - within a few feet of each other.

[174] **Colonel J. A. Crossthwaite** – Regular Officer previously with the Durham Light Infantry. He fell ill on 30th June 1916 as a result of wounds that he received in Ypres in 1915.

[175] **Major T. C. Clough** – Ex Territorial Forces. He left 12th Y&L on 30th June 1916, shortly before the commencement of the Battle of the Somme.

[176] **Major A. Plackett** – Official account states that he acted as Commanding Officer from 30th June 1916 but was wounded in action on 1st July 1916.

[177] **La Signy Farm** – the scene of much bitter fighting, situated on a ridge opposite to the ridge when Serre is positioned.

[178] **Railway Avenue / Railway Hollow** – support trench between front line and Rob Roy trench. Now the site of Railway Hollow Cemetery.

[179] **Louvencourt** – six miles behind the front line lying between Doullens and Albert. From July 1915 until August 1916 British Field Ambulances were stationed there. Buried in Louvencourt Military

twelve miles with only two short halts of a minute or so while the rear closed up.

We got billets in a barn and had an early breakfast, **_July 5 Wednesday_** and a rest all morning. In the afternoon the Brigadier addressed us with the most fulsome praise, saying that never had troops advance so steadily in the face of such a fearful fire. It was like a Guards parade. Then we were marched up to a field to be addressed by General Weston. He repeated the eulogy and said he was proud to salute us all as comrades, which he did. We were then told that although we did not reach our objective, our attack had the desired effect, it held large masses of Germans in hand and a large concentration of guns, thus enabling the French on our right to make such progress in places almost unopposed. Thus our suspicions were confirmed, **_we had merely been offered as a sacrifice_**. No reserves were at hand to follow us up, nor was it ever intended we should ever be reinforced

Sergeant Oakes[180] asked Captain Colley for reinforcements before going over as all his section had been blown up, Colley tried to get him some but couldn't. *"Never mind," he said, just before going over. "We shall all be dead in 2 minutes."* General Joffre[181] confirmed his appreciation and thanks for what we had done, attributing his progress to the same. We were overwhelmed with parcels while at Louvencourt, which belonged to the casualties. As nothing more could be done with these, they were shared out among the remainder of the platoons to which they belonged. Here I put my diabetes to severe test.

The next day **_July 6 Thursday_** we set out for destination unknown. More consideration as regards halts has been shown for us now that **Major Allen**[182] is in charge. We got to Gezaincourt thinking it was our destination but our spirits suffered severely when we doubled back towards Doullens and then right over the hills to the right, on to Longuevillette. It seems that no billets could be found for us nearer, which made the march about 12 miles long. We got some splendid billets though, at a very clean farm in a wholesome barn with the floor covered in luxuriant straw. Eggs could be obtained, cooked at the farm at a cost of 2 centimes each. I had three for tea but afterwards could find room for no more on account of the parcels, which continued to arrive.

The next day **_July 7 Friday_** we were to have moved again but this was postponed until **_July 8 Saturday._** We set out for another destination unknown at mid day, doubling back through Doullens. Our objective turned out to be Frevent. We marched the 14 miles having a good rest with tea half way. We then had two or three hours to wait at the station. We were then loaded into cattle trucks which had not even been cleaned out with heaps of manure being pushed to each end, a general complaint led to this being removed for us and a

---

Cemetery is Lieutenant Roland Leighton who died at the age of 19 as a result of wounds received near John Copse 23 December 1915. He was a friend of Vera Brittain and features in her classic memoir of a lost generation 'Testament of Youth'.

[180] **12/1010 Sergeant S. Oakes** – was a Sheffield University Student and was killed in action on 6th May 1917 whilst serving with the Royal Engineers. He is buried in Beaulencourt Military cemetery in Ligny.

[181] **Joseph Jacques Césaire Joffre** was the French General who served as Commander-in-Chief of the French Army between 1914-1916 during World War 1.

[182] **Major D. C. Allen** – also served with the Tank Corps.

little straw being put where the floor was wettest. We started about 10pm and arrived at Steerboeque via Bethune about 1.30am. Here Oxo Cubes and <u>warm</u> water even was provided by this time. I have commenced to suffer from diarrhoea - the result of too many sweets I think. We were all carrying parcels or portions of the same in addition to the maximum load the Army so far invented. At about 2.30am we set out to march for Merville. We were all exceedingly tired and in the last few miles the men were falling out in batches, absolutely done in. However we managed to stick to the nine miles and we welcomed that full day's Sunday rest. We were billeted in huts, the best we have had in France with wooden floors and benches to sleep on, also plenty of sandbags stuffed with straw.

For three days I was reporting sick to the Doctor with diarrhoea. I was always given **tablets and duty**[183], these or nature eventually cured me. In spite of this I found the time quite enjoyable at Merville. For two evenings I went to the town and had a 'table d'hote' dinner in the evening and bought some strawberries to finish up with, these were rather dry and flavourless though. Captain Cousins, back from his safe job in brigade was in command of C Company, so of course we had a lot of 'smartening' parades. A very clean café nearby provided unlimited fried or boiled eggs at two and a half centimes a time and coffee in a basin. I spent a lot of time there and always supplemented my breakfast and supper with eggs. All the houses round about seem scrupulously clean and the people very pleasant and obliging, markedly in contrast to most of the barbarians in the Artois.

---

[183] **M&D** - Medicine and Duty i.e. a dose of No. 9 (a purgative pill) or other medicine and then back to work.

7
Neuve Chappelle

We left on ***July 15 Saturday*** and made an easy march to Vielle Chapelle which was eight or nine miles away. Our billet here is in the boarded roof space over a house run as an **estaminet**[184] and is very handy for beer, eggs at three centimes each and coffee for one centime. We are in reserve. The Barnsleys went to the trenches right away but I don't think we shall do so. As is usually the case, things begin to get lively with our arrival. The trenches are quite near and the bombardment grows more intense every day. There are strong rumours that the Anzacs are going to attack very soon. By the way, Division General O'Gowan addressed us at Merville. All the usual praise then told us that the Germans had twice the number of guns we knew about beforehand he also added that there was a corps of eight machine guns opposing us that they had no idea of. After our first day here all the estaminets were closed to troops. We managed to find one open however, among the artillery billets, which was a mile away and here we got a very good red wine. A Sergeant billeted here had a piano and two gramophones which he then carted about with him on the **G.S.**[185] wagon. The roads are now policed and we are not allowed far from our billets.

July 18 Tuesday
Whilst washing in the morning down at the brook, I left a new tablet of Pears soap on the bank and a cow came along and consumed it with great gusto, some Beechams! I gave in letters to Mother, Auntie Annie and A.A. and wrote a PC to Doll and Mother.

July 19 Wednesday
Meals: ditto. We attended bombing courses again and were then left alone, doing nothing as usual, so I've been spending time filling in this diary. It has been a very hot, fine day after a cold night.

July 20 Thursday
Meals: ditto. Westby has paid a little more attention today but has not overdone it. After living on rumours of leave and marching to Etaples or Boulogne where our thoughts stray, it's reported that tonight we will relieve A Company on Saturday somewhere in the trenches. My letter to Auntie Annie was returned today, I have rewritten it, so I will try again. I have eggs and coffee for supper from an estaminet.

---

[184] **Estaminet** – tavern.
[185] **G.S.** - General Service.

July 21 Friday

Meals: ditto. We had an hour dummy bomb throwing in the morning and were then dismissed to be ready for a bath parade 12.45pm at the end of bomb course. I did not volunteer to continue, as I prefer to leave everything to fate that has looked after me well so far. I got back from a decent and refreshing bath about 2.20pm and received letters from Doll and Mother of 17th July. I then wrote to Doll. I had some vin blanc at the back entrance of the closed estaminet and a supper of fried eggs, chips, petit buerre and coffee in the evening. We had a Reville at 6am in the morning and were off to relieve A Company at 8am.

July 22 Saturday

Breakfast: bacon. Dinner: Maconochies. Tea: jam and figs. We were awakened about 1am and told to prepare to stand to. There was a great burst of machine gun fire and artillery soon afterwards but no call however. We took over the strong point at Croix Rouge and it looks like being an easy time. We have a table in the guardroom to have meals at, so I made toast for tea, to remind me of home. I handed in letter to Doll. We are now midway between Laventie and Neuve Chapelle on the Estaires to La Bassee Road.

July 23 Sunday

Breakfast: bacon. Dinner: Maconochies and new potatoes. Tea: jam. I was awake all night as corporal of the guard and spent my time reading. Our guns were very busy as usual. There is a large conflagration directly in front of us, apparently over the enemy line and red lights were going up at night. I slept most of the time from breakfast to tea. I received a letter from Doll of 18th. Of course, it was too good to last and we are unexpectedly relieved at night - usurped should be the word and return to headquarters for the night, getting there about midnight and billeted in huts.

July 24 Monday

Breakfast: bacon. Dinner: boiled beef. Tea: jam. We are to go to the trenches today, so bang go the rumours of four days march to Etaples and leave starting. We are to reinforce the Barnsleys. I received a newspaper from Colin. We march off for the trenches at 1.30pm and we all bear trunks. The enemy are shelling pretty hard this afternoon. A few heavy shells have made a pretty mess of the trenches near our post just before we came in. I'm in charge of the post! We are at Neuve Chapelle, the village of which, behind our front line is represented by various heaps of smashed brickwork

July 25 Tuesday

Breakfast: cold bacon. Dinner: cold beef and pickles. Tea: jam. The Germans are badly bashing us in our trenches, so I have eighteen hours guard and work and six hours in operation again. It was a quiet night last night but I got no rest in the morning. They were shelling all round my shelter with high explosive fifteen pounders, one struck a gas tank one yard from corner of same. Then they dropped heavy shells fifty yards behind us all morning and it was also raining

103

Minenwerfers[186] on our right and on our left all afternoon. I was sandbagging all afternoon. Before our Brigade came here, the East Yorks were in for twenty four days and had only six casualties but our brigade changed all of that. The Barnsleys will tickle anything into activity. In spite of the infernal din today, there were no casualties up to 8pm and we had one or two yesterday though. The Barnsleys on our left after all had two killed and two casualties from a **Minnie**[187]. We had one or two casualties.

July 26 Wednesday
Meals: ditto. It was a quiet night. The Germans repeat yesterday's programme identically, except that having smashed up our cookhouse, they continue with minenwerfers on the left after our tea, so we have less tea. Another shelter I happen to be in during the afternoon has the same narrow shave from an **H.E. wizz bang**[188] as yesterday, they also drop on the parapet and parados each side of me. Our total casualties up to 7pm were five. There are good rumours that we are getting relieved tomorrow morning. They continue to shower Minenwerfers on our left till 9pm which is the most fearsome thing they have produced and we had five killed. There were craters twenty feet in diameter, giving fragment wounds to fellows 300 yards away. **Captain Woolhouse**[189] went to the artillery Commander to ask for fire on their mortar. He couldn't do it except by order of Corps Commander and did not consider it worthwhile getting the same, considering numerous channels it would have to pass through. The Brigadier was due to visit the trenches but heavy shelling apparently prompted him to remember another appointment but noticing the Barnsleys dodging behind their parapets, sent a note to their Captain saying it was unsoldierly conduct.

July 27 Thursday
Meals: ditto. We were relieved by the Berkshires at about 11am after a quiet morning. Out of 100 of us who went in, we had about 20 casualties. I received a letter from Doll of 21st. We marched to camp at Vielle Chapelle and are given tea and I get a good dinner of eggs, chips and coffee at an estaminet. We march off at 4pm and have a billet at Le Bourge, Lestrem, which is a comfortable barn. **Hall**[190] has a good parcel of tinned fruit which we have for tea. I bathe my feet in stream nearby. I send a Field PC to Doll and Mother and then go to bed. We hear a fierce bombardment commencing at 9.30pm.

July 28 Friday
Breakfast: bacon. Dinner: good stew. Tea: currants. We have no parade except to have our clothing steam stoved. The Germans raided the trenches that we had

---

[186] **Minenwerfer or 'Minnie'** - a German trench mortar - bomb thrower, also known as flying pig.

[187] **Minnie** – see above.

[188] **H.E. wizz bang** – a high explosive German shell with a flat trajectory which made a *wizzbang* noise.

[189] **Captain E. G. G. Woolhouse** – commanded the Battalion temporarily and resigned. He was left out of the attack on 1st July and at the end of the attack was the only senior officer left standing. He was commissioned on 18th September 1914.

[190] **12/663 Private Herbert Hall** Sniper and Lewis gunner, took part in battle on 1st July 16 and was commissioned to KOYLI.

left last night and the West Yorks had about 60 casualties - the Germans captured and wiped out. I received letters from Doll, Mother and Maggie of the 24th and wrote to Doll. I had dinner in town which was pork chops, potatoes and cauliflower in batter, followed by three fried eggs with salad then pastries, three cups of tea and coffee 2 francs 80. Rumours of England and then Mesopotamia are rife.

July 29 Saturday
Breakfast: bacon. Dinner: mutton stew. Tea: jam. We only had a Bathing parade in the morning and I had a very good bath and a warm, continual shower. I then rested for the remainder of the day until 6.30pm when I'm Corporal of the guard in town. There is an un-napping rumour that a Divisional music hall troupe is being formed and is to carry on through the winter.

July 30 Sunday
Breakfast: bacon. Dinner: mutton, potatoes, cabbage, Heinz beans. Tea: jam. I had a good night's sleep on the floor although I was disturbed every two hours for the changing of the guard. I had a very easy time all day and was relieved at 7pm. I wrote to Maggie, Mr Edwards and the office. I had dinner in the evening which was a veal cutlet, cauliflower and potatoes with wine beforehand and coffee and pastries, supplemented with fried eggs.

July 31 Monday
Breakfast: bacon. Dinner: bully beef new potatoes, Heinz beans. In the morning we paraded and had a wiring demonstration and rifle drill in the afternoon. Major Gurney of the 13th Barnsleys becomes our Chief Officer and gives a nice sermon in the evening. I walk to La Fosse to make purchases at the canteen. I received a paper from Colin and there are rumours that we are going to Egypt now.

August 1 Tuesday
Breakfast: bacon. Dinner: bully beef potatoes and cabbage. Tea: Marmalade. I hear Major Plackett who left the trenches at Serre with what he called 'shattered nerves' after the bombardment, is now convalescing and writing to the papers re the Battalion that he had the honour to command at the time. He has been given three months sick leave on full pay. **Hough**[191] who went mad from the same causes was compelled to go over and was killed. I am detailed for a course at the bombing school at Croix Barbee where we are to assemble at 3pm, thereby getting off the morning route march. I take a C Corps party of eight including myself. We make rather a tired march of it but manage to arrive on time but it was very hot. We had nothing doing for the rest of the day and I have a bathe but am over my knees in mud. I receive a parcel from A.A. which contains a big tin of fruit, tea, lime drops, a tin of cigarettes, mosquito net and magazine.

---

[191] **12/691 Private Ernest Hough** was killed in action on 1st July 1916, his body was never found and he is commemorated on the Thiepval Memorial.

August 2 Wednesday
Breakfast: bacon. Dinner: Maconochies. Tea: marmalade. We parade 9.15am and are all highly cleaned up for the rifle inspection. A short lecture followed then we had throwing practice and another lecture and fall out at 12pm. I received a letter from Doll and there are rumours of leave starting on Friday. We paraded 2pm till 4.30pm in the afternoon, followed by trench fighting, bayonet drill and a lecture on rifle grenades. I wrote to Doll and then visited the haunt near our old billet for fried eggs, chips and coffee for supper.

August 3 Thursday
Our meals have been very meagre. Breakfast: bacon. Dinner: bully beef and potatoes which we have to pinch out of the fields. Tea: treacle! We have had no butter since we came. We had parades in the morning and a bayonet drill and lecture on No.3. In the afternoon we had a lecture on No.19, throwing and a lecture on trench fighting. Half of the class of all the Battalions were unexpectedly sent back to regroup for the trenches after tea, I remained to follow at the end of the course. I went out for a stroll and drink in the evening and met **Walton**[192] the Battalion runner. He tells me that the advance party for relieving the division is already here and they don't even know at headquarters whether we shall go in or not now. I handed in a letter for Doll this morning and also one for A.A. this evening.

August 4 Friday
Breakfast: bacon. Dinner: bully beef stew and potatoes. Tea: dry figs. We paraded in the morning from 9.15am until 12 noon. We were throwing and had a lecture on rifle grenades on No.3 and in the afternoon from 2pm till 4.30pm we had a throwing lecture and rifle grenade practice and trench fighting. I stayed in all evening, wrote to Mother, handed it in and made cocoa and toasted cheese for supper. We expect to go to the trenches on Sunday afternoon.

August 5 Saturday
Meals Ditto but treacle at tea. Our orders are similar to yesterday. I had to go down to the old billet to get water at dinnertime so had two beers and a café au lait. I went to Vielle Chapelle in the evening and had two vin blancs on the way and bought chocolate, spice cake, greengages, biscuits and a cup of cocoa and felt very full up. I saved fifty cigarettes for the trenches.

August 6 Sunday
Breakfast: bacon. Dinner: cold beef, potatoes and haricots. Tea: marmalade. We paraded from 9.15am until 12 noon describing bombs and grenades from memory and we were then throwing live bombs. At 2pm we march off for the trenches, the length of time is to be announced but it can be anything up to sixteen days. We are on the right of our last position on the front line gun positions and so far have been left practically alone but we are in the bay where the Germans entered on their last raid, the night we came out. Our Stokes gave

---

[192] **Private G. Walton** - Battalion runner also served in 94th Brigade.

them a bit of **strafe**[193] on the right but fail to draw their fire. I received a letter from Doll and Mother and I await one from July 31st. Aunt Annie has apparently not received my letter of July 20th. Doll is in too much of a hurry to write much, perhaps she is offended by the stiffness of my censored letters. My party is mostly used up to supplement other bays so I have not one to man at all.

August 7 Monday

Breakfast: cold bacon and baked beans. Dinner: cold beef. Tea: marmalade and butter. The Germans were very quiet last night except for machine gun fire and our artillery fails to move them. Being without a bay to man, I took charge of a working party strengthening Captain Woolhouse's dugout. Our new Chief Officer **Captain Gurney**[194] from the Barnsleys has made trench conditions much easier. The men are allowed to sleep at night on the firestep during their rest periods. One NCO is now allowed to take charge of two bays while the other rests. I have managed to dodge through the whole day with only about one hour's voluntary work, filling sandbags. Our artillery and Stokes have been very productive all day drawing occasional bursts of retaliation from the Germans. I hear that our aeroplanes dropped bombs on to the German lines last night and also what appeared like a huge firework display. I received a letter from Uncle Bob, August 2nd. I was on the working party again tonight.

August 8 Tuesday

Breakfast: cold bacon baked beans. Dinner: cold mutton and tea. Tea: jam. I received a post card from Maud and sent Doll a postcard. It was a quiet night except for machine gun fire until 3.45am and then the Germans exploded a mine on our right and we reply with heavy machine gun fire. I hear that a mine exploded in our wire practically wiping out A Company. The Germans attacked but were caught by our fire and suffered badly. Our Stokes and guns drew retaliation in the form of super mortars, which are worse than the heaviest guns I've seen, one man of D company was killed as he ran up a communication trench for safety! I get three new drafts to help man our bay. Two are taken out with the wiring party right away, so we do not move again. I was revetting the parados until 2am then slept until stand to. Captain Woolhouse tells me we are to be relieved tomorrow.

August 9 Wednesday

Breakfast: cold bacon with baked beans and tomatoes. Dinner: bully beef. Tea: Honey which I find in the dugout, probably rejected as marmalade. We are to be relieved at 10.30am. There is heavy rifle grenade fire on our right and the East Lancs catch it rather badly I'm afraid. We get out after a delay during a quiet spell. Whilst resting on the road, we are suddenly scattered by heavy shelling. Later we are all sent to man different strong posts. I am put in charge of three

---

[193] **Strafe** – to fire upon with rifle or artillery. From the German battle cry, ' Gotte Strafe England' (God punish England). The morning or evening hate was also known as the morning or the evening strafe.
[194] **Major C. H. Gurney** – from 13 Yorks & Lancs took over as Commanding Officer of 12 York and Lancaster from 25 July 1916 until 18 August 1916 and again from 3 October 1916 until 16 October 1916.

men and go to Rue de Petit a rather nice secluded little spot which is in a strong point with good dugouts. One of our own Battalions is quite near and rather tiresome. We had a little machine gunfire and the stray shell or two but nothing much to trouble about. We only mount guard at night and do just enough work by day to make an entry in the log. I received a letter from Doll, August 4th.

August 10 Thursday
Breakfast: cold bacon baked beans. Dinner: cold beef. Tea: currants. The sentry although he was supposed to wake me for stand to takes it upon himself to refrain, so I oversleep until 8.30am. We start work just before 3pm and five minutes later the CO and the **adjutant**[195] arrive but we are busy. What luck! Later **Moxey**[196] comes and credits us with the work performed by thirteen men! We fry onions with baked beans very successfully and make some good tea too. We then visit the estaminets on La Basse Road and drink with the Barnsleys for fellowship and meet the **Manchesters** [197] of 61st Division. I received a letter and parcel from Mother of August 5th.

August 11 Friday
Breakfast: cold bacon and baked beans. Dinner: Maconochies. Tea: jam. I received a letter from Arthur, August 7th and a paper from Colin.

August 12 Saturday
Official meals, breakfast: cold bacon. Dinner: bully beef pickle and baked beans. Tea: raspberry jam.
Sharpe[198] who elected to be the cook was indisposed and lazy, so I took on the cooking and had cold boiled bacon fried with eggs which were very good. I made bread and current pudding for dinner but I'm afraid we shall be milk less tomorrow. I gathered pears and stewed the same in the afternoon, which were very good. The batteries round us have been very active today, but evidently haven't found the German heavy mortars yet, which keep popping up quite merrily. I wrote to Mother and received a letter from Doll, August 6[th.]

August 13 Sunday
The rations are getting topside of us. Breakfast: more very best frying bacon than we can consume, also baked beans. Dinner: cold mutton. Tea: jam, tin of butter, milk, bully beef onions etc. Loaves and loaves of bread are being handed out. The ovens were left on after our stand to and this resulted in our having breakfast at 10.30am, it might be an English Sunday morning. I handed in a letter to Arthur and wrote to Mother.

---

[195] **Adjutant** - a staff officer in the army, air force, or marine corps who assists the commanding officer and is responsible especially for correspondence.
[196] **Captain D Moxey** – Born in Brazil – Machine Gun Officer transferred to Royal Flying Corps in July 1917 he was awarded a posthumous George Cross in World War II.
[197] **Manchesters** - 61st (Manchester University) Battalion.
[198] **Private 12/943 J. T. Sharpe** – he took part in the attack on 1st July 1916.

August 14 Monday
Rations, liberal portions of frying bacon, baked beans, Maconochies, jam, onions, bread, cheese tea and sugar. There was plenty of cold mutton and bacon in hand so there was no need for the Maconochies. Forty boxes of bombs are sent to us today and the stores are renewed and it looks as though we are expecting an attack. I handed in a letter to Arthur and wrote and handed in a letter for Doll. I am continually unimpressed lately with the necessity of mounting sentries carefully, which means that I shall have to awake every two hours to inspect them. Our artillery was very active this evening and the enemy reply with shrapnel and fragments fall in our post. I received a letter from Mother, August 10th.

August 15 Tuesday
Rations, plenty of bacon, baked beans, bully beef, cheese, apricot jam, butter, milk, bread, tea and sugar. It has been a showery day and I was paid 10 francs. There are rumours of a three days march and going to England on Saturday. McCloud tells me we are to be relieved tomorrow or Thursday. I received a parcel from A.A. which contained cake, tongue, lemonade, a writing case and cigs.

August 16 Wednesday
Rations ditto. It was a quiet, idle day but a hail of shell fragments and machine gun bullets fall on our post as a result of the enemy firing on our aeroplanes. It was a showery day but a pleasant cool evening and I listen to a gramophone of the Barnsleys across the road which was a splendid selection of classical pieces and waltzes. It takes me back to Doll and beautiful smooth ballroom floors - visions of dreamy peace on my one hand and heavy guns firing in contrast on the other.

August 17 Thursday
Our rations are as yesterday with dates. I spent the day idling as usual. McCloud tells me we are to be relieved tomorrow. It was another dull and showery day. I send post cards to Doll and Mother and received a letter from Doll, August 12th.

August 18 Friday
Breakfast: bacon. Dinner: stew. Tea: jam.
We were relieved at 2pm by the Gloucesters from 61st Division. The Germans shell the crossroads at Croix Barbee. We have dinner on the way and are billeted again in Lestrem but in those that D Company last occupied, which are very smelly and lousy. We eat fried eggs and enjoy café au lait at the farm that is attached. *I hear that our old trenches at Serre are now 900 yards away from the Germans, both sides having retreated on account of the stench from our dead bodies.*

August 19 Saturday
Breakfast: bacon. Dinner: stewed mutton-chops and potatoes. Tea: jam.

I have a fine night's sleep but woke up with dozens of lice. I wrote to Doll and handed it in. I went to a concert in the Chateau ground and found it was a minstrel troupe composed of the C Company men apparently. They weren't really up to much except for one man but I enjoyed it nevertheless. At 6.30pm and 7pm C and D Companies were ordered to report to their billets respectively and immediately. We called and had the dinner that we had ordered though; pork cutlets, beans and potatoes, café au lait. We found D Company and were ordered to the trenches for a working party to be made up with C Company. I thought that my stripes had saved me but they had to detail me at the last minute to make up numbers after 10pm. I hurriedly got my kit together and marched off at 10.20pm. We turned into our billets about 1am at Richburg Saint Vaast. The rats are worse than anywhere I've been yet and I was awakened in the night by them running over my face. They would sit on it and an ordinary shake wouldn't drive them off, they had to be thrown. **Blacktin**[199] who was at the side of me had moved forward with his face level with my waist. I felt a rat about there and gave a good punch with my fist, getting Blacktin in the face. We had parades during the day and had only one that consisted of a kit inspection in the afternoon and an inspection of billets that was held over us throughout the day. I went to sleep soaked in perspiration and woke up still damp and had a rather chilly night in consequence.

August 20 Sunday
Breakfast: bacon. Dinner: jam. Tea: roast mutton, fried potatoes, onions, baked beans, tea.
I had the best dinner we've been served with since leaving England — all credit due to the D Company cooks, it shows what can be done with rations if they are not as lazy as C Company. The mutton provided is beautifully fresh meat. There is a rumour about Sir Douglas Haig who is going to surprise the world within 96 hours but about two days have gone now. We have the whole day at rest then fall in at 8.45pm for work. I wandered around Richburg St Vaast Church which is a mass of ruins; tombs were broken in by shells, exposing coffins and their contents. A crucifix on the west wall remained absolutely untouched amid the ruins, which was a favourite subject for the photographers in illustrated papers. It was a fine and cool day. There were no letters sent for C Company but of course, D Company got theirs. I wrote to A.A. We paraded at 8.45pm for a night fatigue and we marched to the end of a communication trench and then waited for three hours for a Royal Engineer cart and dug out in parts we had to carry down to front line. Note, why not go late next time and let the Royal Engineers wait for us. We were only employed for about ½ hour and were back at 3.30am. I slept in a ditch, wrapped in an oil sheet while waiting while machine gun bullets were whizzing unpleasantly across the area.

---

[199] **12/596 Private S. C. Blacktin** – a member of C Company.

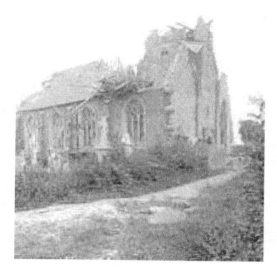

The ruins of Richburg St Vaast Church

August 21 Monday

Breakfast: bacon. Dinner: jam and tea. Tea: roast mutton and onions, really beautifully done and first class fresh meat. We rested till 2pm and then went on working on **travesses**[200] in communication trenches, filling them in with earth which was rather risky as we were well under German observation. There was some heavy shelling on the left but not our way. We worked till 6.10pm and got back at 6.45pm. I handed in letter to A.A. and received a letter from Mother dated August 17th and a paper from Colin. I was reading in the orchard at the back of the billets while machine gun bullets and shrapnel fired at aeroplanes were falling uncomfortably close. I hear that the East Yorks did for 300 Germans last night on a section that we visited. We anticipated the attack and went out into No Man's Land with machine guns and set up barrage with trench mortar fire.

August 22 Tuesday

Breakfast: fried bacon – more than we could manage. Dinner: stew. Tea: jam. We paraded at 8.30am for the trenches and there was no time for a wash or freshen up at all and we didn't get one until after tea. We left the trenches at 1pm and got back about 1.30pm. We had rifle inspection in the afternoon and also a Medical Officer inspection, with gas helmets and particulars were taken of our inoculations. There was no mail today and I was disappointed as I was expecting one from Doll. I hear that we are stopping here until Saturday and are then going into trenches again, what rotten luck. Wrote to Mother and handed it in. One of our aeroplanes was brought down this evening, its petrol tank was hit which set it on fire. It fell in No Man's Land and the two occupants fell out

---

[200] **Travesses** – crossing points.

before it reached the ground. We have to get under cover almost every evening now, to avoid the hail of missiles from above.

August 23 Wednesday
Breakfast: bacon. Dinner: fresh stew. Tea: jam. We paraded at 8am, had the same work as yesterday and got back at 1.30pm, followed by rifle inspection at 3pm. There are eighteen new D Company draft who arrive to replace the C Company men. I, to my satisfaction am left behind. I received a letter from Doll dated August 18th. The weather is still fine and fairly cool. We bombard the enemy very heavily during the night and the East Yorks are to make a raid.

August 24 Thursday
Meals: ditto. The following is printed up with our orders today, which is a translation of a German document dated 20th February 1916 which was found on a German Prisoner;

"Committee for the Increase of the Population" Notice No.13975
Sir
On account of all the able bodied men having been called to the colours, it remains the duty of all those behind, for the sake of the Fatherland, to interest themselves in the happiness of the married women and maidens by doubling or even trebling the number of births.

Your name has been given to us as a capable man and you are hearwith requested to take on this office of honour and to do your duty in right German style. It must here be pointed out that your wife in France will not be able to claim a divorce. It is fact to be hoped that the women will bear this discomfort heroically for the sake of the war.

You will be given the district of …… Should you not feel capable of coping with the situation you will be given three days in which to name someone in your place. On the other hand if you are prepared to take on a second district as well, you will become a 'Decksoffizier' and receive a pension.

An exhibition of women and maidens as well as a collection of photographs is to be found at our office. You are requested to bring this letter with you.

Your good work should commence immediately and it is in your interest to submit to us a full report of results after 9 months.

Signed …………………………
President of the Committee
First Army
21/2/16

Are our Army officials passing it on as a joke, or do they think this leg pulling takes us in too? We had the same work as yesterday, but have very little to do. We have rifles and then rations inspected in the afternoon. I received a letter from Doll dated August 20th and wrote to Doll and handed it in.

August 25 Friday

Meals: ditto. Our work today is similar but further to the west in the old British Line. I got back soon after 1pm to hear we are to move to Lestrem at 3pm and return to the trenches tomorrow. This order was then cancelled and we go to the local baths instead, where I get a good change of underclothing. We are to go to trenches tomorrow though, for an indefinite period. The local canteen opened last night, so I got in the cigs. It is rumoured that this is our last time in the trenches and that we are going to England before Egypt. The latest Barnsley rumour is that they are going on garrison duty in Malta.

August 26 Saturday

Meals: ditto. It was a showery morning. We marched off for the trenches at 1pm and arrived at 2pm. I am in charge of bay 119 near 111 where I was before. No 12 are where the Minnies dropped but it has been very quiet so far today. Some lads in my charge are the last draft of old soldiers from the Yorks and Lancs. We were up above the parapet and firing right away in broad daylight. A pigeon flew over our post to enemy camp with a visible message at 7.45pm. I sent a FPC to Doll and Mother.

August 27 Sunday

Rations very short: bacon, 1/3 of a loaf bread, cold beef and jam. Captain Cousins D and C Company is rather keen on work but not much is being done. It was a quiet morning. It was showery today.

August 28 Monday (Mother's Birthday)

Our rations were meagre again. Breakfast: bacon. Dinner: Maconochies. Tea: jam and butter. Today is Mother's birthday and I wish her many happy returns and us all. The day is celebrated by a pretty decent strafe in the afternoon and our exchange of compliments in the middle of the morning. The Germans are chucking over a lot of heavy Minnies and they dropped a lot just about where we had been working this afternoon, very shortly after we had left. Last night was quite fine and cold and today is warm and bright with slight quiet showers. I can see **Vimy Ridge**[201] very clearly. I received a parcel from A.A. which contained a tin of pineapple, a tin of salmon, a tin of cigs, lemonade, a tin of sweets and a ration bag.

August 29 Tuesday

Our rations were only ¼ loaf of bread each but biscuits to make up. Breakfast: bacon. Dinner: Maconochies. Tea: jam. I received a paper from Colin and then worked in the morning mending trench boards. We rested about 2pm in the afternoon. The weather was wet and then there was a severe thunderstorm at the same time that our trench mortars play hell, which was a contest between man and nature. The rain pours through the roof of my dugout and the floor is soon

---

[201] **Vimy Ridge** - ran almost 12km north-east of Arras. The Germans occupied Vimy Ridge in September 1914 and their engineers immediately began to construct a network of artillery-proof trenches and bunkers.

swimming. I sit huddled on the trench board trying to decide whether to get my tea when Cousins turns us all out to drain the trenches which are getting flooded. Of all the stinking putrid jobs, that was the limit. I got my tea at stand to at 8.15pm and so started with trousers wet through for a showery night's vigil. I tried to get a little sleep on a wet fire-step but it was not very good. Cousins insists on a working party as usual.

August 30 Wednesday
Rations are rather more bread but bully beef and baked beans for breakfast and dinner. I did not want any dinner. Tea: jam and butter, which has been plentiful. I received a letter from Doll, August 25th. I am transferred to another dugout and the old sand bags near my nose stink like an upturned cemetery. We have a rest in the morning and get about two hours but I am disturbed twice as the Brigadier is coming around and everything has to be in 'apple per cider'. D Company in the support trenches, have not clicked so after all. They provide carrying and wiring parties in the front line and today the Germans sent only about six whizz bangs into our line and **killed one**[202] and wounded two and there is one with shell shock. One shell pierced the back the dugout, laying out the two wounded machine gunners. It settled as a wet day. I was revetting the collapsed parapet in the afternoon and it was wet again for a wet night. The Brigadier was very keen indeed on the sand bags being turned inside out, so as not to show the seam. This was his most brilliant suggestion so far, I believe. The night turns out finer.

August 31 Thursday
Rations, ½ loaf to six men, biscuits instead. Breakfast: meagre bacon. Dinner: bully beef and beans. Tea: jam. The day is quite fine and quiet. There are rumours of a naval engagement, 14 Bristol sunk seven of the German fleet.

September 1 Friday
Rations: no bread. Breakfast: square inch of bacon. Dinner: bully, beans and onions. Tea: jam and butter. The weather is dull, fine and quiet. We stood to at 3am and there is a strafe on the right. The Barnsleys are going over but I don't think that they were successful. I received letters from Doll, August 27th. It has been dull with slight rain and the night keeps fine. It is rumoured that we are going to be relieved tomorrow.

September 2 Saturday
The rottenest rations we've had yet – nothing but bully beef, jam and biscuits. It has been a fine and quiet day. We have had no relief yet but may be tomorrow, I think. We are disappointed again – the Barnsleys are only reinforcing us. God knows when we will get out. I am going out on patrol tonight and **Davies**[203] says that he is tired of reporting nothing, so he means to find something. I write and hand a letter in to Doll. The patrol is cancelled for a small bombing raid,

---

[202] **12/1190 Private Albert Cavill** died of wounds on 30 August 1916 and **23246 Private Edward Thorpe** died from his wounds the following day both are buried in Merville Community cemetery.
[203] **39129 Lance Corporal H. G. Davies** – Special Patrol Party.

114

which didn't bomb. A Company patrol throw a bomb to see if trenches are occupied, they have a result and two were wounded. There was then a heavy bombing stunt on the right.

September 3 Sunday
Rations back up again, enough bread. Breakfast: cold bacon. Dinner: cold beef. Tea: butter and jam.

I got no rest last night till 3.30am, we then stood to at 4.30am. The weather is fine but dull. I received a letter from Maggie, August 29th.

September 4 Monday
Rations: Breakfast: bacon. Dinner: bully and a good two teaspoonfuls of potato. Tea: jam. The night was very cold and I slept on the fire-step, from 1.30am to 4.14am. It started to rain at stand down but cleared at 10am. It was a quiet and dull day. I received a letter from Doll, August 30th and sent FPC to Doll, Mother, **F.E.P.E.**[204] and wrote to A.A. and handed in. My one stripe and lack of another seem to save me a lot of patrols and wiring parties.

September 5 Tuesday
Rations: ¼ loaf, biscuits. Breakfast: cold bacon. Dinner: cold beef and onions. Tea: jam and butter. Last night was cold but quiet and I managed to sleep for 2½ hours on the fire-step. I received a paper from Colin. I am taking out a patrol tonight to complete this afternoon's revetting. Cousins then postpones the patrol as it is too beastly wet and it then turns out to be a fine night. I then get from 12 midnight to 2.30am in a beautiful sleep in **Ellison's**[205] dugout.

September 6 Wednesday
Rations, ¼ loaf & biscuits. Breakfast: bacon. Dinner: bully beef, beans, potatoes. Tea: jam. It was a very foggy morning. We stood to till 9am and were then firing at the Germans that we could see out to the right. It was a beautiful fine day but was turning cold this evening. There was a strafe in our front about 5pm to 7pm and it was mostly ours though. The Germans are practically only replying with a few heavy trench mortars on both the right and left. I spend time writing to Doll and send a FPC to Mother. I am to take out the patrol tonight from 11pm to 12.30 with four men, exploring old trenches and ditches in No Man's Land. We all get safely back. I am preparing a plan of the same and writing a report till after 2am and then slept on the fire-step till stand to. Three of my men were old soldiers of the last draft – Salva Bay etc. etc. who were regular blood thirsty fire eaters in the trenches but as soon as they were outside they got the wind up badly. They could see and hear Germans everywhere, even where none existed. They lagged behind all the way and I wouldn't have trusted

---

[204] **F.E.P.E. – Mr F. E. Pearce Edwards** was the City Architect at Sheffield Town Hall. He became a lifelong friend of Franks and also assisted in the design of the City Battalion Camp at Redmires.
[205] **12/910 Sergeant C. Ellison** – took part in the attack on 1st July 1916.

them to stand a minute if attacked. **Marshall**[206] is a better class of fellow, one of the old Draft and was worth a heap of them.

September 7 Thursday
Rations were 1/3rd loaf, plenty. Breakfast: cold bacon. Dinner: cold beef and rice pudding. Tea: prunes

My report had gone to headquarters without Cousins seeing it, so I had to describe my work to him this morning. He said it was just what he wanted to know and asked me to prepare another plan for him, when I had nothing much to do. Sic..! I did it in my working time. It was a fine day again. It was fairly quiet but we had a strafe again this evening as yesterday. I received a letter from Doll, September 1st. I was sent out on the **listening post**[207] with two men from 10pm until 1am, about 100 yards in front of our wire in the open. From 12.15am until 12.45am our artillery open heavy bombardment over our heads. It was very lively indeed with shrapnel bursting short and also heavies, which throw back huge chunks over 600 yards, as was proved by a lump dropping in our trench this afternoon. Ours and the enemy machine guns were whizzing very close too. We all got back safely, then Cousins said he had not intended us to go further than the end of the sap trench. I slept on the fire-step from 3am until 5am then a stand to. Men without shrapnel helmets on C Company say my name and reputation is at stake, as an NCO is to be put under arrest if his men were found without their helmets in the trenches. It is pretty good considering that we had gone out officially without them and came under heavy fire into the bargain. I felt fed up.

September 8 Friday
Rations: 1/3rd loaf. Breakfast: bacon. Dinner: Maconochies. Tea: jam. Everyone was allowed to rest in the morning except the observers. I get down and sleep from 6.30am to 7.30am and from 10am to 21.30pm then again 2am to 4.30am and enjoyed every bit of it, it was badly wanted. I received a PC from Doll, September 2nd. We had the usual strafe tonight from 6pm -7pm. the enemy reply, less even then before and only for one minute. I hear we don't go out till Sunday. It was a fine day and night and quiet in our section, with bombing starts on each side. I get two hours sleep every two hours.

September 9 Saturday
Rations: 1/3rd loaf. Breakfast: cold bacon. Dinner: cold beef. Tea: jam. I rested in the morning after standing to till 8pm, on account of the fog. We had stand to at 11am and as usual there was strafe by our Stokes. The enemy reply with shrapnel. We go up to Ham Corner for sand bags in the afternoon and as there were no bags, we have to carry barbed wire coils instead. I received letters from Doll and Mother, September 3rd and wrote a love letter to Doll which **S.M.**

---

[206] **230744 Private J. Marshall** – killed in action 13th October 1918 and served with 14th and 15th York and Lancaster.

[207] **Listening Post** – a dangerous forward post where two or three men stationed to listen for enemy activity.

Gallimore[208], the censor allowed me to send. I was out on a listening post from 1am to 4am. Our strafe commenced at 1.30am when our Battalion bombing party went over. It was the usual washout and the front line was deserted, communications were barricaded and we hear that **three are killed**[209], including **Blenkarn**[210] and twenty are wounded. I still went to the listening post in spite of the machine guns and shrapnel, which was rather a pinch as we missed standing to with gas helmets.

September 10 Sunday
Rations: ditto but dinner; bully, pickles and beans. I get two hours rest in the afternoon and then stand to for the usual strafe which has a very feeble reply. I sent FPC to Mother. It was a fine day and a very light night. I went out on patrol on a rather advanced listening post from 12.30am to 2.30am with **Johnson**[211] and **Jutson**[212].

September 11 Monday
Cousins details me an NCO out of C Company for wiring and trenching course. I had to report to BHQ, which was forty minutes walk away at 7.30am, so I had to start off without breakfast or rations. I waylaid a breakfast party on the way however and collared cold bacon and tea. We marched straight away to Vielle Chapelle and started right away having a commenced meal on the way. I gathered some more meals on the way, which were very good. The course lasted from 8.30am to 12.30am then finished, we were kept hard at it though. There was no smoking allowed, only during the ¼ hr interval. It is hard to be rather slack, I hear - the Brigadier must have been around. **Thompson**[213] marches us back to Chapelle which is ½ hr away and keeps us hanging about till 5.30pm before finding us a billet. I got a dinner of eggs and chips in meantime. I was billeted in a roof attic over a pub up two long flights of winding stairs. I see **Wood**[214] at Brigade HQ and he proves to be a good friend again and gives me tea and supplies me with rations. He also lends me an overcoat and a bundle of sandbags, so I enjoy a good night's sleep, although I came unprovided.

---

[208] **12/1123 Sergeant R. Gallimore** - a Bank Clerk who was wounded in the attack on 1st July 1916.

[209] **12/1412 Private Hector Atkinson Wilson** was also killed. He threw bombs into the German trench and was killed instantly when he was shot through the head. He is commemorated on the Loos Memorial.

[210] **12/597 Lance Corporal William Blenkarn** – killed in action 10th September 1916 (according to war record) and is commemorated on Loos Memorial.

[211] **24497 Corporal Frank Johnson** – killed in action on 27th June 1917, he is commemorated on the Arras Memorial.

[212] **21890 W. H. Jutson** – served with 12th York and Lancaster on 1st July 1916, also served with 1st York and Lancaster.

[213] **11225 Sergeant A Thompson** – a member of A Company.

[214] **12/559 Lance Sergeant Thomas Harper Wood** – killed in action 2nd November 1916 and is buried in Sailly au Bois Military Cemetery.

September 12 Tuesday

Breakfast: bacon. Dinner: stewed beef. Tea: jam. The course goes down better in the morning. I bathe and change in the afternoon and then go to La Fosse and Lestrem for a good feed in the evening, I was full up. Leaving Fosse on my return at 9.15pm, **RSM Polden**[215] nearly gets me. He was just telling a sentry to take men's names who are out of their billets as I pass. Special reference is made to 'that man in front', thanks to the slowness in his response, I pass. I receive a parcel from A.A containing handkerchiefs, salmon, cream, cigs, toothbrush and powder. I also receive a parcel of papers from Auntie Annie and I was paid 15 francs.

September 13 Wednesday

Breakfast: bacon. Dinner: steak. Tea: jam. We had Cousins in the morning from 8.30am to 12noon. It rained hard so we had a lecture at 11.30am and an early dismissal. I had three glasses of beer and slept till after dinner. I stopped in and read in the evening and received a PC from Doll, September 8th.

September 14 Thursday

Meals ditto but stew for dinner. We had the usual morning and the course was fine. There were slight showers for the rest of the afternoon. I intended writing letters in the afternoon but slept again which was necessary recuperation after the strain of the trenches. I received a letter and PC from Doll, September 7th and a letter from Aunt Annie, September 8th.

September 15 Friday

Meals: ditto but get boned beef in addition. We finished our course in the morning. The most interesting item was an exploding **bangalore torpedo**[216] in the barbed wire. The absolute clearance for a length of gas pipe was 10 or 12 feet wide and not a particle of wire was left. I rejoined the Battalion soon after 6pm. I received a letter from Doll dated September 10th and wrote back to her. We were ordered for the trenches again on Sunday.

I am more shocked at the beastly crime about to be perpetrated that I have been at anything since coming to France...

A fellow[217] in 2nd York came to us as a draft just before we last went into the trenches. He was under open arrest, pending a sentence for four days

---

[215] **12/480 Regimental Sergeant Major C. Polden** – ex Army regular commissioned to 12th York and Lancaster on 20th June 1917.

[216] **Bangalore torpedo** - is an explosive placed on the end of a long, extendible tube. In World War 1 it was primarily used for clearing barbed wire before an attack. It could be used whilst under fire, from a protected position in a trench.

[217] **7595 Private J. A. Haddock** was the 'fellow' in question. He was already under a suspended sentence of 20 years penal servitude for a previous offence of desertion. On the way to the front line on 30th June 1916, his nerve cracked and he went into hiding. He was arrested by the Military Police, probably suffering from battle fatigue some five days later. He was executed on 16th September 1916 and is buried in Vielle Chapelle Military Cemetery at La Coutre. There is no mention of his execution in the Battalion's War Diary and he is not mentioned/commemorated in the publication 'Soldiers that Died in The Great War'. It would appear that the entire matter has been subject to a 'cover up.'

desertion. He had then given himself up, saying that he had only been to see his brother, an old soldier with fifteen years service in India, he was probably a bit touched. He has a wife and three kids. He has been sentenced before for a similar crime and reprieved. He took his wack with us during sixteen days in the trenches; mounted guard, loaded rifles, firing over parapet – practically a free man. He thought he was going to get off again. Today the sentence was communicated **'_TO BE SHOT_'** in the morning. My platoon is guarding him today and B Company will provide the firing party. I have just seen him – he bears himself splendidly.

N.B. In the book 'Shot at Dawn' by Julian Putkowski, and Julian Sykes it states that James Haddock was a regular soldier who was originally posted to the 2nd Battalion but was then transferred to the Sheffield City Battalion. At the time of his posting to the trenches on the Somme, he was already on a twenty year, later reduced to five years, suspended sentence for a previous offence of desertion. Despite this he left again on his way up to the trenches on 30th June 1916, the day before Somme Offensive of 1st July 1916. He went into hiding but was discovered five days later on 5th July by the Military Police, seven miles from the Battalions trenches

At the subsequent Field Court Martial held on 24th August 1916, his defence was that he was suffering with his feet and the medical officer had told him to rest. He had got lost trying to find transport and when he was apprehended, he was actually looking for the police to ask for directions. His orders at the time of his desertion were to follow his colleagues into the trenches and he did not and went missing for five days. When he was found, he was hiding in a civilian wagon without either his equipment or rifle. He had made no attempt whatsoever to rejoin his colleagues.

His past Army service record showed that since arriving in France, he had deserted seven times as well as being charged with being drunk on active service and refusing to obey an order. He was already under a suspended sentence of five years that had been passed by a Field General Court Martial, so the verdict of the Court Martial was inevitable and he was sentenced to death by firing squad. The verdict was then passed and it reached General Douglas Haig on 12th September 1916, who confirmed the verdict and the sentence of the Field General Court Martial. The most likely cause was a form of stress called 'battle fatigue' but in 1916 this was thought of as cowardice. The execution by firing squad took place at dawn on 16th September 1916 and James Haddock was the first soldier from Sheffield to be executed in the Great War.

September 16 Saturday

Breakfast: bacon. Dinner: Roast mutton, baked beans, potatoes, carrots, pickles. Tea: jam. **The sentence on that poor devil was duly carried out at 5.35 this morning. He took it smiling.** We are ordered for the trenches today, packing and unpacking all morning. Our first order is to take our hammocks, our second order is to take everything and our third order is to take our valise and leave the hammocks. I received a letter from Doll dated September 11th and handed in my letters to Doll and Mother. We set off for the trenches in military transport wagons, at last the British Army moves on wheels. We take up action at

Festubert and arrive at our trenches at stand to which was a tidy march to the front after unloading. The frontline was formed of isolated posts and only to be attained at night with any safety. I am put in charge of a sorting group to cover a trench that consists of only three men. We are disbanded at 3am to release two who are sentry men – turncoats! At No. 14 island posts we have **one machine gunner killed**[218] first thing going over the parapet to an island.

September 17 Sunday

Breakfast: bacon. Dinner: cold beef. Tea: jam and butter. **Jukes**[219] is sent to cook for us. The beauty of this post is that there is little chance of unpredicted visits or inspections during the day time. I'm in charge of one group of three, so do my sentry again. We were freely shelled from 10am till mid day. One dugout is blown in just as **Askew**[220] goes in it. **Coates**[221] is just outside too and it is marvellous that neither is hurt. Nevertheless, I would rather be here than anywhere. It was pouring with rain all night. I stood to from 10.30pm to 11.30pm for a bit of a bombing attack just on the right. Cousins then visits us to see what work we are going to do.

September 18 Monday

Breakfast: cold bacon. Dinner: ¼ of a tin Maconochies. Tea: jam and butter. I received a letter from Doll dated September 13th. It was pouring with rain all day again. Cousins makes his way to this ditch to see about work – he would. There was none done though, except cleaning a few bombs. I had a good sleep both during the morning and the afternoon, although the dugout is pretty wet and my feet were in a pool. The weather cleared up at night.

September 19 Tuesday

Breakfast: cold bacon. Dinner: cold meat. Tea: jam and butter. It was a fine morning and a showery afternoon. I received a letter from Mother dated September 13th and sent a FPC to Doll and Mother and wrote to A.A. It was a showery and cold night.

September 20 Wednesday

Breakfast: cold bacon. Dinner: bully and baked beans. Tea: jam. It was a cold and wet day and the night was fairly fine. I received a letter from Doll dated September 15th. The East Lancs machine guns are in support again as last night and they pepper us freely on our side. There is much more danger from our side than from the Germans during the night fires.

September 21 Thursday

---

[218] **12/105 Private Alan Hugh Foxon** - a Sheffield University student who took part in the attack on 1st July 1916 was killed. He is buried in Le Touret Military Cemetery.

[219] **12/1254 Private A. Jukes** – took part in the battle on 1st July 1916.

[220] **12/578 Corporal Herbert Askew** – died of wounds on 25th October 1918 when with 7th Y&L, he is buried in Awoingt Military Cemetery.

[221] **40092 Private W. Coates** – killed in action on 1st October 1917, he is buried in Hooge Crater Military Cemetery.

Breakfast: cold rissoles. Dinner: cold beef – very good. Tea: raspberry jam. Our rum rations commenced at stand to. It was a fine day and the mud is drying nicely. The night was fine and warmer. It was very muddy on the connecting patrol with the East Lancs and they had two men sniped today, one man was killed and an officer was wounded. *I was made a Corporal today.*

September 22 Friday
Generous rations. Breakfast: cold bacon. Dinner: Maconochies. Tea: jam and butter, also a present of fruit salad. Today was beautifully fine and it is drying up splendidly. Our aeroplane drops two bombs just in front of our parapet. I received a letter from Doll dated September 17th and sent Doll an FPC. It was a very cold night with a damp mist.

September 23 Saturday
Breakfast: cold bacon. Dinner: cold beef. Tea: jam. It was a hot, fine day and was very quiet. We are to be relieved tomorrow night. I wrote to Doll and handed it in. It has been a very foggy night.

September 24 Sunday
Ample rations. Breakfast: cold bacon. Dinner: bully beef and baked beans. Tea: jam and butter. We stood to till after 8am. It was very foggy at first but then it was a bright hot day. I rested previous to relief and received a letter from Doll dated September 19th. We were relieved at about 9.30am and I followed the cover trench up to the north and west out by Rope Trench. There was two feet of mud and water a great deal of the way and I'd blackened my boots before going out. **Another man**[222] was sniped today, making only our second casualty killed here, Grant was also sniped in the arm. We arrived at our billets in Festubert at 12.30am and were very tired, where tea and a very nice stew were provided. They are the best billets that we have had, stable stalls with a boarded floor and new straw. It was a very cold night and blankets were served out.

September 25 Monday
Breakfast: Maconochies. Dinner: roast beef, baked potatoes, carrots, turnips, onions, cabbage. Tea: Hartley's strawberry jam and butter. We cleaned up in the morning and I had a bath in the afternoon and a clean change. I received a letter from Mother dated September 20[th,] a PC from Doll dated September 21st and a parcel from A.A. which contained cake, potted tongue, chocolate, cigs, soap and a novel. I sent an FPC to Doll and Mother. I was on 24hr guard at 7pm, I would have previously slept in the billets but RSM Polden makes duty billet the 'hovel' guard room with a mud floor. **QM Charlesworth**[223] however, gave us

---

[222] **12/2047 Private Joseph Seamore Fairclough** – killed in action on 24th September 1916. He is buried at Le Touret Military Cemetery, Richebourg.

[223] **12/561 Company Quartermaster Sergeant F. Charlesworth** – was commissioned to West Riding on 31st July 1917.

plenty of straw, so we are comfortable. Everyone is very **windy**[224] about the thought of gas.

September 26 Tuesday
Breakfast: bacon. Dinner: Maconochies. Tea: jam and butter. It was a fine and bright day and Poulden is finding trouble as usual. I receive a 'Passing Show' from Colin and was in a working party tonight, as we missed it we have to continue until 9am tomorrow. I wrote to Mother and handed in.

September 27 Wednesday
Breakfast: bacon. Dinner: stew. Tea: treacle. There were slight showers but it has been generally fine. I was in a working party at 6pm and excused duty for relief at 9am. I wrote to A.A. and handed it in and received 15 francs pay. We paraded for the working party at 6pm and I got to work at 8pm, finished at 2am and was back again at 3.30am. It was a fine day, but foggy later. Rissoles were served for B Company on their return.

September 28 Thursday
Dinner: stew. Tea: treacle. I slept till about 11am, just in time to clean up for dinner we then parade at 2.30pm for a rifle and gas bag inspection. It was a fine day. I received a letter from Doll dated September 22nd. I fell in at 6pm for the working party as usual which was led by an officer on a circular route which took 2½ hours to get to the trenches. We commenced at 9am and I worked as before, filling in the parapet on the old British line working under machine gun fire. The weather was showery. We knocked off at 2am and were taken back the longest way out of the trenches, through water with each leg up to our knees, walking off trench boards in the dark. We arrived back at 4am where breakfast, bacon, was awaiting us.

September 29 Friday
Dinner: stew. Tea: treacle. I was up at 11.30am and there was no time for a proper clean up. We had dinner and then fell in at 12.55pm for a flammenwerfer display. We marched to Burvey, then the next three miles taking a London motor bus to the Pacaut Divisional School near Merville. We had a flammenwerfer display as usual but with the most interesting equipment which were 3" tubes of ammonal laid in shallow grips, which exploded from the sap trench. 100 yards is considered by the officer as far enough away from the explosion but we go 120 or more. The sky is obscured by falling debris, two of our chaps have temporary 'lune de combat'. The trenches formed were four or five feet deep by eight or nine feet wide. We march by the inspection of 18lbs and 4.5 howitzers. Major Gurney says we must hurry back for the working party at 6.30pm and we have a heavy load of anticipation. We go back to Burvey in another direction, via Bethune and then march back from Burvey and arrive at our billets at 7pm. There is much relief that the working party is off. We have

---

[224] **Windy** – Fear, not be confused with 'cold feet' which means to back out of duty through fear. To 'have the wind up' implied no disgrace.

tea and I then sew my stripes on to my tunic, first chance that I've had of doing anything for myself for ten days, than bed time and lights out at 9.15pm. It was a wet morning but then the rest of the day was fine. What a pleasure to undress to go to bed.

September 30 Saturday
Breakfast: bacon. Dinner: stew. Tea: prunes. We had a brief inspection this morning to attend to some cobbles for slight repair and filling in last few days of this dairy while I wait as there has been no chance before, not to mention letter writing. There is no working party tonight but they cannot really let us rest, so we fall in at 12.55am for a route march that was rather forced, with only one break in 3½ hrs. We get an extra hour's rest tonight owing to the clocks being put back. I received a letter from Doll dated September 22nd and then sent a PC to Doll. It has been a fine and bright day.

October 1 Sunday
Breakfast: bacon. Dinner: stew. Tea: jam and butter. We are going into the trenches again today, so we were packing our kit and cleaning up in the morning. We parade at 1.30pm with absolutely everything we have and waders chucked in as the last straw. It is the same sector as before but this time I am in charge of a central bombing group in Bay 15. There was just time to get tea before stand to and the tea itself arrives about 8pm. It was a quiet night and I get some sleep in the dugout from 12 midnight – 4am and then stand to. It was a fine day.

October 2 Monday
Breakfast: cold bacon. Dinner: Maconochies, carrots, turnips and rice pudding. Tea: jam. There is a change of working parties in the morning and afternoon and I am to get a whole nights rest and not stand to till stand to. The Germans sent baby Minnies over our dugouts just in front of the parapet that I'm standing in. A little later one blows up our spade dump, from which we have just drawn. Our waders are a blessing as the mud is over our knees. It has been a fine morning and a wet afternoon and raining. I must really make an effort and write to Doll in the morning. It is rumoured that we go out tomorrow marching and training to Abbeville next, then Salonika or Egypt.

October 3 Tuesday
Breakfast: cold bacon. Dinner: cold beef and tea. Tea: blackcurrant jam. I was left undisturbed from 7.30pm till 4.30am in the dugout, I did not sleep very soundly though, took off my gum boots and put on underwear and puttees. The Colonel and **Lieutenant Colonel Fisher**[225] were sniped this morning and both were killed. The former was going on his rounds to the islands and the latter was looking over the parapet as usual. I took the working party down to the left

---

[225] **Lieutenant Colonel H. B. Fisher** Served 12 Y&L from 18 Aug 1916. He is buried in Le Touret Military Cemetery in Richebourg. He had just returned from a conference at 1st Army School. He was touring the Battalion's position in the early hours of the morning to get to know the layout and to visit his men.

front line but we were sent back after half an hour as the new artillery was going to register this morning. We were back again in the afternoon with the artillery registering and narrowly missing our parapet. It was a wet morning and a fine afternoon. I wrote to Doll and handed in.

October 4 Wednesday
Breakfast: cold bacon. Dinner: bully beef and pickle. We expect to go out this afternoon, so we work and I get packed as best I can. It was a wet morning and I received a letter from Mother dated September 28th. We did not get relieved by the West Kents till 9pm. We had no tea and were back in the old billets by 11pm, where we received a first rate stew and tea for supper and we then had a clean up this evening.

October 5 Thursday
Breakfast: bacon. Dinner: stew and rice. Tea: prunes. We were cleaning up and had a rifle inspection and an inspection of C Company in the morning. We are leaving the district; Salonika, Egypt and the Somme are surmised, it is sure to be the latter. We marched off at 2.30pm and are billeted at Verdin les Bethune on the outskirts of Bethune. I went there in the evening and had steak and chips for supper, coffee, vin rouge and three cream buns. There were some very fine pastry cook shops there and I returned hot and tired. The weather has been fine. I sent an FPC to Mother and Doll.

October 6 Friday
Breakfast: bacon. Dinner: stew. Tea: butter & jam. I woke up feeling very done in with a thick head and a sick feeling. I had a little breakfast and then dozed all morning and couldn't touch dinner. I had eggs and milk just before we started off at 1.30pm, which agreed with one. I received a letter from Doll dated September 28th. We marched to Robecq and managed a little tea and dozed as far as duties would allow till bed time. We had clean good straw in our billets but passed a restless night. The weather has been fine.

October 7 Saturday
Breakfast: tinned hot bacon. Dinner: stew and rice. Tea: jam. I felt better today but my appetite not completely restored. We had a short inspection in the morning and slight musketry in the afternoon. I feel a complete mug giving orders on parade, I am much more at home in the trenches. **Leaman**[226] tells me I must buck up. It was a wet afternoon and evening during which I rest again. I received a letter from Doll dated October 1st and a letter from Mother dated October 3rd with a keen blow – the news of Maggie's death at 1.45am on October 3rd. I sent an FPC to Mother and Doll.

---

[226] **Captain R. W. Leaman** Served 12 York and Lancaster from February 1915 to September 1917.

8
Return to the Somme

October 8 Sunday
Breakfast: Maconochies – I was not up to it, so I bought eggs. We marched off on a showery day, carrying extra iron rations and jam at 8.30am. We reached Berguette, a further six miles at 11.15am. I bought buns, nuts and apples and we were entrained as usual in crowded cattle trucks and departed for Doullens at 12 noon and arrived there about 5pm. We marched straight away without replenishment for Marieux, a further 7 miles and arrived about 8.30pm. We billeted in incomplete huts that were so crowded that there was not sufficient floor space for each man. I got down and was asleep when tea was brought around about 10.30pm. I rested better than I've done for the last two nights as I was tired out.

October 9 Monday
Breakfast: bacon. Dinner: stew. Tea: jam and butter. We were turned out of our billets immediately after breakfast and new billets subsequently were found which were dirty hovels with no straw. I have been acting as Platoon Sergeant so the whole of my spare time has been taken up. No time to write again to Mother or Teddie. I am fed up. We are told that we are advancing in a few days but I don't think so personally, as we are the last reserves, I believe. Anyway we are in for hard preparatory training.

October 10 Tuesday
Breakfast: bacon. Dinner: stew. Tea: jam & butter. We had a stiff morning parade, followed by artillery formation and extended order and attack, doubling up hill. My legs were like lead at the end of the day. We had a bombing lecture in the evening followed by a pint of good strong ale. Received a letter from Doll dated October 4th and a paper from Colin and Auntie Annie.

October 11 Wednesday
Breakfast: Maconochies. Dinner: stew. Tea: jam. Today has been an easy day. We had a short NCO conference in the morning, which was artillery formation and an extended order attack and in the afternoon we had communication with aeroplane signalling. The weather has been fine except for slight showers lately but fairly cold and windy. I'm beginning to pick up again but have not yet regained my appetite. The Sergeant Major is back tonight, so Ellison will come back to the platoon, for which there is much relief and thanks. Leaman distributes 10 francs for our good work yesterday morning. I wrote to Mother and handed in and Teddie ditto.

October 12 Thursday

Breakfast: bacon. Dinner: stew. Tea: jam & butter. We had a morning parade and an extended order for attack and ditto this afternoon and bayonet fighting. Sergeant Major is still sick and is on light duty, so I am still run off my legs as Platoon Sergeant. I snatched sufficient time to write to Doll and hand in. It has been a fine day but dull and cool.

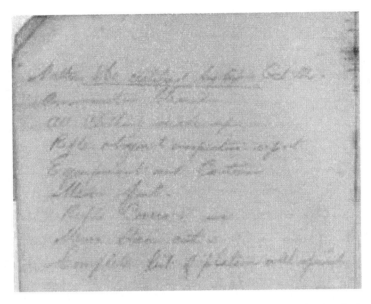

An extract taken from Frank's Diary which also included at the back, lists of his platoons and duties

Matters to be certified by 5pm on October 12th:
> *Ammunition cleaned*
> *All clothing made up*
> *Rifle and bayonet inspection report*
> *Equipment and canteen*
> *Men's feet*
> *Rifle covers*
> *Men's hair cut*
> *Complete list of platoon with specials*

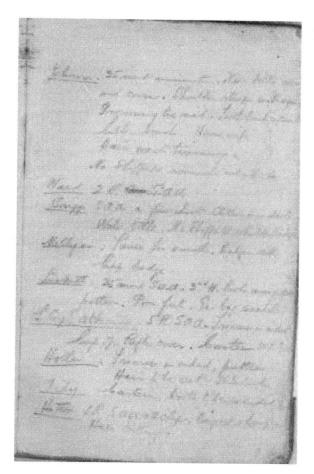

An extract taken from Frank's Diary which also included at the back, inspection notes as follows:

<u>Johnson</u> *25 rounds ammunition, new billy can and cover, shoulder straps wet edging, in growing toenail, toothbrush and comb, lather brush, housewife, hair wants trimming, no Sheffield numerals, only Y&L*

<u>Ward</u> *2R SAA*

<u>Briggs</u> *SAA a few short, clothing on indent, water bottle, no Sheffield shoulder badge.*

<u>Nelligan</u> *Tunic too small, badges ditto, cap badge.*

<u>Lockett</u> *25 ward SAA 2nd H, boots uncomfortable, puttees, poor feet, gas bag satchel*

<u>L Corp. Atkinson</u> *5R. SAA, trousers an indent, cap 7 Rifle cover, canteen WBC.*

<u>Hollis</u> *trousers an indent, puttees, hair to be cut, WB Cook*

<u>Tidy</u> *Canteen, boots to be mended*

<u>Hatton</u> *1R SAA + 2 clips, bayonet sharpen, hair cutting*

October 13 Friday
Breakfast: rissoles. Dinner: steak, baked beans, fried potatoes, rice pudding, a very good dinner. I was up at 6am, getting out lists and so manage to hand in on time. We got off the parade in morning for a boot repair and a bath. This afternoon we had an eight mile route march under the new Colonel as Gurney has gone for two months instruction. I have been docking out indents all night.

October 14 Saturday
Breakfast: bacon. Dinner: boiled bacon, haricot beans, potatoes. Tea: jam. I am Corporal of fatigue parts at Divisional HQ with only half an hour loading in the morning and afternoon but I managed to dodge the parade.

October 15 Sunday
Breakfast: bacon. Dinner: stew. Tea: jam and butter. We had a Church parade in the morning and bayonet exercise in afternoon. On our return I saw a soldier in the entrance to our billet and took no notice of him. He came up to me and then it was quite an interval before I grasped it was Arthur. It was as good as a bit of leave. My spirits went up immediately. I bought a tin of peaches to celebrate. He had tea with me and we had till 7.30pm together. I was paid 20 francs and I gave Arthur 5. My leg is very painful all day and I wonder if it is rheumatism. I received a letter from Doll dated October 9th.

October 16 Monday
Breakfast: bacon. Dinner: stew. Tea: jam and butter. My leg ached too much to sleep and I am up for half of the night, also a lot of new chaps came in the middle of the night. My leg felt better in the morning and I woke in quite good spirits again, a result of Arthur's visit, he was looking fine. It was splendid weather and wonderfully clear. It was a Brigade field day and we were kept out until 2pm. We were told we had parading in the afternoon, then we turned out at 3pm for a short spell of bayonet drill and night manoeuvres in the evening from 6pm – 8pm with hot tea on our return.

October 17 Tuesday
Breakfast: rissoles. Dinner: stew. Tea: jam and butter. It has been a showery day. We are getting ready to move our billets in the morning, so there is nothing doing. We march to Flamechon in afternoon which is only about three miles away. We get awarded the first floor and I go out and get eggs and coffee after tea. I buy a bale of straw and get down very cosily and am then fetched out for guard. I received a letter from Doll, October 11th and sent a FPC to Doll and Mother.

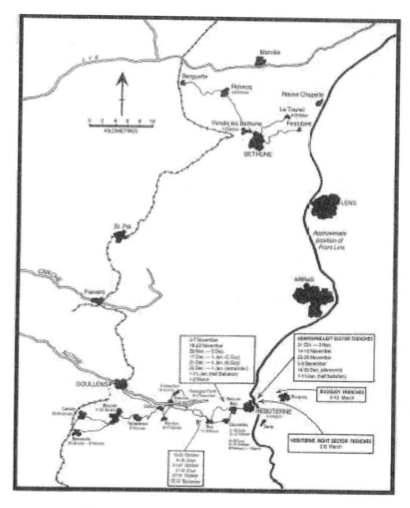

Map showing the City Battalion's position on their return to the Somme

October 18 Wednesday

Breakfast: bacon. Dinner: stew. Tea: jam. We made a good night of it in the tent. I was fetched to take charge again of **Minney**[227] and Johnson and I let them down as softly as possible as they were refusing to obey orders. They were let off with light punishment. We were ordered to pack valises ready to move with half an hour's notice given. We fall in at 2pm and march to Authie Wood and are herded into dilapidated huts on the north side of those we left prior to July 1st. There are no beds, a rough earth floor and the sides are torn and partly open. We got tea about 6pm and the whole Battalion was out for most of

---

[227] **36058 Private H. A. Minney** – also served in 6th York and Lancaster.

evening, carting stuff up from the road to QMS, being Corporal of the guard, I touched.

October 19 Thursday
Breakfast: bacon. Dinner: bully beef stew. Tea: jam and butter. It was a very wet night and is continuing today and many fellows got flooded out in the hut. The Battalion paraded but soon returned to the hut to get out of the wet. I was in charge of the draining party. General O'Gowan looked in and was very affable as he was before last sending us to our slaughter. We had an extended order drill in the afternoon. We walked into St Leger les Authie in the evening through mire and muck in the dark. The eggs were off when we got there. I handed in letter to Mother.

October 20 Friday
Breakfast: bacon. Dinner: roast beef, cabbage, potatoes & rice pudding. Tea: dates, butter & 1/6 loaf
We had a drilling party from 9.30am – 12noon. I handed in my application for a commission to Leaman. There was no parade in afternoon as the working parties are expected tonight and A and B Company are to go. The NCOs of C Company parade for a night marching. It has been a fine and a cold day.

October 21 Saturday
Breakfast: bacon. Dinner: stew. Tea: jam & butter. The A Company march was cancelled in the morning and we pack up and march for billets at Courcelles. No arrangements have been made when we get there, so we are forced into a bivouac between there and Bertrancourt with six under a tarpaulin. It was worse than anything we've touched yet with six men to four blankets. I went into Bertrancourt, there no eggs and the church hut was the only place that sells anything. I bought chocolate and cigs and obtained coffee in the village. We then passed a very cold night – freezing.

October 22 Sunday
Breakfast: bacon. Dinner: Stew. Tea: Jam and butter. We turned out 6.30am for breakfast, paraded at 7am and marched to Hebuterne which was about five miles. We had a working party dressing roads with no warning for lunch. We ceased work after some heavy shelling nearby at 2.30pm and returned to camp. We had tea at 4pm closely followed by stew. I received a letter from Mother dated October 13th with a funeral card (Maggie's funeral) open notice. It has been a bright frosty day that turned drizzly in the evening and later with fog.

October 23 Monday
Breakfast: bacon. Dinner: stew. Tea: jam and butter. We paraded again at 7am and commenced work on the roads, returning to Colincamps at 8am. We had a half hour break at 12 noon for dry biscuits then worked till 5pm and got back at 5.30pm to a combined dinner and tea in drizzle and darkness. It was a foggy day that was fine until the evening. I handed in green envelope to Doll at last, which I wrote on October 20th. I went to Bertrancourt in the evening and packed away

petite beurre biscuits and four basins of coffee. I felt really full up, on top of a big dinner and tea. The night party turned out at 11pm, so I had a whole bivouac to myself. It poured with rain all night with a pool of water in the middle of bivouac.

October 24 Tuesday
Breakfast: bacon. Dinner: stew. Tea: ¼ loaf ration. We had breakfast at 6am and then paraded at 6.30am as we were yesterday. We then fell out till 6.55am with time for breakfast in consequence but I took it with me for lunch. We were filling sand bags in at Hebuterne which ran out about 11.30am so we had a good long break. I was narrowly missed by a heavy shell in the meantime. It was drizzling all morning and we paraded in the afternoon. I was superintending covering the roof and floor over at the pumping station with sand bags. There is not much chance of a shell dropping here. We finished at about 3.30pm and went back to the camp through pouring rain about 5.15 pm. The new recruits get rather panicky at the shelling en route. We had combined meals as usual in the mud, rain and darkness. I received a letter from Teddie and Doll (Cat 17018). The rain ran through the tarpaulin in streams. I stopped under and read. The night was fine and cold.

October 25 Wednesday
Breakfast: bacon that congealed in a minute. Dinner and Tea: stew, jam and butter.

We paraded at 7am for Hebuterne again, going on with the same job. It was fine but cold and dull, which turned to rain in the afternoon. The Germans start shelling about 3.15am and we chuck it in at 3.30am and march back through the pouring rain. I went to Bertrancourt for coffee, biscuits and chocs in the evening and received a paper from Colin.

October 26 Thursday
Meals: ditto. We were loading stone onto the siding at Colincamps for repairing roads. A fool of an RE takes the first load by mistake to Hebuterne where he dumped it. I followed on foot endeavouring to catch him which was a three mile squelch through unutterable mud. We ceased work at 4pm. It has been a fine and bright day with much aerial activity and several Bosches appear to be have been brought down. We were back at 4.45pm and had dinner almost by daylight. I had written a letter to Mother of 18th which was handed back to me as Cloud has censored the words 'mud and darkness'. I erase the paragraph and write a postscript and give it in again. I went to Bertrancourt as usual. The rum ration that I had when I got back was very sparse for six but divided between two of us had a cosy appreciable effect. It was salvation after soaking our feet for days.

October 27 Friday
Breakfast: bacon. Dinner: stew and tea. No tea ration. It has been the wettest day and was particularly heavy in early morning. We return to Authie Wood via the baths at Couin in a full pack. I had a good hot shower but we were very

exposed to the cold wind and there was no change of clothing. We were left alone for rest of day, except for recreational fatigues and mud scraping. I'm in charge of No.9 Platoon. There are 36 men in one hut which is just comfortable. I got my application for R.E. (Royal Engineers) commission returned from Mr Leaman yesterday with the intimation that he would deal with it in about a fortnight. I had a good stiff rum ration last thing tonight and was very comfortable.

October 28 Saturday
Breakfast: bacon. Dinner: stew. Tea: jam. It has been a fine day but a wet evening. There is a change of trench consolidation party and we finished at 2.30pm as it is probable that we are the working party tonight. We are likely to go in the trenches on Monday, we are all told. I sent an FPC to Doll and then settled down to rubbing my feet and legs with anti-frost bite. I was called out for working party at 7.30pm and marched to the Hebuterne trenches which were eight miles away. The men were taking one pack to three shovels on way. The first surprisingly incompetent officer of the Royal Engineers that I have met, leads us to a very deep trench in shocking conditions. We are over the knees in glutinous mud and slush and he casually is telling us to spread out and clear it. It is an impossible task without scoops, buckets and scaffolding, entailing a throw of over 15 feet. We stood nine or less shivering in despair for four hours, then marched home again arriving at 7.30am. Going we had seven casualties from shell fire on the crossroads at Hebuterne, **one killed**[228], one dying. The net summary: 16 mile march, 4 hours starvation work, **2 dead**[229], 5 wounded. Average work about 1 shovel full per man as the picks are useless

October 29 Sunday
Breakfast: bacon. Dinner: stew and figs. Tea: jam and butter. We had a rum ration on our return and then we had partially cleaned up and breakfasted by 9.30am. We rested but there was no sleep till dinner. In the afternoon we were detailing working parties, drinking rum rations etc. I was paid 10 francs. We are going to the trenches tomorrow. I received a letter and parcel from Mother dated October 22nd and sent Mother an FPC.

October 30 Monday
Breakfast: bacon. Dinner: bully beef. Tea: jam. We were roused at 6.30am and were told to be ready to parade for the trenches at 7.30am. We had dreadful heavy, rolling blankets and packing valises to hand in and were putting up equipment. We all scramble to grab breakfast and bolt the same. We march straight across the country to Hebuterne trenches and arrive at 11.30am. We have a fine **elephant dugout**[230] in support. It was a fine morning but it poured

---

[228] **31342 Private Robert Henry Yelf** – killed in action on 28th October 1916 and he is buried in Hebuterne Military Cemetery.

[229] **38042 Private James Pownall** was also killed, dying from wounds on 29th October 1916. He also served with the Lancashire Fusiliers and is buried in Couin Military Cemetery.

[230] **Elephant dugouts** were normally built using a specially curved (rolled) heavy gauge corrugated iron sheet which when bolted together formed a large curved roof shelter. Grey, when viewed from a distance

in torrents in the afternoon and the trench was a river, flooded in places. I draw given lots; wherever you sit you wipe yourself on a muddy score. I lost .75 at Solo and had a comfortable night.

October 31 Tuesday
Breakfast: bacon. Dinner: bully beef. Tea: jam and butter. We were drawing stores from the RE dump in the morning and there was some lively shell fire. We paraded the men at 2.30pm from B Company's tea and drew the same at 4.30pm. As we got near the destination we got men stuck all over the place. I was busily engaged pulling them out leg after leg. B Company gets its tea at stand down but it was cold. One fellow got stuck again on the return journey and leaves his gun book which I make him retrieve. We got back about 9pm and I knock up tea and a rum ration. I received a letter from Doll October 24th which was dated 21st. It was a fine day and I had a comfortable night but my diabetes symptoms are very troublesome.

November 1 Wednesday
Breakfast: rissoles and bacon. Dinner: stew. Tea: jam and butter. I was detailing men for the ration parties and we move off at 1.45 am to relieve B Company in the front. We were under heavy shelling as we approach. I was posted on the entrance to the left of our position and the deep dugout is just a particularly muddy trench with a roof. The NCO went to sleep and I explore the trenches to the right of B Company, which was successful after much trouble. My gum boots are just long enough and the water and mud are up to my thighs. The tea arrives at 11pm and I get warned of it at 12 but I am too late. B Company have found a much better way. The rats are very audacious, one runs over my face with muddy feet which is very objectionable. I sit filling in this diary in the mud, slushed up to my eyes.

November 2 Thursday
Breakfast: bacon. Dinner: bully, tea, Oxo, potatoes. Tea: jam and butter. We rest during the day and we are on duty after stand to. It was a cold and frosty night, we were always going to send gas over but the conditions were never just right. C & B Company send fighting patrol over as usual – wash out. 10 minutes machine gun fire and rifle rapid ditto with heavy strafe. The Battalion Head Quarters are blown in with **2 killed**[231] and some wounded. We get a little rum ration at night.

---

they did not look unlike elephants and were often assembled above ground in rear areas before being dropped into holes or pushed up against banks and covered over to form dressing station or other larger shelters. A typical example could hold maybe twenty men but they could be bolted together to form much longer "tunnels". Most seem to have been about twelve feet long. They appeared on the Western Front from about 1916 onwards.

[231] **12/559 Lance Sergeant Thomas Harper Wood** and **12/889 Private Charles Frederick Chamberlain** were both killed. Wood is buried in Sailly-au-Bois Military Cemetery and Chamberlain in Hebuterne Military Cemetery.

November 3 Friday

No Breakfast – spare rations we have by. Dinner: bully. Tea: bacon. We are relieved in the morning and are given boots which are handed in before we leave for the front lines. We are over our thighs in mud and going out many fellows get stuck. There is a fleet of enemy aeroplanes having it their own way over Hebuterne and are going over, flying very low. I never saw the fellows so jiggered and it was mostly the new draft. We get to our billets about 3pm in Sailly which are a weather proof room in a Mairie but we are on a tile floor and it is very crowded. We are constantly being shelled with heavies all round and there are six killed[232] and one wounded in the billet just before we arrive. I lost 7 centimes at Solo this evening. I had very good night's sleep with an extra blanket as I am Corporal in charge of the billet.

November 4 Saturday

Breakfast: bacon. Dinner: stew. Tea: jam. We have been cleaning up all day and had an inspection in evening. I have just seen **two killed**[233] and two injured on road outside. There is an old woman with a bed-ridden man actually remaining in this place selling cakes, chocolate, milk and eggs, which I purchase. I am on a working party tonight at 6pm which was delayed at the start while stretcher parties attend to the casualties. **Cowen**[234] rushes off and loses connection and 3 Platoon who turn up after the delay. The farce of picks carried for mud pushing is repeated. It is pouring with rain and we cease work at midnight. Cowen rushes away as before with a following of four or five. The remainder of us go out another way and find Cowen and his party lost on the plain. He takes command and presently I notice we have faced about. Having lost us he loses himself and we take about one hour to find him. I then suggest a direction which proves correct. We march right in to rest of the battery and hear the fire order given, just in time to lie flat, so avoid a full blast. We get back to the billet at 3.30am. I received letters from Doll, October 28th and 30th and a paper from Colin. I am sludged up head to foot, so undress and have a sound sleep.

November 5 Sunday

Meals: ditto. The whole day is spent cleaning up shells which are falling at intervals very near to our billets. I lose about 1 franc in one hour's Solo. We fall in at 5.30pm from the working party again. There are about fifteen shrapnel shells which are put directly over one's head and the men bolt like rabbits. I find that I have only three of my party of twenty left when we have got down to our trenches. I ascertain where we were working and then return and am successful in finding my party. About ¾hr after our return we are sent back. B Company has disappeared under Captain Woolhouse and I find the messenger to my Company is lost with a link to C Company. I decide to manage it myself,

---

[232] **12/647 Acting Sergeant Major F. L. Faker** was one of those killed. He is commemorated on the Thiepval Memorial.

[233] **12/1668 Private George Henry Bramham** was killed in action on 4th November 1916, also killed was **16879 Private Charles Paling**, both are buried in Sailly au Bois Military Cemetery.

[234] **Captain J. C. Cowen** – was commissioned on 15th July 1915 and was Adjutant from December 1917.

so they work till 1.30am instead of midnight. On our return we meet a portion of B Company, who we guide back again. I eventually start to clear out at 2am and direct various remnants on the way. We get back alone to the billet through pouring rain at 4am and I am thoroughly done in. I had been on the working party in the trenches for nine hours. The rum ration and tea were very comforting.

November 6 Monday
Meals: ditto with the addition of pickle. The C Orderly Sergeant tells me that I am let off the working party tonight but eventually they are all cancelled as we are moving tomorrow. The Barnsleys are raiding tonight and there is to be some strafe on. I sleep till about 11am then we are cleaning up till tea time. Afterwards have a long night at Solo and I lose about 1½ francs. Only twelve of us are left in the billet, the rest taken out to cellar somewhere. We are to go in on our own should the Germans retaliate to our strafe. They send over no more than usual, so we remain as we are until 2am then go to sleep. I receive cigarettes from Arthur. It is a showery day and a bright clear night turning to rain next morning.

November 7 Tuesday
Meals: ditto, bacon very plentiful. We prepare for the morning off at 10.45am and march about one mile outside Sailly, then halt in the driving rain. We wait for some time, then to our impossible relief, we hear it's for the ration buses which turn up after 1½ hours delay. By a devious route we arrive at our billets in Thievres. The machine gun sections who dragged their own carts, arrive just before us. We are in a comfortable billet in barn but it is very crowded. I received a letter from Mother, November 1st and won 1.80 francs at Solo.

November 8 Wednesday
Meals: ditto. It has been a wet day. I have been cleaning up and had an inspection. I received a letter from Doll, November 4th and wrote and handed in a letter to Doll and sent an FPC to Doll and Mother. I had three eggs, petite beurre and cafe au lait for supper.

November 9 Thursday
Breakfast: bacon. Dinner: rissoles, potatoes & pickles. Tea: jam & butter, ¼ of a loaf. We had parades from 9.15am till 12.30pm and various drills from 2pm to 3.30pm and then bayonet drill and instruction. It was a fine day and I won three francs at Solo. I went to Famechon for eggs and chips. The chips were off so I returned to Thievres and had three eggs, bread and two coffees.

November 10 Friday
Meals - Breakfast: bacon. Dinner: stew. Tea: stewed dates and raisins. We had bayonets, physical and company duties from 9am till 12.30pm and a route march from 2pm to 4.45pm, in which our gallant officers get completely lost three miles from our billets. I won about five francs at Solo. It has been a fine day.

November 11 Saturday

Meals - Breakfast: bacon. Diner: stew & pickles. Tea: jam and butter. We parade at 8.30am and have a Battalion drill under the Colonel all morning till 12.30pm. The Colonel is a tartar. We paraded again at 1.30pm and have bayonet fighting and are back at 3.30pm. The night positions are in order but are cancelled as we move tomorrow. I gave Mr Leaman my application for permission to apply for a commission in RE again. He shilly-shallied again and said trampers were not allowed, he had already spoken to adjutant. I must see Ward myself soon. I walked to Famechon in the evening for eggs and chips again. Chips were off but I had three eggs and coffee. I received a parcel and a letter from Doll, apparently a tin of sludge, which was postmarked November 1st. I identified a bunch of grapes by their stalks, the tomatoes a bit by their colour and the rotten pears were just recognisable. I salvaged from bottom two stale sausage rolls and most of a cake, all with a strong winey flavour. We are all worried to death by the Colonel and officers' rare smartness of clothes and polish, boots buttons etc. and all of our spare time is preoccupied with the same as we are continually getting sludged up to neck. We had a rum ration and cake goes well with it. I had a good sleep and the weather continues fine. The prospects for an advance are looking up.

November 12 Sunday

Meals - Breakfast: bacon. Dinner: stew. Tea: jam and butter. I spend the morning cleaning and packing up for the move as usual on a Sunday. We fall in 1.10 pm and arrive at old hut which is an encampment in Warnimont Wood. We are near to Authie soon after 3pm. There is more mud than ever and as usual No.9 Platoon are on bare ground and the remainder have wire beds. We can hear the heavy bombardment which continues all day. The weather is damp but fine. I must ask Doll to send another diary. *I thought that the war would have been over by the time I finished this.*
> *(He then begins a new diary which is a small note book.)*

November 13 Monday

Breakfast: bacon. Dinner: stew. Tea: Hartley's blackberry and apple jelly. I slept in my boots and puttees last night as the push was coming off this morning. We hear that right and left of Serre has been successful and the 3rd Division on Serre was a failure but this was heavily bombarded all day and they are expected to be evacuated today. They close the order and we have an extended ditto drill all morning from 9.30am – 12 noon and then from 2pm to 3.30pm we then had bayonet fighting and a battle order. We then had quick preparation for an inspection. **Jowett**[235] went on leave this morning to get married. No one allowed out of camp not even to YMCA. We are in the trenches tomorrow. No letters accepted although I have one to Mother and AA ready, also FPC for Doll. I lost 9 Francs at Solo.

---

[235] **31632/ Private A Jowett:** Sanitary Man, also served in 3/5 North Staffs and 13 Y&L.

November 14 Tuesday

Breakfast: bacon. Dinner: stewed beef, potatoes. Tea: jam and bread. We were up at 5am and paraded for the trenches and at 6.30am were relieved by the West Lancs. I am Corporal of the guard at the entrance and follow the line to Hebuterne. I am on guard from a corrugated tin hut which gives very little protection, even from shrapnel. The Germans drop heavily round us and are very close with **Taube**[236] very close hovering us over all afternoon. There was almost a constant string of East Yorks that were wounded and being carried out. They took the second and third lines and had to abandon the same at 4pm yesterday owing to intense fire, so the advance on Serre had failed. The dugout in Cateau was blown in and ten were killed. We are bringing them to the cemetery here to bury. I gave **Miles**[237] an FPC for Doll en route. We had **3 killed**[238] and 2 wounded almost as soon as we got in who were blown up while dinner was served in Givenchy. I made a fire in the brazier in the tin hut which was very smoky and I had to periodically revive it, while we recovered. I had frequent and copious doses of water and pinched a **sleep skin**[239] from the stock by the Guard Room. It has been fine but foggy.

November 15 Wednesday

Breakfast: bacon. Dinner: stewed half potatoes, baked beans. Tea: butter and jam. It has been a very cold morning and a fine and dull day with fog. We hear that the Germans pinched a Lewis gun from the East Lancs on the left, during the night. The afternoon turned out bright and frosty. We were relieved at dinner time and paraded at 5pm to relieve B Company, who have only been in front line for a day but we are to prepare for a stunt. We are put in old Serre's end fusilier the old dug out has been blown in and the original post is very exposed now and unsafe. The Germans have it well marked and we have to remain in the open bay, nearly up to our knees in mud. I make a bit of a shelter at one end. The night is very cold, turning frosty in morning but with no rain.

November 16 Thursday

Breakfast: cold bacon. Dinner: Cold beef, pickles, cheese. Tea: jam and butter. There were no dugouts available for a rest during the day time. I catch a fitful sleep on the fire-step for an hour or so in the morning and have mud in the bay cleared. We are relieved after tea and get the best dugout in the neighbourhood with a brazier. We crowd in twelve where four could fit comfortably. I slept fairly well in instalments, in a half upright position. The Germans shelled along Serre pretty hard during the day. The day has been bright and frosty.

---

[236] **Taube** – Germany's first practical military aircraft, **the Taube**, meaning Dove, was used for virtually all military aircraft action including fighter, bomber and surveillance applications.

[237] **12/731 Corporal A. B. Miles** - also served with 2nd Y&L and was commissioned to Lancashire Fusiliers on 28th May 1918.

[238] **19224 Private Henry Martin** and **38034 Private J. Millership** were both killed in action and are buried in Sailly au Bois Military Cemetery **31558 Private John Barlow** and **12/100 William Edgar Ford** both died from their wounds the following dayand are buried in Sailly au Bois Military Cemetery.

[239] **Sleep skin** – It is possible that this was a WW1 sleeping bag. They were sometimes referred to as 'blanket bags' at the time. Officers could, and did, have any kit they liked as it was privately purchased. Such blanket bags were available well before the Great War.

November 17 Friday

Breakfast: cold bacon. Dinner: bully and cheese. Tea: three dates and two chestnuts. We have reduced rations but they have improved while in support to ½ loaf per man. We touched lucky for rations and chased in our usual rations for twelve and then afterwards drew a share in Corporal's rations. I received a letter from Auntie Annie dated November 12th and stood to at 5.45pm. We had a rum ration and a sip apiece. After breakfast the men were turned out of our comfy dugout for a unit to make room for the machine gunners. I get them started and then we all squeeze in again and I fill in this diary for last few days. The Germans are shelling around us pretty hard and an aeroplane comes down in pieces over the German lines, which side I don't know. We hear a rumour that the B Company stunt is off, if so as they will have trenched for only in one day. No.9 Platoon are in the advance trench tonight. It is a very frosty last night and has been a bright, cold day. I continue with this diary under the most miserable conditions I have yet experienced, i.e. if my fingers consent to write. We returned to cosy dug out about 1pm turning the machine gunners out and make the most appetising dish by frying together Bully, cheese and onion. We use up all of the remaining water available and are making tea. The brazier also proved very handy last night and this morning, in warming up our tea ration. B Company are very lax in supplying us with rations and there is no water available in the line. I spent the afternoon thoroughly rubbing into feet and legs whale oil and anti frost bite. I then have tea with tea, bacon, pickles which I have found in a blouse in dugout and some dates. Nine others and I share remaining three Corporal's rations, as some has not been claimed. We fall in at 4.45pm to proceed to the advance post and are told that we are in for 24hrs (damn). We are in rottenest of the lot with no fire-step and no shelter whatsoever. I curse Ellison who has posted us here. He poor fellow is almost beyond same I hear later, with shrapnel in his back and shin and he has also had a thumb off. The night is very cold and frosty. I suck ice that has been broken off from a muddy shell hole. Our artillery strafe the Bosche in front of us very hard. All my men are conscripts and seem absolutely daft - don't just blast them.

November 18 Saturday

Our rum ration is inadequate as usual and was brought to us 2pm. Our rations arrive at 4am and there is no provision for dinner or breakfast. There are three tins of army meat and veg between seven and two loaves and one tea and jam for all. It is the idea of the Quarter Master evidently, luckily we are relieved in the morning. We have to stay here till dusk tonight as the communication trench is impassable and the only way out is by is going over the top. The rain and thaw sets in about 5am and I gather more ice to thaw into my billy can. The Bosches in front of us are heavily strafed at about 6am and then the most infernal bombardment opens on the right. I wonder if it is another attack on Serre as it is the most intense that I have yet witnessed. Tea had arrived previously that was icy cold, so we save it till after breakfast. I pour muddy ice water into the same and save it for later consumption. The Bosches have been heavily firing on our right all day, perhaps we have occupied Serre or the trenches in that direction again? They also don't forget us and rifle grenades are very frequent and close. It has been raining almost all day and I catch fitful naps under a groundsheet and am thankful for the fur coat that I've pinched. I send a guide over the top at dusk to go and bring relief. He does not **return**[240] with same who lose themselves, so we get relieved about one hour after everyone else at 6.30am. It is an awful business getting out over top, I was tumbling over barbed wire and into shell holes and I rolled over in the mud twice. Everyone had gone when we got back to our Headquarters. I went out by Serre Road and came under some pretty hot machine gun fire at the Hebuterne end. I was absolutely jiggered and rested for several times on the road and stopped to change my gum boots. I had to enquire in Sailly when the Battalion were last in the vale. The East Lancs cooks gave me a cup of tea and I got down eventually in wretched sandbag huts with six men where two might exist. After all we were here an hour or two before the rest of the Company, who had been brought out by **Jena**[241] and over the plain. We had tea and stew on arrival.

November 19 Sunday
Breakfast: bacon. Dinner: Roast beef (bone), soup, boiled beans. Tea: jam and butter, 1/3 loaf. We were cleaning up all day and I was paid 20 francs. I received a letter from Mother dated November 10th and she hasn't received my letters since the middle of October. I received a paper from Colin and visited the canteen for stout, chocolate, biscuits and candles. No letters or PCs were collected again. It is fine but fearfully muddy.

November 20 Monday
Breakfast: cold bacon. Dinner: stew and rice pudding. Tea: jam and butter. We have been cleaning up all day again except for ½ hour in morning when we had inspection and physical. We paraded for the baths at 3.45pm which was off as the water pipe is burst. Our letters are off and C Company collected them but only two each letters are allowed, they are the first to be collected since we left Warnimont Wood. I handed in letters to Doll and Mother and FPCs to each ditto. I take poor old **Johnson**[242] up to see Leaman about the leave that he had applied for as his two children have died within a few days of each other. We have no satisfaction. The weather has been fine.

November 21 Tuesday
Breakfast: bacon. Dinner: bread and cheese. Tea: stew, jam and butter. We roused at 6am to hear that we are to move to Courcelles at 8am. There was the usual commotion rolling blankets and packing up. We march to Courcelles and report at the RC dump and are then sent to Colincamp sidings with a full pack as a working party, unloading ballast off trucks. We are finished before 12 noon

---

[240] **38036 Private James Mulchrist** did not return and he died on 17th November 1916 and I commemorated on the Thiepval Memorial.

[241] **Jena** – a town near to Hebuterne and Serre.

[242] **Private 31631 T Johnson** also served in 3/5 North Staffs and 13 Y&L.

and have lunch and then march back to our bivouacs. I nearly pull a corn stack to pieces for straw. Being only two at our end we make ourselves very cosy with two blankets a piece. The adjutant sends for me. A Sergeant and eighty NCO men are wanted from the Battalion for a Brigade Support Company. He is therefore making me Company Acting Lance Lieutenant unpaid, while with the detachment, which will probably be for four or five weeks and I am to report Sailly at 10am next morning. I sew Sergeant stripes over the Corporal stripes accordingly. There is a nasty shock for the Battalion to hear that they are to go into the trenches again in the morning, it is only four days since they came out and were put in those wretched dugouts. I select Johnson T, as one of my party. It has been a fine day.

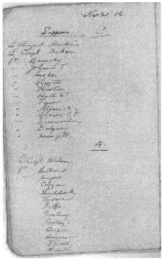

Extracts taken from Frank's notebook giving the names of those in Platoons A & C on 21ˢᵗ November 1916

<u>Sappers</u>
<u>C</u>   <u>A</u>
L Sergeant	Meakin		
L Corpl	Askew	L Corpl	Wilson
Pte	Barnby	Pte	Holland
Pte	Johnson T	Pte	Hague
Pte	Cook	Pte	Coggan
Pte	Clayton	Pte	Haddock
Pte	Hooton	Pte	Howson
Pte	Hall S T	Pte	Jeffs
Pte	Tyson	Pte	Gosling
Pte	Moore A	Pte	Golby
Pte	Clarke C F	Pte	Cooper
Pte	Simmonds	Pte	Harrison
Pte	Dodgson	Pte	Hall
Pte	Horsfall	Pte	Smith

November 22 Wednesday

Breakfast: bacon. Dinner: bully. In orders we are rationed until 24th but can only obtain tin of bully beef and biscuits. My party are generally the most wretched collection of conscripts I've ever set eyes on. We parade late so make them leg it to make up. There is much groaning and grumbling and there are cries for a rest after twenty minutes. I give them five minutes eventually. **McCran**[243], the pioneer officer to whom we report, turns out one of the best and fires us up in the billets very comfortably in Sailly. *He then tells me that I am the Acting Sergeant Major* over the whole Brigade Company and will billet at the Headquarters, so no more trenches for me, or very little. I get a comfortable wire bed next to the Officers one. I report the shortage of rations and he then gets ample rations from the Brigade in time for tea and also the dinner for men. I'm kept busy but the men are only on small unloading fatigues. I appoint Johnson T as my orderly and he makes himself wonderfully useful, especially at carving a quarter of beef with an axe and saw that he finds, he is very attentive to me. McCran's servant goes on leave, so I give him a letter to Doll to post in England with the good news. We hear that leave will be granted to one Company and I'm to get out a list of the men who went to Egypt and also the other soldiers with twelve months **FS**[244] and no leave. I put in a word for Johnson. McCran gets blankets for the men sent from Battalion and McCran's servant lends me his two, sewn together to form a bag. I have a restless night which is very chilly with much water. It has been a fine day and a frosty night. Those poor devils in the front line...

November 23 Thursday

Breakfast: fried ham ad lib, bought 2 fried eggs, porridge, bread, butter and jam, buttered toast. Dinner: steak, mashed, beans in gravy, which were all lovely with tinned peaches and tea ad lib. Tea: Honey and butter. Supper: Steak ad lib with pickles, stewed figs and custard and tea. This is like living at the Savoy in ordinary times by contrast. Johnson has a cup of tea for me before I get up - this is absolutely the fat of the land. I handed in a letter to the A.A. with my new address. I have a busy day again making lists and detailing guards and working parties, but I'm happy. The men are only working a four hour night shift and the Barnsleys are only just out of the trenches and still resting. My letters are handed in with the usual instruction and censored and sent to the Brigade on the same night, what a contrast to our officers who take a fortnight to gaze at them, on the rare occasions when they are accepted. The after midnight working party are not yet back, they were expected at 10.30pm and returned at 2am. It has been a fine day.

---

[243] **McCran** – The Pioneer Officer.

[244] **FS** – Full service.

November 24 Friday
Breakfast: early cup of tea in bed then bacon and eggs. Dinner: first rate seasoned stew, stewed figs, rice and custard. Tea: honey and blackcurrant jam. Supper: steak and pickles, fried onions and potatoes, figs and custard. It has been a busy day taking indents for clothing. It was a frosty morning and then thawed. The leave starts with men from the East Lancs. A cook was sent to us from ditto.

November 25 Saturday
Breakfast: bacon and fried bread. Dinner: steak pudding, suet dumplings with jam and Ideal milk. Tea: jam and honey. Supper: stewed beef, potatoes and onions, tinned peaches and custard. I have had a busy morning. I couldn't get breakfast till 10.30am and we were then clearing up in the afternoon, which was rather slack. I got to bed before ten but was up about four times to water. We received a few parcels and letters for the Barnsleys but nothing has turned up for us yet. It has been a very wet day. There were no working parties tonight and we start day work tomorrow.

November 26 Sunday
Breakfast: porridge, bacon, toast. Dinner: stew and mashed, also cold beef, figs and custard. Tea: cold beef, jam. Supper: roast Beef, cabbage, mashed potato, fig duff pudding. Tea was available all day. I was up at 5am to see off the working party at 6am but it was wet, so there were no working parties all day. We hear the one man each from 12th and 13th Battalions are to go on leave. I received letters from Doll dated November 16th and 19th and a letter from Mother dated November 18th and a letter from Arthur of November 23rd.

November 27 Monday
Breakfast: bacon and eggs. Dinner: hotted up beef and cold mashed, rice and custard. Tea: jam. Supper: currie and mashed potatoes. It has been an easy day. I went to see **Jimmy Wood**[245] at BHQ, where he gave me half a glass of whiskey to celebrate my promotion. I received a letter from Jimmy Hill of November 16th. It has been a busy evening detailing working parties and a fine day.

November 28 Tuesday
Breakfast: bacon and eggs. Dinner: Maconochies, potatoes, rice and custard. Tea: dripping, toast and jam. Supper: tinned salmon, roast beef, potatoes, cabbage, pineapple fritters. I was up early in morning seeing the men off. I went to the baths and had a hot shower all to myself with clean changes. I did some clerical work in the afternoon, followed by three hours detailing men and having a 'frightening out of wits' parade in the evening. It has been a fine day

---

[245] **12/828 Corporal J. S. Wood** – took part in the attack on 1st July 1916 and was a member of C Company.

142

November 29 Wednesday

Breakfast: bacon. Dinner: Maconochies, mashed carrots, cold beef, pickled walnuts. Tea: dripping, toast and jam. Supper: roast beef, cabbage and mashed, boiled jam roll. I was up early seeing men off. I cursed the East Lancs to eternity as they reported **Watson**[246] for inefficiency. I did some clerical work and had general slackness during the day. The weather has been fine and slightly frosty and I received a letter from Doll of November 22nd. I was busy from 7.30pm to 10pm detailing the morning parade.

November 30 Thursday

Breakfast: bacon and porridge. Dinner: stew and cold beef, cabbage and mashed. Tea: dripping, toast and honey. Supper: roast beef, cabbage, mashed potato, stewed figs. I was up at 6am rushing around detailing and altering last night's work for an additional sand party. I reposted two men for dodging and one is to be returned to the Battalion. I visited Corporal Wood at BHQ, who gave me a delightful glass of whiskey and I bought a packet of Quaker Oats from him for my breakfast. I also visited the Battalion in the Dell (i.e. Sailly Dell) and they all seem to have heard that I'm the Sergeant Major. I wrote to Mother and handed it in. I found a hive in the garden containing some of the purest honey. I managed to get some rum off of **Parker**.[247] The Bosches are dropping considerable heavy strafe around us at bed time. It has been a fine and frosty day.

December 1 Friday

Breakfast: porridge and bacon. Dinner: cold beef, pickles and mashed. Supper: Soup, currie, mashed potato, figs and custard. I was told last night that but for a rifle inspection, that it would be a holiday today. At 9.15am we had to parade every available man for the trench parties. I received a parcel and letter from Doll dated November 22nd and it has been a fine day but foggy and frosty in the evening.

December 2 Saturday

Breakfast: porridge, bacon, fried potato cake. Dinner: stew, stewed figs. Tea: pork pie (Doll's), dripping, toast, jam. Supper: Fried beef, thick gravy and mashed. This morning, all available men are for the trench working parties. Three men go on leave. I wrote to Arthur and handed it in and wrote to Doll and gave the letter to **Askew**[248] to post. I hear that **Sergeant Brooke**[249] of 12th Yorks and Lancs has been to see McCran asking if he can join our Company.

---

[246] **23165 Private J. Watson** – also served in 13th Y&L.

[247] **12/744 Private R. Parker** took part in the attack on 1st July 1916 and is brother of **12/743 Private John William Parker** who was killed in action on 1st July 1916 and is buried in Queens Military Cemetery, Serre.

[248] **12/578 Corporal Herbert Askew** Died of wounds on 25th October 1918 whilst with 7th Y&L. He is buried in Awoingt Military Cemetery.

[249] **12/317 Sergeant Brooke** Served with the Battalion on 1st July 1916 and received Commission for West Yorks Regiment on 30th October 1917.

He is after my job I suspect and seems to be a friend of **Evans.**[250] At Evan's suggestion have to prepare an absurd crime sheet for tomorrow, which is a list of unshaved and duty rifles from yesterday's parade and two men and **Corporal Taylor**[251] are to be sent back to the Battalion after orderly room tonight. It has been frosty all day.

December 3 Sunday
Breakfast: Quaker Oats and bacon. Dinner: roast beef and mashed, sago pudding. Tea: dripping, toast, jam. Supper: soup, steak and kidney pudding, mashed, cabbage, pineapple and apple fritters, pancake. There was no working party but we parade in the morning. I was paid 30 francs and sent a letter to Arthur. The weather is thawing.

December 4 Monday
Breakfast: bacon, egg, Quaker Oats. Dinner: steak and cabbage, mashed. Tea: dripping, toast. Supper: steak, carrots, soup, plum pudding, sardines on toast. I received a letter from Doll and Mother of November 25th and 24th respectively. I visited the Battalion found a big pile of letters still uncensored and rescued letters to Mother and Doll of November 12th and 15th. I handed the same in here and also sent a letter to Auntie Annie. I had a nasty blow this evening. Sergeant Brooke who came here cadging my job, has got it and I return to the Battalion tomorrow.

December 5 Tuesday
Breakfast: Quaker Oats, bacon, toast. Dinner: stew. Tea: dripping, toast and Jam. Supper: cold steak and onions. McCran said that he had hoped to keep me as well and still hoped to have me back again soon. I handed over to the cad Brookes in morning and told him that he had done the dirty on me and was near civil. He admitted asking for the job and appeared to be too ignorant to appreciate his actions. McCran told me not to go till the afternoon. I left at about 6.30pm to join my Company in Fellow Line Trench, reported and told the Adjutant and Captain Leaman of Brooke's underhanded practice. I gave in letters to Doll, Arthur, Auntie Annie and cash in some insurance cards before leaving. It has been a wet morning and a fine afternoon. I am transferred to No. 11 Platoon while I am in the trenches. Brookes was sent to trenches right away at 3pm and he would get back about 11pm. My short wish for him is a speedy Blighty, like having missed pre-permanent too! As I expected, Leaman asks me if the job was too big for me. I expect that I shall have to give up my stripe and am uncertain whether at the present I'm Sergeant or Corporal. I find my capes and this how Sergeants now so look.

---

[250] **12/912 Sergeant C. C. Evans** – he took part in the attack on 1st July 1916.
[251] **12/1997 Corporal E. Taylor**, served with the Battalion on1st July 1916.

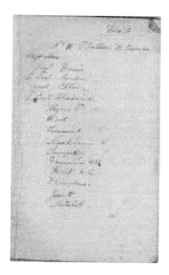

Extracts taken from Frank's notebook giving the names of those in No 11 Platoon in the trenches

Sergt	Davis
L Sergt	Meakin
Corpl	Ellis
L Corpl	Chadwick
	Myers P.
	West
	Bestwick
	Neadham
	Timperly
	Greenwood W.H.
	Holt S. C.
	Flunders
	Jowitt
	Mitchell

December 6 Wednesday

Breakfast: bacon. Dinner: soup, rice pudding. Tea: butter. I supplemented the meals with a huge slab of cold beef steak that I bought and also apple jelly. I was an easy day. I superintended a working party for about two hours in the morning. I then took tea and a water ration party down to the Fusiliers and return and took them to fetch water from a well half a mile away with a crazy windlass which required refining every two turns. I filled two diners and eighteen two-gallon petrol cans, by means of jars and a tin with a hole in the bottom as there was no suitable dish. We discovered the East Yorks canteen down a dark cellar which was very reasonable. A soup kitchen has also been started since I was here last. Any solider can obtain soup, tea or cocoa here.

Whittaker's[252] brother in **RAMC**[253] discovered me and says that Whittaker wants to hear of me. It has been a fine day but raw and dampish. We go in to the front line tomorrow after all.

December 7 Thursday

- Breakfast: bacon. Dinner: stew and rice pudding. Tea: jam and butter. I had a good night's rest and no duties all day so I slept and dozed the morning through. I rubbed feet before going to sleep last night and also this afternoon with whale oil. The latest injustice is if so many in the platoon get **trench foot**[254] the platoon have us stopped, if more, the Company or whole Battalion, besides the individual gets a Court Martial. We were left of the Yellow Line for the front at 5pm and found the posts improved beyond recognition, ours is quite cosy in fact. I was wiring with my workers all night.

December 8 Friday

Breakfast: stew brought down in thermos. Dinner: cold bacon. Tea: strawberry jam and margarine. What a difference in the morning, set in for a wet day. The cosy shelter leaks like a sieve and now contains six where three were just comfortable before. I take the usual refuge under my ground sheet. The weather clears up in the evening and we are relived about 5.45pm, just as the **Bosche**[255] strafe CHQ. Some fellows wanted to shelter in No. 2 post but I had them out and a little later the whole post got laid with shrapnel. We get it pretty hot though and take to the trench again. In a few of the bays before reaching the lines, three shrapnel bullets almost shave me and embed themselves in the parados by my face. Our old cosy dugout with brazier is vacant. The men have to be in post all night but I have the fire going with some coke we bought. Then one man at a time whale rubs his feet and this fills up the entire night, thus enabling me to remain in comfort - while I ask that they do it.

December 9 Saturday

Breakfast: cold bacon and tea or soup. Dinner: stew. Tea: strawberry jam and margarine. Raining again all day, our dugout gradually floods, fuel only enough to just warm up food. It has been another miserable day awaiting relief. We were relieved about 5.15pm and march out with our gumboots off and proceed straight to Sailly where we give the same in. We fall out for valise at the Pioneer HQ but find I have enough to carry without it. A portion of the contents are; trousers, puttees, towel, vest and pants. I receive a parcel and letter from

---

[252] **12/265 Private George W. Whittaker** – wounded on 16th May 1916 and died of wounds on 2nd December 1916 serving with 13th York and Lancaster.

[253] **RAMC** – Royal Army Medical Corps.

[254] **Trench foot** is a medical condition caused by prolonged exposure of the feet to damp, unsanitary, and cold conditions and occurs when feet are cold and damp while wearing constricting footwear. If left untreated, it results in gangrene and possible amputation. It was easily prevented by keeping the feet warm and dry and changing socks frequently. Soldiers often wrote home asking for more socks and were provided with whale grease and told to apply it to their feet to make the feet waterproof. This often made the condition worse as it made the feet perspire and absorb even more water. The most effective preventive measure was regular foot inspections by officers.

[255] **Bosche** – the Germans.

Doll, November 29th and parcel from A.A. I also receive letters from Doll of November 28th and December 2nd and from Mother of December 3rd. The cook gives me tea and a good supper of roast beef, mashed and tinned French beans. We set off about 8.30pm for a march to Rossingnol Farm near Coigneux which is large enough to billet two Battalions. Our quarters are a big barn fitted with wire beds. I find Jimmy Wood who is another comrade in distress. He has had a final flare up with **Berry**[256] and has left the BHQ.

December 10 Sunday
Breakfast: bacon. Dinner: stew and rice pudding. Tea: jam and margarine. We have been cleaning up and had a red tape inspection. It has been a very wet day and my worn out boots sop up mud like a sponge. I am feeling pretty miserable. We are to parade at 8.30 with uniforms all cleaned up. I receive a parcel from Doll which is all smashed up in spite of a wooden box and calico and it contains a cake and mince pies in crumbs, some chicken and a tin of salmon. I also received a parcel from A.A. which contained a tinned almond cake, ten eggs, a ration bag, tea and a soup square. I send off PCs to Doll and Mother.

December 11 Monday
Breakfast: bacon. Dinner: stew. Tea: jam and margarine. It has been a fine and cold morning and was then wet for the rest of the day. We parade from 8.30am till 12 noon and then have a close order and bayonet drill. Captain Leaman had me out practising a communication drill. I've reverted to Corporal again as all the promotions were made while I was away. I am absolutely fed up. I was superintending draining for an hour in the afternoon and get a pass for Sailly in the evening to fetch my valise. There was not enough time to stop for dinner but I managed to get a sandwich. I sent an FPC to the A.A. and received a letter from Doll of December 7[th,] who has had no letter from me yet. I got pair of new boots, thank goodness.

December 12 Tuesday
Breakfast: bacon. Dinner: soup, boiled beef, rice pudding. Tea: jam and butter. It has been snowing all day and all parades are cancelled. We were cleaning up, as we had a kit inspection in the afternoon. I felt very fed up. **Herbert Hall, Blacktin**[257] and I went to Coigneux in the evening. Hall and I shared a bottle of champagne and a bottle of white wine, which were 5 francs and 3 francs respectively. Blacktin had one glass out of the former. It was absolutely rotten champagne but it rebuilt my spirits. Hall goes on leave on Thursday and has a glut of parcels with which I assist.

---

[256] **Lieutenant R. D. Berry** – killed in action on 12th May 1917, he is buried in Albuera Military Cemetery, Bailleul.
[257] **12/596 Private S. C. Blacktin** a member of C Company.

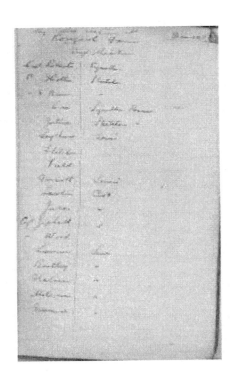

Extracts taken from Frank's notebook giving the names of those in his billet at Rossingol Farm on 10th December 1916

Sergeant Meakin	
Captain Roberts	Signaller
Pte Hollis	Stretcher
Pte S. Brown	Stretcher
Pte Cox	Signaller Rescue
Pte Jutson	Stretcher Rescue
Sergt Thorne	Lewis
Fletcher	Lewis
Field	Lewis
Garratt	Lewis
Lawton	Cook
Jukes	Cook
Cpl Jephcott	Cook
Cpl Wood	Cook
Cpl Lamin	Lewis
Cpl Bentley	Lewis
Cpl Gladman	Lewis
Cpl Mileman	Lewis
Cpl Greenwich	Lewis

December 13 Wednesday
Breakfast: bacon. Dinner: stew. Tea: blackcurrant jam and butter. Parade 9 – 12. We have a close order drill and Sweedish and bayonet all the time and I am absolutely fed up. We then had trench digging nearby in the evening. I had a pass to go into Couin in the evening and went to see 'Pop Offs,' which was very good and had fried eggs and coffee after. I received the 'Passing Show', the Christmas number from Colin.

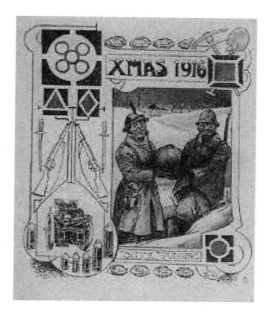

Passing Show Magazine, Christmas Edition 1916

December 14 Thursday
Breakfast: bacon. Dinner: stew and rice pudding. Tea: jam and butter. We parade at 8am and then have trench digging for water pipes and worked till 12 noon then from 2pm – 4pm. I managed most of a letter to Doll while ganging. It has been a fine day with a wet evening. We had a Battalion concert in billet, the result of which was broken beds.

December 15 Friday
Breakfast: bacon. Dinner: stew. Tea: figs. The Battalion marches for about 9 miles in either fine rain or drizzle followed by a foot inspection in the afternoon. I hand in a green envelope for Doll and also enclose letters to Mother, Aunt Clara and Tony. I have also sent Happy Xmas FPCs to Messrs Meakin, Mr and Mrs R Meakin, John Edward, Auntie Annie, Frank Lavin, F. E. P. Edwards, Teddy and J B Mason. I went to Couin in the evening only to find no one there, so had a drink, some eggs and coffee.

December 16 Saturday

Breakfast: bacon and beans. Dinner: mutton, carrots, onions and beans. Tea: jam. We had a parade from 9am – 12.30pm and were then trenching for water pipes again. I went to the Battalion in the afternoon and sent Happy Xmas FPCs to Kniveton, Widdow, Frank Wright and Mr Shand. I went to see the Whiz Bangs at Souastre in the evening, which was an altogether delightful entertainment and was better than most that I have seen at home. I got back to hear that we are to leave for the trenches at 8am in the morning, so sit up late sorting out and packing up. I received an unreasonable, jealous and peevish letter from Doll dated December 10th. She expects me to write love letters for young sobs to read. She makes no allowance for any letters which may have gone astray including two especially nice ones, in which I let myself go and opened out. I should have written some bitter things, had I replied on the spot. I received also a packet of eggs from Auntie Annie.

December 17 Sunday

Breakfast: bacon. Dinner: bully beef and beans. Tea: blackberry jam and butter and stewed figs. We left for the trenches at 8.30am and we marched all the way without a rest and drew the usual wet gum boots at Sailly. We were taken through the trenches up to our knees with ordinary boots which was quite unnecessary, then we went back again with our feet soaking. We were put in the most wretched dugouts that I've experienced and then fetched out to something less secure but much more cosy. I have a frame bed and change my boots and dry my socks at the brazier. We are in the **supports**[258] near to Hebuterne village and we are to take soup to the firing line at 8pm. We arrive at HQ at almost 8.45pm to find the front line garrison having evacuated for strafe which we had passed through at starting out. **CSM Everatt**[259] insists on the soup going to the front, all the same but as the men have just had their tea, they are not ready for soup. The men hang about till 9.45pm and they are then told to evacuate again at 10.45pm, meanwhile I am to take the soup all along the line. The men all declare that they don't want any as they have wind of casualties in No 6. I remonstrate with the CSM but to no avail so follow the garrison. My party are tumbling all over the place as it is fearfully slippery with gum boots. I miss the way and find myself among the Barnsleys, so carry on to the end and all the way back myself, just meeting the garrison returning. I fall full length twice in same shell hole and am staggering and muddy head to foot. I return to our HQ to find only a few pints left, then have to beg the men to have it but they won't come out of their dugouts for it. I get back to my own dugout at 12.30 midnight and make buttered toast and then have a very comfortable night's sleep with a good fire.

---

[258] **Supports** – support trench.

[259] **Company Sergeant Major T. Everatt** – a Sheffield University student. He took part in the attack on 1st July 1916 and was commissioned to Y&L on 29th May 1917.

December 18 Monday

Breakfast: cold bacon, boiled. Dinner: stew. Tea: stewed figs and currants ad lib. I am on Headquarters guard at 11am so have to clear out of my comfortable quarter for a half finished mucky crowded deep dugout. B Company has wangled it yet again, so we are set out to relieve them at 5.15pm. I'm in charge of No 6 fire line end of Serre's which has been abandoned all day by B Company as untenable. One end is blown in but then it is alright. We dug out the rubbish down to the trench boards and make it fairly decent. We are ordered to evacuate twice back to the Fusiliers. This and patrols to adjoining posts and drawing soup and tea make the night pass very nicely.

December 19 Tuesday

Breakfast: cold rissoles. Dinner: stew. Tea: jam and margarine. We get a fire going and so warm up our food. There is no water so I am thirsty all day and doze for most of the morning. We are shelled by trench mortar pretty freely. The adjoining traverse is blown in which drives the water back into our post, so I bale out again. The Germans are getting very tame and I suspect them to feed out of the hand soon. At 4pm about thirty of us walked over the top from their front line and back up the full side apparently to get our tea. They must be able to see us too, as the blown up trench leaves us half exposed. Here we are actually on each side spending thousands of pounds over killing each man, when we soldiers could get the same result for 2d. The Germans drop new incendiary shells in our trench which burns fiercely for hours. We are relieved at about 6.30pm and return to the Fusilier A post which is the most wretched situation trench where we are up to our knees in slush and have only The shelter steps a of blind dugout which are a foot to 18" deep in thick mud. I crushed a steel helmet in the same and sit in the pit and starve. There is no water and we fall back on frozen shell holes again. There is slight snow and a thaw in the morning, then a frosty afternoon and a frosty night.

December 20 Wednesday

It was a beautiful, bright, frosty morning and we had small rum rations. I was told at 7.30am that I and three others are to visit the Battalion Orderly Room at 9am with everything. I had delightful conjectures, is it leave or a cushy job? I find that it is only to look after the new draft of billets etc. There is no time for breakfast and I am fed with a few bits of boiled bacon and bolt a mouthful of bread. Following the example of the Germans, we go out over the top and up Serre Rd in broad daylight and there were no shots. I walked to Coigneux with **Mr Crawford**[260] and get some coffee, biscuits and chocolate at canteen. Jimmy Wood at the HQ gives us a fine dinner which is a lovely stew and rice pudding. I went back to Sailly with Charlesworth and arranged billets and helped to unload the stores and acted as Director to returning C Company who are coming out in the evening. I got some tea and nibbled some biscuits and cheese and then went up to Pioneer HQ at night and got candles and some dinner which

---

[260] **Captain S. Crawford** – Commissioned on 26th September 1916 and served in 12th Y&L from 25th November 1916 and also served with 7th Y&L.

was boeuf sauté with mashed and tinned French beans and plum pudding and sauce. I received a letter from Doll of December 15th and letter from Mother of December 14th. I had a good night's sleep although we did not bother about a fire.

December 21 Thursday

Breakfast: bacon. Dinner: stew. Tea: jam. The new draft arrives in the pouring rain and our billet is swamped out with them. We have an issue of clean underclothing and a bath at Sailly Dell. I have two additional pieces given to me - new socks. The showers are boiling. I received a parcel from Mother which contained a lovely rich Xmas cake with almond icing, a delightful pork pie, chocolate, almonds and raisins and gingerbreads. I started in with a high appetite as I was just longing for some tuck. The billet much more cosy with a crowd in and the brazier going and I had a very comfy night.

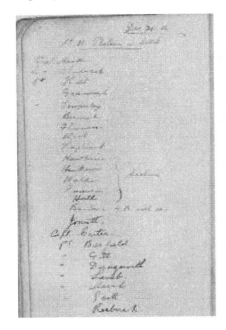

Notes giving the names of No 11 Platoon in the billet

Corpl	*Meakin*		
L	*Chadwick*	*Pte*	*Holt*
Pte	*Greenwood*	*Pte*	*Timperley*
Pte	*Beswick*	*Pte*	*Flounders*
Pte	*West*	*Pte*	*Hazlehurst*
Pte	*Hawkins*	*Pte*	*Hickson }*
Pte	*Walker } Machine*	*Pte*	*Inman }*
Pte	*Hall }*	*Pte*	*Barlow SB with 10*
Pte	*Jowett*	*Corpl*	*Carter*

Pte	Busfield	Pte	Gill
Pte	Dungworth	Pte	Lamb
Pte	Marsh	Pte	Scott
Pte	Roebuck		

December 22 Friday

Breakfast: bacon rations were very meagre. Dinner: stew. Tea: stewed figs and rice and also eat tomorrow's jam. It was a wet morning and early in the afternoon and then it cleared up later. I am in charge of the Sergeant Major's fatigue party and worked from 9am – 12 noon and from 2pm – 3pm cleaning out the ruined billets for repairs. I am Corporal of the gas guard tonight and tomorrow and have been marvelling that we are not on these working parties before now. I received a letter from Arthur dated December 13th and a parcel from A.A. which was sent to the Pioneer HQ which I fetch. It contained some tinned haddock, potted beef, cigs, candle and a book. I am still eating Mother's parcel, although it is now disembellished. I handed in a letter to Arthur.

December 23 Saturday

Breakfast: bacon. Dinner: stew. Tea: jam and butter. I arranged an easy day by acting on my own as I am Corporal of the billet and gas guard. It is a wet day and I miss the trench working party, who were setting off at 1pm and 2pm returning at 9pm and 10pm. I get down about 7pm, just in time for a rum ration and have been clearing up most of my tins of gifts. I received a parcel and a letter from Auntie Annie containing a plum pudding, biscuits, Camp Coffee, cafe au lait, salmon, meat squares, soup, crystallized fruits, pears and apples.

December 24 Sunday (Christmas Eve)

Breakfast: bacon. Dinner: stew. Tea: jam and butter. We were raised at 5.45am for an early breakfast. The new draft, who came in from trenches at 9pm and 10pm last night, are sent back again at 7am this morning. I'm Corporal of the Sergeant Major's fatigue again, cleaning up old buildings for billets. I receive a letter and cigs from Doll, dated December 18th and Xmas cards from Doll and Auntie Annie. It has been a showery morning and then in the fine afternoon and night. I am Corporal of the gas guard in our billet again.

December 25 Monday (Christmas Day)

Breakfast: bacon. Dinner: stew, plum pudding and rum sauce. Tea: jam and butter. It has been a wet and miserable day. Our guns have been straffing intermittently. I still am feeling off the mark and could scarcely eat any pudding, so I read and dozed. Our Army parcel does not turn up and I receive a Xmas card from Elsie Mosley and a letter from Aunt Clara dated December 20th. Leaman comes in at about 9.30pm to ask if we are all happy and comfortable. We have not had a drink to cheer us all day, we couldn't even buy it.

153

December 26 Tuesday (Boxing Day)

Breakfast: bacon. Dinner: stew. Tea: jam and butter. There were no parades today but it was very wet although it commenced with a bright and frosty morning. I received belated army parcels at about 2pm which contained cakes, sardines, packet of cigs, socks and bottle of beer. I handed in green envelope with a letter to Doll and Mother and received also an Independent Boots' Parcel of Soldier Comforts which contained tea tablets, peppermints, quinine tablets, Oxo and some shaving soap. I handed in a card to MS Osborne of Rutland Park in Sheffield. I am still feeling fed up.

December 27 Wednesday

Meals: ditto. This morning we had working parties and I was put on RSM's NCO's class. I wonder if the working parties are not better. The Sergeants seem the biggest major of the lot but personally I feel that this is the meanest class for recruits as it lasts from 9.15am to 12.15pm and from 2pm – 4pm and we are at it without a break except for ½ hour in the morning. I wonder if I shall survive? It has been a fine day.

December 28 Thursday

Meals: ditto. We have some respite in the morning and parade with the Company till 11am for box separation. It is very cold and frosty. RSM has us doubling till we nearly drop. A thaw sets in at night. I received a letter from Mother, dated December 21st. **Herbert Hall**[261] returns from his leave and brings me a pen knife. There are rumours about that we are not going in the trenches again but on working parties instead.

December 29 Friday

Breakfast: bacon. Dinner: rissoles and beans. Tea: jam and butter. It has been a wet and drizzly day. I am still going through it. I go to a 'Pop Off' Concert at the Church Hut in Sailly Dell. It is crowded out and I see nothing and come out at the interval. I am always too tired at night to write letters but I know that I ought to. I have got a tremendous appetite back which I put it down to exercise. I wish I could start on those parcels over again. I received a letter from Doll of December 24th.

December 30 Saturday

Breakfast: bacon. Dinner: stew. Tea: jam and butter. I was turned out with working party at ¼ hour's notice at 8.20am, so cannot go in to my class. I was

---

[261] **12/664 Private Herbert Hall** - was a sniper and Lewis gunner. He took part in the attack on 1st July 1916 and was later commissioned to Kings Own Yorkshire Light Infantry. In the book, Sheffield City Battalion by Ralph Gibson and Paul Oldfield he is quoted as saying: 'the food at first left a lot to be desired, after all the cooks were learning and it was 'Hobson's Choice' if it was edible or not. There was a chap in our hut at Redmires who seemed to be continuously hungry, always asking if you had any spare food, he must have had hollow legs. Even when in the trenches he was a fearless scrounger, always on the lookout for food. His name was 12/729 Francis Meakin'.

given the job of deepening the cable trench by **Revill**[262] at Hebuterne. It is full of water, so we stand for hours awaiting instructions. It is to be deepened from 5 feet to 8 feet, so a feeble attempt was made but the sides keep collapsing, so the cables were laid right away. We finished at 2pm and were back at 3pm. I received a letter from Doll dated December 27th. I went to the Battalion Concert in the Church Hut at the Dell in the evening which was good and much appreciated by all inside, although I was standing all of the time which was rather uncomfortable. I had some plum pudding at dinner time which was very good. A man in our billet had a fit during the night.

December 31 Sunday
Breakfast: bacon. We turned out for a working party at 10.45am and we carry on trenching carrying out excavated earth and chalk from RC dugout to **Hope Street**[263]. We finished 4.15pm and were back at 5.15pm. It has been fine generally but windy and with occasional drizzle.

1917

January 1 Monday (New Year's Day)
Breakfast: bacon. Dinner: stew rice and currants. Tea: jam and butter. Fritz woke us up as usual with a few heavy greetings which were dropped close to our billet. There was no parade or working party today. The roast pork for dinner proved only a rumour and we are to go into the trenches tomorrow. I sent a letter to Doll enclosing letters to A.A. Aunt Pollie, Aunt Annie, Aunt Clara, Mother and Teddie. The weather was wet and windy again.

January 2 Tuesday
Breakfast: bacon. Dinner: stew. Tea: jam and butter. I was up at 5.30am and had breakfast at 6.30 am. The Platoon set off at 7.15pm on a working party in the trenches. **Carter**[264] and me were let off till 10.30am then went straight to the trenches. We have an Elephant dugout in Pelisier, which is fairly comfy. I scooped out the muck and cleaned it up and drained it. I had a comfortable rest till 3.30pm and was then in charge of a carrying party. There was the usual lack of method and disorganisation on part of A Company, which resulted in most of the tea and stew for the advanced posts missing its destination and being wasted. I was back by back 8am on Wednesday. The Germans were shelling pretty heavily in the afternoon. It has been a fine day generally with slight drizzle in evening.

---

[262] **12/1264 Private A. Revill** – was wounded during the attack on 1st July 1916 and was later commissioned to 10th Y&L.

[263] **Hope Street** – a communication trench.

[264] **12/1323 Private W. R. Carter** –Batman to 94th Brigade.

January 3 Wednesday

Breakfast: bacon. Dinner: stew. Tea: jam and margarine. We had a rum ration on return from the carrying party. We were left alone till the middle of afternoon and were then on working parties etc and arranging to go up to front line i.e. Hope Street. There were fourteen men besides servants to carry three officer's rations and effects. I received a letter from Doll, dated December 29th and a parcel from F. E. P. Edwards which contained a tin of shortbread, cafe au lait, Davies polony and cake and eggs. We are in the machine gunners dugout which is damp and muddy. I am on the wiring party from 10pm – 1am. I slept well and my feet were just a bit cold till stand to. It has been a drizzling day.

January 4 Thursday

Breakfast: bacon. Dinner: stew. Tea: jam and butter. We received More Xmas Parcels with rations. My share included; 1/3 cake, about 50 cigs and a tin of tea tablets. There was nothing more doing all morning as it was wet. It cleared up in the afternoon and I detailed my men for Post No. 10. We stood to at 4.45pm and left for fire line at 5.30pm. I found the post rather cosy but a little crowded for nine. Morris[265] was on inspection and he seemed favourably impressed. We had some stew and a good rum ration at night. The night was cold and a bit frosty. I left my billy at our last dugout but Hall says he would look after it for me.

January 5 Friday

Breakfast: cold bacon. 1/3rd loaf, bread and cheese, all rations provided. The tea and stew were sent down at 5.30am. I make a warm camp fire and make some cafe au lait for dinner. It is a fine day and the Bosche pepper us all around with whiz bangs early in the afternoon. I prepare a range card in the morning to send with the guide for relief at 5.30pm. We are relieved at 6pm, when our artillery commence to strafe the Bosche heavily on our right. The Bosche retaliate ditto on us and as a result we are not allowed to go over the top along Revel, so we have a horrible squash getting through.

January 6 Saturday

Breakfast: fried bacon. Dinner: stew. Tea: jam. We receive a good rum ration after stand to and are not interfered with till stand to at night. There are rumours of an attack, so we are to sleep in our equipment all night. We make sandbag steps to assist in a quiet exit. I sent an FPC to Doll and F.E.P. Edwards. Have been sleeping all day, so don't sleep so well at night and I have cold feet again. My PH gas helmet[266] has been pinched by the working party in the morning

---

[265] 12/735 Lance Corporal H. Morris – a Sheffield University Student, commissioned to the Royal Fusiliers on 25th September 1917.

[266] P. H. Gas Helmet is a Phenate-Hexamine Goggle Helmet – An early respirator compromising a felt hood with eye pieces, impregnated with chemicals.

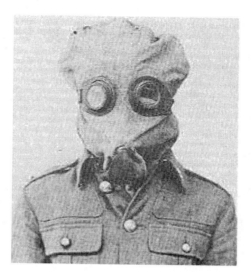

A Phenate-Hexamine Goggle Helmet

January 7 Sunday

Breakfast: fried bacon. Dinner: bully beef stew. Tea: jam and marg. We stood to in our dugout and there has been no rum ration today. I turned out with No.11 at 8.45am and was on a working party on dug out in **Vercingetorix**[267]. It was a fine, bright and rather frosty day. We got back at 2.30pm and take down rations to Hope Street at 7pm. I rested all night and was fairly comfortable.

January 8 Monday

Breakfast: bacon. Dinner: stew. Tea: Hartley's blackberry jam. We stood to in the dugout in the morning. I got two good rations and slept again till 11am, then had a short fatigue cleaning and we were then moving six carts. I got to the front line at 5.30pm and I am back with Herbert Hall and the machine gunners which was crowded and draughty. I am on patrol with two men from 10pm until 1am to locate German sentry posts. There are no stars so we failed to steer a proper course and found that I have carefully neglected the wire to approach one of our main trenches again. I made a fresh start landing too far and nearly ran into German patrol of five. At the flash of our guns and one of our periodic bursts of bombardment going on all night, they jumped up, ran back and suddenly disappeared. We returned about 1.30am as our objective was unattained. We made our supper in the comfort in Cowen's dugout and slept fairly well till stand to, in spite of a cutting draught. It has been raining off and on with a little snow about 2am. I received a letter from Mother of December 31st.

---

[267] **Vercingetorix** is a communication trench near to La Signy Farm.

January 9 Tuesday

Breakfast: boiled bacon. Dinner: bully beef stew. Tea: jam and butter. We had no rum ration at stand to and felt very cold and miserable. It was rain and drizzle for most of the day. The front posts were evacuated at 5am as we are to bombard all day and for most of the next three days. The front posts are only to be occupied for about three hours at night. I'm left alone all day till 1.15 am, when I take charge of the trench working party till 5.15am. I received a letter from Doll dated January 2nd.

January 10 Wednesday

Breakfast: boiled bacon. Dinner: stewed mutton. Tea: jam. I am left alone all day till 5.30pm when I take charge of the party from No. 10 post and occupy the same for three hours. The day is fine and overcast and there is an intermitted bombardment all day and retaliation by the Germans. I am living on stairs of a dugout in progress of construction for the remainder of our stay in the lines. It is safe but comfortable. There is a rumour that the second line of the Quadrilateral[268] was taken by us last night. We have a rum ration on our return from our post.

January 11 Thursday

Breakfast: bread and butter. Dinner: stew. Tea: jam and butter. There is a heavy bombardment at stand to and a rumour that we are attacking Serre on the flank from Beaumont Hamel. The Germans reply with a lot of heavy stuff. I have just heard that the machine gun dugout which I left last night has been blown up. Shells are falling around, thick and fast but I feel very secure down here. On emerging, I find that the trench is badly smashed up and most of the shutters have blown in. I am detailed to guide relief to No.10 fire post. They arrive about 3pm and are Royal Welsh Fusiliers. I wait till about 6pm before starting out. Slight snow obliterates the tracks and I nearly miss the way. I feel very done in and I am invited on returning, into the Royal Welsh Fusiliers dugout to change my gum boots. They are very hospitable but the RE keeps spitting on my equipment and tin hat that is lying on the floor. I get to Sailly Church where we are to assemble at 9am. Cold tea awaits me and I get to sleep about midnight in spite of a continual chorus of songs from the party that has crowded around the brazier on the church floor. We fall in and march nearly to Coigneaux and await the motor buses.

January 12 Friday

Breakfast: bacon. Dinner: stew. Tea: jam. We start off at about 1.30am in a motor GS wagon fitted up as a charabanc. We have a rough passage, it is very bumpy but I am asleep on arrival at Beauval, all the same. We are quartered in the most wretched billets we have yet struck, I have been much more comfortable in the trenches. The beds are screened rabbit wire on untrimmed

---

[268] **Quadrilateral** - The 'Heidenkopf' was a large German Redoubt near to Serre Road. It was arrow head in shape and consisted of deep wide trenches and barriers of barbed wire pointing at the British front line on the opposite side of the road. Serre Road No.2 Military Cemetery now stands on the site of the Quadrilateral which is the largest cemetery in the Somme area with seven and a half thousand graves.

poles, two deep and three high with the merest gangway between, creating a hopeless crunchy, muddy floor, with walls in holes and the usual filthy animal yard. We slept after breakfast till about 1.30pm and then cleaned up a bit and had dinner at 3pm, then rifle inspection and tea. I went out in the evening after our feed and had three fried ages, bread and butter, chips and coffee for 2.5 francs and also bought some ginger cake for 1 franc. I tried to get into see the 'Shell Shifters' after but was turned away before we got to the door. I slept well in spite of the conditions and received a letter from Doll, dated January 7th.

January 13 Saturday

Breakfast: bacon. Dinner: stew. Tea: jam. We were cleaning up then we had a rifle and equipment inspection in the morning. We paraded for physical and football in afternoon from 2pm – 4.30pm in a field about ½ mile away. I was excused participation in either on account of my boils that are gathering and with which I am consumed. I had reported sick for the same in the morning but only got **M&D**[269] and no medicine and only bandages and cold tea and bacon in consequence after wasting an hour. I went to the 'Shell Shifters' in the evening and got just inside the door when the house was declared full. I Almost did an about turn but **Carter**[270] and I hung around with a small crowd until only eight tickets more were announced. I nearly got shoved over at the Ticket Office but I secured for the two. It was a very good show indeed with some exceptional talent and better than we get at home collectively. I went drinking afterwards with **Sergeant Bourne**[271] and **Hacking**[272] and we agree to share a bottle of Muscat for 7 francs. The wretched stuff was diluted with vin ordinaire I fancy. Bourne goes away early in the morning for his commission without settling up, nor does Hacking take the hint to pay, so I shall have to stand the damage with Carter.

January 14 Sunday

Breakfast: bacon. Dinner: stew and rice pudding (no milk). Tea: jam and butter. I miss the Church parade by request but drop in for the horrid business of preparing billets for a CO inspection, which is all a farce. We have an overcoat inspection at 3pm and are then at mine all the time after dinner. I am handicapped with gathered hands and I am very fed up and have never felt more miserable. I went out for tea which was very enjoyable and had two sausages, chips, bread and butter and coffee for 1.5 francs. Thence I went to YMCA, intending to write to Doll and F.E.P. Edwards but our table is removed just as I sit down, to make room for chairs for the service and the sing song which I stick, thinking to continue after but communion follows, so I'm done again. I received some 'Passing Shows' from Maud.

---

[269] **M&D** - Medicine and Duty i.e. a dose of No. 9 (a purgative pill) or other medicine and then back to work.

[270] **12/1323 Private W. R. Carter** – Batman to 94 Brigade until September 1915 then was a Pioneer saddler. He took part in the attack on 1st July 1916.

[271] **31348 Sergeant W. K. Bourne** – also served with Northants and 7th Y&L.

[272] **38057 Sergeant William Hacking**- Died of wounds on 11th May 1917 and is buried in Duisans Military Cemetery. He also served with the Lancashire Fusiliers.

January 15 Monday

Breakfast: bacon. Dinner: stew. Tea: C&B lemon marmalade and butter. We paraded from 8.50am till 12.30pm which is about half an hour's march away overlooking the ground where we practiced our advance last June. We have a Platoon drill and physical all morning and we get let off for most the part again by **Crawford**.[273] We fall in at 1.45pm and have a clean fatigue and then march to the same spot for Sweedish, games and football in which I do not participate again. We got back at 3.45pm and go out for food again at 5pm to the same place as last night. I spoilt it by a previous round of bread with butter and marmalade. Last night the old girls made Hall fetch two tins of water from the village well. Tonight she sits there and watches us unloading a cart full of sacks of potatoes. I have an omelette of two eggs, chips, bread and butter and two 2 glasses of coffee for 1.70 francs. Carter also provides a sponge sandwich but I am too full up and thirsty after. I went back to the YMCA to write letters again but there is a band concert and it is packed tight. I received a letter from Doll, dated January 9th.

January 16 Tuesday

Breakfast: bacon. Dinner: roast beef and rice pudding. Tea: jam and butter. We were up at 6.30am preparing for a parade in spite of which, I go on parade with a muddy groundsheet and belt unbuttoned and I am pegged by the Colonel himself. We then have bayonet fighting and a close order drill on the parade ground in the morning. I return for football in the afternoon but as a spectator. We have found a really decent place next door for washing and getting our tea in the evening, with coffee and bread provided. We took our own butter, marmalade, sardines and apricots. I get a shower and a haircut at the same place and are then cleaning up till 7pm and lights out. I received letters from Doll and Mother both dated January 10th. The weather has been frosty and dull.

January 17 Wednesday

Breakfast: bacon. Dinner: stew. Tea: marmalade and butter.
We were up at 5.30am and were cleaning up. I was warned for the orderly room at 8.30am and was remanded by the CO. The parade then dismissed to prepare for the CO's inspection at 2.30pm. Before the CO at 12.30, I explained the handicap of my gathered hands and being generally done in with boils but my whole story was treated with contempt. I was severely reprimanded and told that if I appear again I shall be reduced to a Private. The weather has been sleeting all day. We paraded for a preliminary inspection at 1.45pm and returned at 2.30pm. We were kept standing for over one hour in the bitter cold before it was our turn to come around for inspection. I am fed up more and more and feel that the boils are taking a fresh hold. I go next down for tea again and take butter, salmon and peas and compote pomme which proves bad.

---

[273] **Captain W. Crawford** – served with 12th Y&L from 25 November 1916 and also served with 7th Y&L.

January 18 Thursday

Breakfast: cold boiled bacon and pickles. Dinner: stew. Tea: blackberry and apple jam with butter. I am up at 6.30am and parade at 9am for a route march. We look like getting back at 11am when the Colonel leads us back to the parade ground and then explains that the Brigadier was justified in A Company yesterday returning before time, therefore in spite of the snow, we've got to continue till 12.30pm. We make preparation for a rifle and ammunition inspection in the afternoon. I have tea again next door which consists of tinned sausages and peaches and the total cost with coffee and bread is 1.5 francs. The weather is fine and bright generally but with some snow. I receive a letter from Doll, dated January 11th and wrote to Doll with an enclosure in a green envelope for F.E.P.E.

January 19 Friday

Breakfast: bacon. Dinner: stew and rice pudding. Tea: marmalade and butter. I was up at 6.30am and I paraded sick to get the sores on my legs properly dressed again. I dodged the general parade and took M&Ds up to the parade ground about 1pm. We had an inspection by 5th Army General Gough of the Battalion at training and I was interrogated by him as section commander. We were kept at it till 12.45pm by order of the Brigadier and this is to be the rule in future. We paraded again at 2.30pm for football in the training ground. I had tea next door as usual, which was sardines and peas and the total cost with coffee and bread was 1.2 francs. I received a letter from Doll posted in Liverpool on January 13th. I reply by return in a green envelope. It has been a fine and frosty day but my feet are very wet with standing in the snow all day.

January 20 Saturday

Breakfast: rissoles and onion sauce. Dinner: stew. Tea: marmalade. We were up at 6.30am and I reported sick for redressing, thus I managing to dodge about half an hour of the parade. We paraded at 12.35pm and we were back at 1.15pm. We paraded again at 2.30pm and had a glove and overcoat inspection followed by an NCO's lecture. We then had an address by General O'Gowan at 5pm. I made a big effort at a good feed and seven of us had a big pork chop each, a sausage and fried onions. The total cost including cafe au lait and French bread was 2.5 francs. It has been a fine and frosty day. I received a letter from Frank Wright, dated January 22nd.

January 21 Sunday

Breakfast: bacon. Dinner: stew and rice pudding. Tea: butter and marmalade. We had an overcoat and kit inspection in the morning and the afternoon we actually had off. I went to the YMCA and consumed coffee and a large amount of a raspberry sandwich. I had tea next door again which consisted of salmon and peaches with the total cost as before: 1.20 francs. I had a last shave by mine host, to whom I have entrusted myself lately on account of a sore chin and dull razor, he sets the latter. The weather has been fine and frosty.

January 22 Monday

Breakfast: bacon. Dinner: stew. Tea: marmalade. We were up at 5.30am preparing and had breakfast at 6.30am. We fall in at 8.45am and leave at 9.20am and we arrive at Candas which is about four miles away at 11.30pm. We are billeted in **bow huts,**[274] which are crowded but preferable to the last billet. I was on the lookout for feeding and washing accommodation with success. I had two fried eggs which were newly laid and a delicious pomme de terre frit for 1.10 francs. I was warned for guard, so I was back early and was then cleaning up till after lights out. The weather was frosty with a slight thaw in the afternoon and a frosty night. I was up several times in the night, my bladder seems very weak. I ordered herrings and fried potatoes for Wednesday.

January 23 Tuesday

Breakfast: bacon. Dinner: stew. Tea: Chivers blackberry jam and margarine. I am for headquarters guard, so I am up at 6.30am cleaning. I am complimented for my clean guard by the adjutant but subsequently constantly bullied by RSM. It must be good for the liver though, as I feel much better today. The guard was cold and draughty but get the brazier going. I found the Madame of the billet very amiable and she is ready to prepare coffee and also boils me three eggs which are 3½ centimes each for six. We have a rum ration served at night and it has been a bright and frosty day. I receive a letter from Doll dated January 17th and some 'Passing Shows' from Maud. I also received a parcel from A.A. which contains an apple pudding, cigs, milk, cocoa, pencil and magazine. The cocoa is very opportune. There is hot water for shave and a wash for nine at our eating abode this morning.

January 24 Wednesday

Breakfast: bacon. Dinner: stew. Tea: jam and butter. I slept well between relieving the guards during the night. My guard was relieved at 9am this morning and the RSM actually leaves us to it. My guard is immediately set cleaning out huts but I manage to dodge the morning off. There is a communication drill for the NCOs in the afternoon. I have tea at the cottage in the evening which consists of two smoked herrings, chips and tinned peaches which are frozen. The weather is cold and frosty. General Wanless O'Gowan looked into our huts in the afternoon and exclaimed 'it's very cold in here lads. I've just been to the German camp, why they are better off then you.' Wasn't it tactful ...

January 25 Thursday

Breakfast: bacon. Dinner: stew. Tea: marmalade and margarine. The NCOs class under the RSM in the morning catch him in much happier view than usual and I rather enjoy it. At the afternoon parade at 2.30pm, I am sent with **Ballard**[275] to

---

[274] **Bow Huts** - During the First World War, tens of thousands of corrugated iron huts were constructed by the armed forces - the Nissen Bow Hut could be constructed almost anywhere.

[275] **12/582 Private E. Ballard** – took part in the attack on 1st July 1916.

sketch the bombing trenches which we have first to find. After wasting 1½ hours by taking the wrong road, we get there at about 3.45 pm. Bombing is in progress, so we are handicapped and find about 1500 yards of trenches. I hand in fair sketch of the same about 7.30pm then proceed for tea at the Cottage and have fried eggs, chips and coffee. I fill in a form for the Inland Transport RE and hand in to Charlesworth. There is a hard frost all day. I receive a letter from Frank Irwin, dated January 19th, his address is now P.O. Assistant Surgeon, Portsmouth.

January 26 Friday
Breakfast: bacon. Dinner: boiled beef, potatoes, baked beans. Tea: marmalade. Parade at 8.45 to proceed to bombing trenches, about 1½ miles away to practice attacks. Fearfully cold and we are kept standing about considerably. Back about 1.30 and fall in again at 2.30. We take the lame who do not desire football on a short march. Resort again to our cottage for fried eggs, chips and coffee. A very hard frost continued all day. I see that my name is on a list of those who have not had leave for nine months, only two left in the Company to go before me. Rum ration, which we partake with coffee at our cottage stove. Letter from Doll, January 20.

January 27 Saturday
Breakfast: bacon. Dinner: stew which was rotten. Tea: marmalade. I reported sick to get my leg dressed and show the Medical Officer the eruptions on my neck too, just casually and get neck dressed. He refuses to dress my leg as all MDs are to get on parade quickly. We had a short lecture by the CSM in the afternoon. I hear two fellows who were going on leave straight from line have died from exposure this morning as they went to sleep in nothing but their overcoats on the platform. I had tinned herrings and chips at the cottage and received letters from Doll dated January 22nd and Mother dated January 17th.

January 28 Sunday
Breakfast: bacon. Dinner: boiled mutton and broth. Tea: marmalade. I reported sick again and got my leg dressed. We had a kit inspection in the morning and then rested in the afternoon. I had egg and chips at the cottage and then was writing to Mother and Doll. I hear that we are moving tomorrow.

January 29 Monday
Breakfast: bacon. Dinner: boiled mutton, broth and mixed veg. Tea: marmalade. I go sick again and hear that it is **Gamble**[276] who has omitted to put me on, so the Doctor in consequence refuses to attend to me. We parade from 9.45am till 10.45am and have dinner at 11am and fall in at 12.40pm and march to Bonneville. The Corporals are billeted together fairly cosily or would be if there was plenty of fuel. The shops and estaminets here seem very scarce. I finish my letters to Mother, Doll and A.A. but there is no collection and I received a letter from Doll sent on January 24th.

---

[276] **39135 Corporal F. Gamble** – also served with 7th and 10th Y&L.

January 30 Tuesday
Breakfast: bacon. Dinner: stew and boiled mutton. Tea: marmalade. I missed about two hours parade by going sick to get my leg dressed. We had a bit of bayonet and musketry drill at 11.30am and at 12.30pm we were practising an attack. I was excused the afternoon parade to rest my leg and I am disappointed at receiving no pay or rum ration.

January 31 Wednesday
Breakfast: bacon. Dinner: stew. Tea: marmalade and margarine. We hung about starving and perishing all morning and afternoon waiting to fire ten rounds at 50 yards. The second group fired sixteen out of twenty. We are given a rum ration and the weather is still freezing hard.

February 1 Thursday
Breakfast: Maconochies. Dinner: bully beef and clear stew which was rotten and jam roll. Tea: marmalade and margarine. I reported sick to get my leg and gathered finger dressed. We then marched for about an hour parade and then had a charge of barrage and ½ hour attack is all that I did. In the afternoon we had a fatigue marking out an extension to the trenches for the Battalion attack tomorrow. I was paid 25 francs and received a parcel from A.A. which contained cake, humbugs, soup square and a book. I then shared a tin of herrings for supper. I have had a complete change of underclothing, which is about time, as I felt overrun with lice and my blanket must swarm with them. There were signs of a thaw at midday but the weather has turned to hard frost again.

February 2 Friday
Breakfast: Maconochies. Dinner: stew. Tea: marmalade. We parade at 8.15am and I am in charge of the platoon. We practice the attack in the second half of the morning and parade for our inoculations at 2pm. The hypodermic needle seems very blunt and rusty and feels like sticking a skewer in and it breaks in the next man. My breast gets painful towards the evening but I go to Candas to feed at our cottage and have eggs and chips, sausages and rabbit and I then have biscuits, sweets etc at the YMCA. We have a rum ration on our return and I received a letter from Mother sent on January 29th.

February 3 Saturday
Breakfast: Maconochies. Dinner: stew. Tea: biscuits and raisin snack, butter. I lie abed imagining we are really entitled to 48 hours complete rest as in the Battalion orders. At the last ¼ hour we are ordered for a parade and inspection are then to be dismissed but are sent back by the CSM soon after we appear. I get some tinned sausages warmed for breakfast, which are very tasty and then get back to bed for the rest of the morning. Crawford asks me to write my name for a draughtsman suitable for water points but I decline on the grounds of the I.T.[277] jobs that I was previously entitled for. I read in the afternoon and then get

---

[277] **I.T. jobs –** internal transfer.

back to bed after tea for some warmth. I received a letter from Auntie Annie, of January 28th.

February 4 Sunday
Breakfast: rissoles. Dinner: bully stew and biscuit and raisin snack. Tea: figs and margarine. My breast feels better today but I report sick again to get my leg dressed and some of the sores are drying up. The 48 hours rest does not finish till 2pm but the billets have to be specially cleaned up for the Brigadier's inspection and we all have to clear out while same takes place this morning. I did a bit of reading in the afternoon and warmed up a tin of rabbit for tea. I put my name down for a Field Survey Observer for the 5th Company, someone of superior intellect and education is required, especially Architects, Engineers and School Masters. I should get out of this **bally**[278] Battalion somehow. I started a letter to Mother in the evening but left it to do the Orderly Sergeant for Carter. I get in a bottle of vin rouge which was three francs, and the same was hot.

February 5 Monday
Breakfast: bacon. Dinner: rissole and tea. Tea: marmalade and margarine. I did the orderly sergeant again for Carter in the morning, so I missed the parade till 11am, which was bayonet-sticking at sacks and a platoon drill. We had a football match in the afternoon which I dodged and finished my letters to Mother, Doll and to the A.A. which I give in. I received a letter from Doll of January 31st and papers from Auntie Annie. I share a bottle of vin rouge chaud for 3½ francs with Carter and Ellis[279] at the estaminet and also some coffee which was very cosy.

February 6 Tuesday
Breakfast: Maconochies. Dinner: stew and marmalade roll. Tea: marmalade and margarine. We paraded at 8.45am and then marched to the bombing trenches between Candas and Beauval, which was three and a half miles to practice an attack and we were back at about 3pm. I had coffee at the canteen after dinner then had an NCO's conference and lecture by the Colonel on various subjects including the attack. He mentions heavy slains coming in for damage whilst getting forward. Breaths and threats but there are no suggestions as to how the troops are to keep warm. I have never known a CO to take less interest in the comfort of troops. We are back for tea at about 7pm and I then had a glass of beer at the estaminet for sake of warmth in same. I got a dressing and some ointment for my feet and attended to my leg myself to save time going sick. I sent Doll FPC and the frost is holding hard. The two last men in C Company; **Lockett**[280] and **Hills**[281] go off for their leave tonight. We had a rum ration.

---

[278] **Bally** – euphemistic word for bloody.

[279] **12/644 Private J. S. Ellis,** served in C Company and took part in the attack on 1st July 1916.

[280] **12/717 Private G. Lockett** – took part in the attack of 1st July 1916 and also served with 9th Y&L.

[281] **12/678 Private A. J. Hills** – took part in the attack of 1st July 1916 and also served with 13th Y&L.

February 7 Wednesday

Breakfast: rissole meat, icy cold. Dinner: stew. Tea: marmalade and butter. We paraded at 8.45am and marched five miles to practice the attack, it was a long climb and we are in an absolutely exposed position. We did it three times and then finished at 2pm. We returned which was mostly downhill and were back at 3.15pm. I went to the canteen after dinner for coffee which was wet and milk-less but hot. It is frosty and it is still holding hard. I am warned for another NCO conference under the Colonel our return and we don't get our tea till late again as a consequence. The Colonel turns up late with news that the Brigade attack operations are cancelled and we march off to Courcelles in the morning. We stay the night at Terres du Mesnil which is about ten miles away. He has also been instructed to lecture and appeal to the officers, NCOs and men to consider new war loans. There won't be a very hearty response from the men I think, on five or ten francs per fortnight. I received a letter from Doll, dated February 1st and received a 'Public Opinion' from Maud.

February 8 Thursday

Breakfast: bacon. Dinner: stew. Tea: marmalade and margarine. My pack is very full and heavy with four tins of tobacco and an extra fur jerkin. We paraded for twenty minutes before moving off at 9.30am. Had frequent halts and very pleasantly surprised to find that Terres du Mesnil was only about eight miles away, which was quite enough nevertheless and we arrived about 1.30pm. We are billeted in a roof floor over a farmhouse. I then went out and consumed coffees till dinner at 2.30pm and went to the estaminet for warmth and vin rouge, chaud which was very good. The weather is bright and frosty.

February 9 Friday

Breakfast: bacon. Dinner: stew. Tea: stewed figs. We marched off for Courcelles at 9.20am with 14½ miles reported to be ahead via Beauquesne, Louvencourt and Bus. We had frequent short rests again and my feet are sore but they are not blistered. I stuck it much better than I had expected and think the distance was 12 – 13 miles after all. Our billet is in a canvas hut with a Sergeant's brazier going. We are on wire beds, so it looks like being fairly cosy. Courcelles seems much improved as regards canteens and I had a mug of good cocoa for 2 francs. There was some heavy strafe in the evening. I had a very comfortable night and I was only up once. The weather is still freezing hard and bright.

February 10 Saturday

Breakfast: bacon. Dinner: stew. Tea: stewed figs. I stayed abed till about 8.30am and there were no parades in the morning just cleaning up around and then about one hour's parade drill in the afternoon. I received a letter from Doll, dated February 4th with a 10/- enclosure. I had a rum ration and secured enough to get a little effect. I had a more comfortable night than ever and was only up once towards the morning. The weather is bright and frosty again. I am getting a big appetite which Army fare fails to satisfy but it is expensive satisfying same on chocolate and biscuits at the canteen.

February 11 Sunday
Breakfast: bacon. Dinner: stew which was good. Tea: stewed currants. We had another restful day and only paraded at 11am for a gas helmet and boot inspection. I read in the afternoon and went to Bertrancourt after tea and bought some biscuits, cake and chocolate at the **RAFA**[282] Camp canteen, which was much more reasonable than the Divisional Canteen. The chocolate at the former was 7½ francs and at the later 1 franc. We had a white frost last night which was thawing in sun during the day and then freezing hard at night but misty. I received letters from Mother dated February 5th and A.A. and make an enquiry to see if any parcels have been received. I was only up once in the night and there was some heavy strafing during the night too.

February 12 Monday
Breakfast: bacon. Dinner: only tea. Tea: stew. We paraded at 8am and marched to the railway which was about ½ hour away and were kept standing about till nearly 3pm before any work was found. We get over chlorinated tea at dinner time and were back at 5pm. I sent letter to A.A. and went to the Chaplin's quarters in the evening and got let in for a short service. I wrote to Doll in a green envelope. Our rum ration is now every other night. I was up twice in the night. The weather has thawed during the day and the evening was cloudy.

February 13 Tuesday
Breakfast: bully beef. Dinner: stew. Tea: stewed currants. I was freezing in the morning again. We paraded at 7.45am and were kept waiting for ½ hour before having the morning off. The weather was thawing during the day with a raw wind. There was little impression made with the ground as it is still covered with explosives. The guns were strafing pretty hard all day.

February 14 Wednesday
Breakfast: bacon. Dinner: stew. Tea: jam and margarine. We paraded at 7.45am and were kept standing for about ½ hour. We had a chin inspection and many men pulled up as unshaven, fortunately I was alright. It put the wind up most of us though and there was much cleaning of boots and buttons that evening - we shall now win the war. Then instead of spending ½ hour taking tools right back to the dump, we leave them on the job and cut straight through areas to home. It has been a frosty morning with bright sun but a cold raw wind in the afternoon.

February 15 Thursday
Breakfast: bacon. Dinner: stew. Tea: jam. We had railway fatigue as before. It was a frosty morning with warm sunshine later. I was paid 50 francs and went to the Division Follies at the new YMCA hut in the evening, I have seen better. I received a letter from Arthur, dated February 7th.

---

[282] **RAFA** – Royal Air Force Association.

February 16 Friday
Breakfast: bacon. Dinner: stew, good. Tea: stewed figs. A few shells dropped quite close to us before we got up this morning and I was on railway fatigue as before. The Bosche start shelling up both heavily and accurately at tea time and several were killed and wounded, chiefly in our **Battalion**[283] which really is hard lines when we should still be on a Divisional rest. Two aeroplanes came down this morning, one of the enemy and one of ours, it was all very active. It was a frosty morning, with slight rain in afternoon and then a thaw set in. I received a letter from Doll, dated February 6th and bought at the canteen some good beer for 1 franc. Our rations are getting meagre with only ¼ small loaf per man.

February 17 Saturday
Breakfast: bully beef. Dinner: stew. Tea: jam and margarine. Two more fellows are wounded this morning from the German shells, making the total here about twenty casualties and six killed. **RFA**[284] say that they have retaliated with thousands of tons of shells on two villages that they have left alone lately. Our Mid day stew did not turn up till time to start work again and Moxey said that we will get it one or two at a time but we had it in sixes and it was pretty cold for the last men. Another indignity, the Colonel does not wish us to return till 5pm. That is another ½ hours work although the Canadian officer does not wish it. Carter procures bloaters for tea which were very fine. I received a letter from Doll, dated February 13th and a parcel from 'Xmas Gift for Soldier's Friend' containing a tin of herrings and tomato, two slabs of medium chocolate, packet of dates, butterscotch, tea, milk, soap, candle, coffee, tea, Vaseline dubbing, spearmint. I went off to a concert at the YMCA from 8pm – 10pm and found it splendid.

February 18 Sunday
Breakfast: bacon. Dinner: stew. Tea: jam and margarine. We had a day off except for rifle inspection. I was eating biscuits, sweets and the contents of my parcel all day and sent a card with thanks for the latter. I played chess in the afternoon and I lost to **Davis**[285] and then played Solo in the evening and won .75 francs. I also wrote to Mother and Doll. It has been a fine day but dull and very muddy.

February 19 Monday
Breakfast: bacon. Dinner: stew. Tea: jam. We had a parade as usual for work, the ground is very wet and muddy now and I have very cold feet. The weather is fine but dull. I received letters from Doll and Mother, both dated February 14th and I sent a letter to Doll with a green envelope with one enclosed to Mother.

---

[283]**Lance Corporal 40185 Cyril Appleton** and **Private 31641 Edward Leadbetter** were both killed in action and are buried in Courcelles Military Cemetery Extension.

[284] **RFA** – Royal Field Artillery.

[285] **12/916 Private L. Davies** – also served with 13th and 14th Y&L.

February 20 Tuesday
Breakfast: Maconochies which was bad. Dinner: stew. Tea: jam. It has been a wet day. We walked till 11.30am then returned for our dinner and paraded for baths at Sailly at 1pm. There was just a trickle of scalding water for the showers to wash under but the whale oil and rum ration countered the effect. The roads are very flooded. We have a disquieting order that we are to move at any time and also names for a sapping company are being taken. I also saw a Battalion of 31st Division returning to the line.

February 21 Wednesday
Breakfast: bacon. Dinner: stew. Tea: strawberry jam. We have been working as usual and it has been a fine day. The Canadians say that we are to be kept on the job and there is a report that leave started yesterday but nothing has been heard of in it in this Battalion.

February 22 Thursday
Breakfast: Maconochies. Dinner: stew. Tea: stewed figs. We march to the old working ground for tools, then to the new section past Mailley Maillet. The big guns, the 9.2s are firing nearby which is very disturbing. The weather is dull with slight drizzle and the roads are like butter. Our rum ration was very comforting.

February 23 Friday
Breakfast: bacon. Dinner: stew. Tea: stewed figs. I am at work at Mailley again and the air rings from the big guns, 9.2s, close at hand and some came to earth amongst us, hurtling on the ground like heavy whips. I spent two francs at dinner here on beer and chocolate. We get back again after an hour's march at 5pm. There has been no mail to speak of for several days. The Follies are back and I endeavoured to see them but there was a queue 150 yards long. The weather is fine but damp and foggy.

February 24 Saturday
Breakfast: bully. Dinner: stew. Tea: jam. I am working near to our original section again and the weather is fine but dull. Just before we should go home, the Canadian officer sends for us to unload coal from the trucks. **Morris**[286] objects and marches us home but not before many of us had secured a sackful though. The first English mail for many days arrives but there is none for me.

February 25 Sunday
Breakfast: Maconochies. Dinner: stew. Tea: jam and margarine. We have the day off but the whole morning is taken up with inspections etc. There was a slight frost during the night and it is a bright spring like day with a cold nip in the air. There are rumours of the Germans evacuating round Serre and also a big

---

[286] **12/735 Lance Corporal H. Morris** – a Sheffield University Student, commissioned to the Royal Fusiliers on 25th September 1917.

advance at Ypres. Before tea I walked over to the RAFA Camp Canteen at Bertrancourt and got a good supply of coffee, chocolate, biscuits and sausages and it is two francs per tea. I received a letter from Doll sent on February 18th. I sent Doll and Mother FPCs and whilst writing to Doll I was interrupted by an order to report to orderly soon in the morning to proceed to Boulogne and report to Troops Transportation Officer, an RE job at last?

February 26 Monday
Breakfast: bacon, took bread, bacon, bully and jam rations. I reported orderly at 9am and set off about 10am. I arrived at Acheux station about 11.45am and was told to be ready for the train at 4.30pm. I waited in the YMCA and got sardines at 6½ per tin as I found out that tea wasn't due till 5.30pm. I got away about 6pm in the usual cattle truck and arrived at Abbeville at 3am. The weather has been cold but bright.

February 27 Tuesday
I slept in the YMCA hut at Abbeville till 6.30am and got a brew fired on the railway brazier. Rations were dished out to those who wanted them bit I did not trouble, else I might have got bread and milk and also butter which would have been very useful later. The cattle truck for Boulogne left at 10.30am and arrived in Boulogne at about 4pm. 113 of us marched up to the Transportation Camp above the town which was 2.5 kilometres out. We were given soup and allotted tents. I got some very good beer at a cafe nearby for one franc per glass and prime stout was 75 centimes. We were allowed out after 4.30pm but after clean up but I wasn't ready till 7.15pm so there no time for the town. Three new blankets were given to us and I spent a very comfortable night with wooden floors to tents. It has been a bright and fine day.

February 28 Wednesday
Breakfast: bacon. Dinner: stew. Tea: cheese and pickles. The meals were very disorganised. The crowd that I turned up with were turned away as there was no more bread. I found **Chadwick**[287] employed in a men's tent so touched him for a good breakfast and had a bit of bread, so I got about ½ lb of bacon with it and tea. We paraded at 9am and I was allotted to 113 RE Company and was disgusted to find that I am put down as a plate layer and I also hear that we shall all be reduced. I got a bath and a change in the camp. There is no bread with dinner stew and we have a kit inspection in the afternoon and indents were taken and we then paraded again for a roll call. There was only dry bread, cheese and pickles with tea. I went down town with **Dunne**[288] for a cinema show and a feed. The cinema was not open today and any decent restaurants were difficult to find. I eventually took 1½ hours to get a bit of fish, three little potatoes and bread and

---

[287] **38013 Lieutenant John Henry Chadwick** – also served with Lancashire Fusiliers. He died on 18th February 1918 and is buried in Great Harwood Cemetery.

[288] **38016 Lance Corporal Thomas Dunne** – killed in action on 16th June 1917 and is buried in Bailleul Road Military Cemetery, brother of **38015 Private J. E. Dunne** who died of wounds on 7th November 1916 and is buried in Warlincourt Halte Military Cemetery. Both had previously served with the Lancashire Fusiliers and did not take part in the attack on 1st July 1916.

butter for 1.5 francs and a glass of beer for 4 francs – robbery. I noticed a fellow dining alone who got as much as we had put together. I got some beer for 1½ francs per glass which was very good. I sent a green envelope to Doll and wrote to Arthur and Carter. I have been changed into 113 lines. It has been a fine day and warm in the evening with slight showers.

March 1 Thursday
Breakfast: bacon. Dinner: stew with ghastly meat which was uneatable. Tea: jam. We parade at 9am for a roll call, then we have another parade at 10.30am for a medical and the CO's inspection. I was asked by the CO how long I had been out here and if I had been ill. Indents were taken and we parade at 2pm for a roll call. There is a rumour that we may move off in the evening and that we should have to stand to but no order was given just cleaning out at 4.30pm when I was collared for orderly sergeant. I should have been off, if I had not waited for Dunne. I had to hang about the camp all evening with nothing to do till seeing all present at 9pm and then the staff parade after. Dunne said that the pictures were very good. It has been a bright and fine day.

March 2 Friday
Breakfast: cold bacon. Dinner: bean and bully beef soup and cold beef. Tea: jam. We are kept pretty busy as the orderly sergeant and various parades for indents and inspections. We finally paraded in full marching order, presumably to move off but found only for inspection with two blankets included. We are not allowed out of the camp, so spend the evening at the canteen over beer and biscuits. The draft who parade for moving away at 1.30pm, we don't move off till about 7.30pm. We hear we are for Doullens district and I write to A.A. notifying them of my change of address. It has been a beautiful bright and warm day. Our rationing is very meagre all the time we are here and we are ordered to sleep in our clothes and be ready to move. This was rescinded at about 10.30pm.

March 3 Saturday
Breakfast: cheese and pickles and margarine. Dinner: soup and cold beef (good). Tea: jam. There are no parades for the draft, so we are standing to all day. I am sent for by 1st Lieutenant and I asked how I came to be a plate layer and he remarked that it was the usual Army way. I was told that I should go in the office all right as a draughtsman. He wanted me to draw out some schemes for scratching off a rope railway. I criticised each one, so he said that they would require further consideration and he wanted to know if I had my instruments with me. We have nothing to do but sup beer at the canteen as long as it is open. It has been a frosty morning and a bright, cold day. There was a report that we are moving off at 11pm but nothing happened. It has been rather cold with only one blanket as the other one is packed up with my kit.

March 4 Sunday
Breakfast: cold bacon. Dinner: soup and cold beef. Tea: jam. There is no parading not even for a roll call now. We are taken on a route march quite unburdened along the coast and back behind via the monument at Wimereux

which was most enjoyable, fine and bright. It is hazy over the sea, which made one long for a sight of Blighty. It is rumoured again that the train goes at Midnight but again I settle down for the night as I am confident that we shouldn't be going. The only recreation once again is beer, biscuits and chocolate. I sent a letter to Mother.

March 5 Monday
Breakfast: cold bacon. Dinner: stew and beans. Tea: lobby roast beef. Two inches of snow has fallen during the night but it had almost disappeared by the morning and there was a heavy shower at 4.30pm. We had another constitutional march in the morning to Wimille and then back by Wimereux station and the monument. We had a decent tea as above at 3.30pm and fall in and out again for a shower at 4.30pm and then marched off at 5pm for the train due at 6pm.The latter eventually crawled out at 8.45pm and arrived at Etaples at 12 midnight and to our surprise were disembarked to rest there for a day. We have a pack on again with the two additional blankets and arrived at the tents at 12.45pm. Only thirty kilometres of our alleged journey to Doullens is accomplished.

March 6 Tuesday
Meals: Bully beef, cheese and biscuits. I slept comfortably till after light. We are not allowed to go in to Etaples or Paris Plage and must only stay in the camp area which is vast. We spent the morning cleaning up and sewing and getting our hair cut. In the afternoon I walked around the camp which was rather picturesque and novel, with high sand hills covered with trees growing directly out of the sand which was a strange contrast of colour. I saw some Portuguese troops about who were very inferior looking and who especially contrasted with the New Zealanders and Australians who were remarkably fine looking fellows. I took tea in a Tipperary Hut served by ladies and I had three hard eggs, two rounds of bread and butter and a basin of tea for 1.20 francs. Afterwards I went to the cinema which was a long five part western drama. **Napoo**[289] beer.

March 7 Wednesday
Rations: bully beef, cheese, margarine and biscuits. Breakfast at 5.30am and fell in at 6am for the train due at 6.30am. I did not leave until 9am, had a free tea at YMCA and I also bought sausage rolls and cakes. Got a brazier and tea made in a truck. It has been a very cold and windy day. We arrived in Doullens at about 7pm, our tents were about ½ mile from the station. We got tea and cheese and bread served at 9pm. Slight snow fall.

March 8 Thursday
Breakfast: bacon. Dinner: fresh meat stew. Tea: jam and margarine. I slept till about 8am and got breakfast at 10am and fifty cigs were served for our tobacco ration. I did about 1½ hours fatigue in the morning, shifting sleepers and had dinner about 3pm. I went into Doullens after tea and the cinema was full, so I

---

[289] **Napoo** – From the French 'Il n'y en a plus' – there is no more. The word was later applied to mean 'there is none'- thus 'Napoo beer'.

had a feast consisting of a pork cutlet, chips, cafe au lait and a tumbler of vin rouge for 2.35 francs. The snow thawed during the day and it was frosty in the evening.

March 9 Friday
Breakfast: bacon. Dinner: stew (fresh meat). Tea: jam. We moved after breakfast to another part of the line, which was about the same distance from the town, about a quarter of an hour's walk away. We are billeted in trucks fitted up with berths. We started work straight away putting up a marquee and tents and ceased work at 4.15pm. I went into Doullens and saw a picture show which I had to come out of in the middle of 'Charlie (Chaplin) in the Park' to get in by 8.30pm. We hear that the NCOs have had a lecture and were all told that there would be reduced threats of being sent back to respective Battalions if they don't do their whack. I sent an FPC to Doll. It has been snowing for most of the day and is still frosty.

March 10 Saturday
Breakfast: bacon. Dinner: roast beef - a wacking ration and potatoes. Tea: jam and cheese. We commenced work at 7am after breakfast at 6.15am and had tea and lunch from 12 noon to 12.30pm and then finished work at 4.30pm, putting up frame tents. I then stopped in the evening and was writing to Doll. The weather thawing and it is very muddy.

March 11 Sunday
Breakfast: bacon. Dinner: stew. Tea: cheese and sardines and marmalade. We were working as yesterday and there is no difference as it is Sunday and I sent a letter to Doll. I am Corporal of the night guard and clinch a considerable rest which is scarcely interfered with and I also have half a day off tomorrow. It is a fine and bright day, so the mud is drying up. We had lightening at night and rain later. We are having to clear out of the van, as the original occupants are coming back.

March 12 Monday
Breakfast: bacon. Dinner: fresh meat and stew. Tea: sardines, cheese, marmalade and 1/3 loaf. We had the morning off after the guard and we then moved into the tents. We continued with huts in the afternoon and Caplain took particulars of my occupation and entered it as Surveyor and Draughtsman. It was a bright morning and a wet in the afternoon. I was paid 15 francs.

March 13 Tuesday
Breakfast: bacon. Tea: marmalade, cheese, margarine and sardines. Dinner: roast beef and potatoes, very good. I am in charge of the hut erection as before. It was a very wet day and my overcoat was soaked. We had a rum ration before dinner and I then went to the cinema in the evening. I received a letter from Doll dated March 5th, enclosing 5/-. I was off at 8am till 11.30am reporting sick to get some glasses for drawing and I got an order to attend hospital at Frevant for an eye examination.

March 14 Wednesday

Breakfast: bacon. Tea: marmalade, cheese and margarine. Dinner: stew, fresh meat and peas. We parade as before and I am in charge of working on the huts and. I was soaking wet all day and my feet were wet through. I went to the cinema in the evening and the road was so bad that I saw a motor lorry up to its axles in mud and abandoned.

March 15 Thursday

Breakfast: cold bacon. We paraded at 6.30am for work as the French Line was to be cut and then the French did not allow it after all. I had to go to Frevant for my glasses by the 9.19am train, so I spent the interval cleaning up. I got to the hospital at about 11am and was fortunate in getting attention almost right away. The Captain eye specialist was a fine set up fellow, a perfect gentleman, in fact I might have been a private patient with a big fee. He puts drops in my eyes and went into a dark room and then tested them properly. I was told to stay in rest hut and come at 10am in the morning for my glasses. My eyesight was as blurred and strained as the blind drunk for about six hours. I got bully, cheese, pickles, bread and tea for dinner and fried bread and marmalade for tea. I went to the cinema in the evening and could see well enough and a pianist played just like I used to. I must still owe my existence to the great forbearance of my family and friends. Two blankets were served at night and it was a fine day.

March 16 Friday (My 36th Birthday)

Breakfast: good helping of bacon. Dinner: tin of Maconochies and tea. Tea: fresh meat stew and potatoes. I had a very good night and I did not get up once. My eyesight is still blurred and I cannot read. I went to the hospital at 10am and the MO said that my eyes had not sufficiently recovered to try the glasses and to come again at 12 noon. I went into town and had half a dozen pastries, ½lb dates, three oranges, chocolate bonbons and some coffee. I returned and got my glasses which were very satisfactory. I had dinner at the rest hut and caught the 2.23pm passenger train which arrived at Doullens before 4pm and I was back in the camp for dinner. I stopped in for the evening and wrote to Doll, Mother and Carter and also sent an FPC to Doll. The weather has been a beautifully fine day.

March 17 Saturday

Breakfast: none served except tea and were made to do with cheese, marmalade, bread and marg. Tea: ditto. Dinner: roast beef and onions. We hung about half of the morning and then I surveyed the camp and started to plot it by the end of the afternoon. I went to the 'Fancies' in the evening which was pretty good but not up to those I've seen lately. I handed in the letters written last night first thing this morning. It has been a beautifully fine day.

March 18 Sunday

Breakfast: bacon. Dinner: bully stew. Tea: as usual. We had breakfast at 7.15am and then paraded at 8am. I plotted the camp survey in the morning and then read in the afternoon waiting for MO inspection at 3.45pm. This was postponed pending his arrival to stand to. I wrote to Arthur and sent an FPC to Mrs Headland and went to the pictures in the evening.

March 19 Monday
Breakfast: only tea served, eat general rations. Tea: sardines. Dinner: bully stew. We had parades as usual and I reported sick as I am verminous, in order to get a bath. I took my own change and got a splendid hot bath at Northumbrian No. 2 Hospital. I left my clothing in town to get a wash and then finished plotting the camp survey in the afternoon. I had a very quiet evening and stopped in and had an undisturbed night and a rum ration.

March 20 Tuesday
Breakfast: bacon. Dinner: stew. Tea: as usual. I was supervising the **Chester's**[290] levelling sites for huts and then went to the pictures in the evening. It was a wet, cold day again with sleet.

March 21 Wednesday
Breakfast: bacon. Dinner: roast mutton. Tea: as usual and I obtained some dripping from the cook house. We have parades as usual and I am levelling sites for the huts and supervising the Chesters on the same and making paths round the Officer's quarters. We had a big mail in and I received letters from Doll dated February 20th, 21st and March 9th and a letter from Mother of March 9th. I went to the pictures in the evening and tried to buy some bread but couldn't. We had a rum ration in the evening and I feel that I'm starting with a cold and have an irritating cough. The weather is fine generally but cold. I heard that the 12th Yorks and Lancs Division have been passing through Doullens on their way to Neuve Chapelle – I am sorry to have missed them.

March 22 Thursday
Breakfast: bacon. Dinner: bully stew and desiccated veg. Tea: as usual. There was no bread ration today and only about three biscuits apiece. We handed in our rifles, bayonets and scabbard with sling and bolt cover in the morning parade. I have never given up a best friend more cheerfully. I then finished levelling the huts in the morning. The weather a little snow. I wrote to Doll and then went to see the Archies at the cinema, Napoo as we are going away tomorrow. I heard that the 12th Yorks and Lancs were camping near Doullens last night.

March 23 Friday
Breakfast: cold bacon. Tea: sardines and as usual. Dinner: bully stew, desiccated veg and rice and currant pudding. I am in charge of the Chesters again who are putting up a latrine for the ASC. I was paid 20 francs and went to the pictures in the evening. It has been a bright, fine and cold day and we have changed huts again.

---

[290] **Chesters** - 12th (Service) Battalion Cheshire Regiment.

March 24 Saturday
Breakfast: bacon. Tea: as usual. Dinner: fresh meat, stew and potato. There is nothing much to do except watch the Chesters. In the afternoon saw 'Damn Daphne' and then was suddenly called out to be tested in levelling and a pretty mess we made of it, with strange staff level and officer flurrying us. I got my washing back in the evening and then had a rum ration. It has been a fine and cold day.

March 25 Sunday
Breakfast: bacon. Tea: roast beef. Tea: as usual. Summer time started today, so breakfast was really at 5.15am, so it was semi darkness. Our working hours today were from 7am – 12.30pm and then the afternoon was a holiday. I had nothing to do, so I helped to put the floor in the hut. I slept after dinner and went to the pictures in the evening. The weather was beautiful and the wind has gone down.

March 26 Monday
Breakfast: cold boiled bacon. Tea: as usual. Dinner: fresh mutton and stew. I had nothing to do all day and I am afraid that I shall be reduced to working on the line. I wrote to Teddie expressing my regrets at his loss of his Father. I was a wet day and I went to see the Archies in the evening, who have returned, they were rotten. I received letters from Doll and Carter both dated March 15th and a letter from Mother of March 16th. The Battalion (12th Yorks and Lancs) evidently went into advance soon after I left. They have had two of my parcels from the A.A.

March 27 Tuesday
Breakfast: bacon. Tea: as usual. Dinner: mutton stew. Today I had a rum ration and was putting up the hut. The weather has been cold with a little snow. I received a letter from Doll of March 22nd and I stopped in for the evening except for a late visit to a nearby estaminet for two hours where I had coffee and cake.

March 28 Wednesday
Breakfast: bacon. Tea: as usual. Dinner: roast beef which was very good, cauliflower and potatoes. I spent the day carpentering on the hut. I signed a form to transfer to the Royal Engineers and went to the pictures in the evening. It was a frosty morning afterwards, thawing and showery.

March 29 Thursday
Breakfast: bacon. Tea: as usual. Dinner: fresh meat stew. I spent the day carpentering followed by a rum ration. The weather was very wet. I hear indirectly that they are trying to transfer me elsewhere as an architect.

March 30 Friday
Breakfast: cold ham. Tea: as usual. Dinner: roast beef and boiled chestnuts. I spent the day carpentering in the hut. It has been a very wet day and was then

fine in the evening. I went to the pictures. We have had no bread for two days, so bought some at the YMCA. I received a parcel from the A.A. forwarded from Boulogne.

March 31 Saturday
Breakfast: bacon. Tea: as usual. Dinner: fresh, meat stew and boiled chestnuts. I spent the day carpentering in the huts again and there was hail and a thunderstorm in the afternoon. I received a letter from Carter, dated March 26th and they have received Mother's birthday parcel which was pronounced splendid. I sent a letter to Doll and A.A. and was on guard tonight and then read until 2am. I was very warm with both the brazier and lamp stove going.

April 1 Sunday
Breakfast: cold ham. Dinner: fresh meat stew. Tea: as usual. I was excused duty till 10 am and then we had a holiday in the afternoon except for a clothing parade. I went to the pictures in the evening and the weather was mostly fine with some showers.

April 2 Monday
Breakfast: cold ham. Tea: as usual. Dinner: roast beef and desiccated vegs. We had parades as usual. Last night was very frosty with a thaw in the morning and snow in the afternoon. I received a large belated mail with letters from Doll of February 26th and March 4th and 5th and letters from Mother of February 24th and March 3rd and a funeral card from Teddie of March 4th.

April 3 Tuesday (Our Second Wedding Anniversary)
Breakfast: bacon. Tea: as usual. Dinner: fresh meat stew. There was very little to do today, I am to join my platoon on the line till future orders in the morning. There was snow and some frost in the night and it was bright and warm in the afternoon. *Today is the second anniversary of my wedding - the best thing I did in my life.*

April 4 Wednesday
Breakfast: bacon. Tea: bread, marg and cheese. Dinner: roast beef and desiccated potatoes. Today was my first day back on the line; taking up points, crossing and replacing them and packing and heaving on crowbars and carrying rails and sleepers. It was the hardest and seemed to be the longest day's work I've done for some time. I did not leave till about 5pm and then went to the pictures in the evening. We were allowed only ½ hour for lunch, which we get on the job. It brought on my little weakness again akin to rupture. It has been a wet day.

April 5 Thursday
Breakfast: tea only served. Lunch: as yesterday. Dinner: unlimited fresh meat stew. I have been working on the line again as yesterday but decided to take it easy and assist the blacksmith in holding a striker. My sprain is now much better. I start taking a crossing out at 3.45pm so have to stop till 6pm to finish

replacing and I will get an hour off tomorrow for it. I received letters from Doll of March 20th and 21st and from Mother of March 25th and April 1s. It is almost bedtime by the finish of dinner and I clean up. It has been a beautifully fine and bright day.

April 6 Good Friday
Breakfast: bacon. Lunch: as before. Dinner: roast beef, cauliflower and roast chestnuts. We paraded at 8am and were then back on the line as before and I assisted the blacksmith again. It was a fine bright morning and was showery in the afternoon. I was paid 20 francs and then went to the pictures in the evening.

April 7 Saturday
Breakfast: bacon. Lunch was as before with strawberry jam. Dinner: roast beef, cauliflower and chestnuts. It has been an easy day and I have been flagging most of the time. I had a bath and changed into my clean washing. The weather is fine but there is a cold wind. I sent FPCs to Doll and Mother.

April 8 Easter Sunday
Breakfast: bacon. Dinner: fresh meat stew. Tea: strawberry jam, marg and cheese. There are no working parties today. We had breakfast at 8am and paraded at 9am for a gas helmet, groundsheet and steel helmet inspection and I then had to scrub the huts out afterwards. I sent letters to Doll and Mother and a green envelope to Doll. It was a perfect day; warm and bright.

April 9 Easter Monday
Breakfast: bacon. Lunch: as usual. Dinner: roast mutton and cauliflower. I had a nasty shock. I was fetched from the working party to be told that I was being sent back to the unit. The endeavours that had been made to get me on at Headquarters as an Architect have come to no avail. I was rationed for three days and exported **RTO**[291] to Doullens at 7pm. I was sent to Abbeville at 8.15pm to arrive at midnight. I had some cocoa at BEF and slept on the floor for the night. I sent a letter to Doll, Mother and A.A. It was a showery and cold day. My three days rations are not very appetising, they consist of loaf of bread, a of chunk of cheese, marg, three tins of bully, one tin of jam and a packet of tea. I make out at the canteen with buns and biscuits and I bought dates for 8 francs in Doullens, which always cost 1 franc before.

April 10 Tuesday
I arrived at an estaminet in Abbeville at 10am and got off about 11am and arrived at Etaples at 3.30pm and am taken to a rest camp. I go to the cinema in the afternoon which was a splendid show but am left in doubt as to the fate of 'Peg 'o the Ring' as she and her lover, after disposing of about ten villains are left facing a den of lions – further adventures are tomorrow. I get poached eggs

---

[291] **RTO – Road Traffic Officer** whose duty it is to direct the transport of troop movements and to assist soldiers who were returning to their units from leave.

and some beer at the canteen and have a comfortable night in a tent. There are bright spells during a cold day that are interspersed with blizzards.

April 11 Wednesday
I was roused at 5am with a mug of tea served and then went off for train at the station, which was said to be due at 6am. I eventually get off at 10am. There is free tea served at the YMCA. We stop at Calais, the nearest I shall be to dear Doll for some time, I fear. We also stop again outside St Omer. The weather is raining and sleeting diagonally. I'm glad that I'm not in the line today anyway. Reinforcements for the 31st Division were turned out at Lillers. It is wretched weather and I'm not having any, so go on to Bethune arriving at 9pm. The RTO comes around in trucks to inspect movement orders and sends me up to YMCA for the night to report at 10am in the morning where I got tea and beans and a kip on the floor. It was so crowded, there was only space to put only a foot in between. There was some heavy snow late in the afternoon, which then turned to sleet.

April 12 Thursday
I got shaved and washed at the YMCA and had bread, jam and cheese for breakfast and reported to the RTO at 10am and was told to stand to, awaiting further instructions. I had a vain search for a paper boy and return to find that the 31st Division had paraded, with transport to be found for them. I was ordered to stand to again, so go into town to get a paper, only to find on my return, that the 31st Division have gone off in motors. I join forces with three of our hospital cases that are returning and I am sent on 13th Corps motors to Verdun to find the Battalion that left yesterday. We meet our transport fetching our blankets and I hear that the 12th Yorks and Lancs are at Labourse, so I get another motor back to Bethune station. I go to the YMCA and make dinner from rations and tea and then wait at Charing X for a motor to Labouese. The Bosche are shelling Bethune meanwhile. One of our transport carts comes along, so we load our packs on it and walk behind it and we get to the Battalion at about 5pm at Sailly Labouese. It was nice to see the old Pals again. We had very leaky and draughty billets in a roof over the barn and I booze up with the boys in the evening. The weather is cold and bright during the day mostly, with rain in the morning.

April 13 Friday
Breakfast: bacon. Dinner: boiled mutton, broth and desiccated potatoes. Tea: jam and marg. I get my boots repaired at the cobblers in the morning and we have only about one hour's parade in the afternoon, passing messages. The Bosche are sending occasional shells all day at the coal mine nearby. We have drinks in the evening again and three fried eggs for supper. It was a fine and bright day. I sent FPCs to Doll and Mother and am given a rum ration and three blankets, so have a warm and cosy night. I did not get up till about 7.30am this morning which was rather a treat after late early rising. We paraded at 9.30am just for a rifle inspection. Sailly Labourse is a mining village with a YMCA. The 12th Yorks and Lancs band give a concert this evening.

179

April 14 Saturday
Breakfast: bacon. Dinner: fresh meat and bully stew. Tea: as usual. I got up at 6.30am and paraded at 8.40am for marching off and set off at 9am. It was good marching weather, cool and bright but my feet got rather sore in consequence of their two months rest. We arrived at our destination sooner than expected and as usual and were billeted at Hermin, a rural village and I am in a barn with plenty of dirty straw on the floor. I get three fried eggs for tea and stop imbibing coffee for the rest of the evening. My money is getting alarmingly low and I shall have to get Doll's 5/- changed as soon as possible. I sent my letters to Doll, Mother and Murvell. We passed through the dirty mining district at first on the march and crossed several ridges into hilly rural country.

April 15 Sunday
Breakfast: cold ham. Dinner: stew. Tea: treacle and marg. We were cleaning up and had a rifle inspection in the morning, followed by a first aid lecture by the Medical Officer. I have listened to many of these before almost unmoved and have waded among the dead and gore undeterred but today I first felt sick and then felt very much like fainting. One fellow did and this short excitement quite restored me. I had the A.A. pudding for dinner and spent the afternoon in the adjoining farm, hither sipping cafe nous and reading. It was a wretchedly wet day. I received a letter from Doll dated 5th April, a parcel from A.A. of March 28th and a letter dated April 5th. I wrote to Doll in a green envelope with enclosures for Mother and Mr Burke and also wrote to A.A. We could hear a heavy, distant bombardment going on this morning.

April 16 Monday
Breakfast: bacon. Dinner: veg soup, date pudding, tea. Tea: jam and cheese. We paraded at 9.30am and spent the morning getting our clothing and blankets fumigated, followed at 2.30pm by an inspection by the Medical Officer for scabies and then afterwards a firing and platoon drill till 4pm. I handed in my letters written yesterday. I went to the farm kitchen for coffee in the evening and then fried eggs with my A.A. sausages. It was a fine morning, which turned out wet at the end if the afternoon which then set in for the evening. We paraded first thing in the morning at the presentation of RSM Poulden with a Military Cross for nothing exceptional at all. My faith in the Military Cross is down.

April 17 Tuesday
Breakfast: bacon. Dinner: rissoles, breaded mutton and rice pudding. Tea: jam. We had field operations on the programme to parade at 9am. It was a wet morning so we stood to. We fell in at 1am and marched for about ½ hour through frequent hailstorms and then turned back and were dismissed at about 2.15pm. I was paid 15 francs and was imbibing coffee and fried eggs in the evening. The weather has been rain, hail and snowstorms all day with bright intervals.

April 18 Wednesday

Breakfast: rissoles. Dinner: mutton and boiled Maconochies. Tea: minced bully and jam. We stood to in the morning and had a lecture in the billet till about 11am and then went to the parade field for bayonet fighting. In the afternoon we marched to the Labourse range where we had firing and advancing by platoons and the rifle grenadiers and bombers did not take part at all. I received a letter from Doll dated April 11th and from Mother dated April 9th. The weather has been showery all day. We received a rum ration at night and I was sent for by Captain Leaman to consult with **Mr Pimm**[292] about the string point to be constructed tomorrow. I then went for coffee and eggs in the evening.

April 19 Thursday

Breakfast: bacon. Dinner: stew. Tea: ham and ham. We paraded at 8.45am and then stood to for about ½ hour. I started on the string point which was to be finished in two hours, which was done and gained approval from the powers that be. We had a gas helmet drill for ¼ hour and then only a parade in the billets in the afternoon. I received a letter from Mother of April 15th and then had coffee and eggs in the evening. It has been a fine morning with a little rain in the afternoon.

April 20 Friday

Breakfast: cold bacon, ample. Dinner: stewed mutton and beef with boiled chestnuts and pork and beans all in abundance. Tea: currant bread pudding. We had a morning route march from 9.30am till 12 noon which was about six miles and then a good rest. In the afternoon we paraded for drills with an extended order for the outpost. It was a beautifully fine day. I had coffee and eggs in the evening and received a letter from Doll dated April 15th and had a rum ration.

April 21 Saturday

Breakfast: bacon. Dinner: roast mutton, boiled Maconochies and beans. Tea: stewed currants and bread and currant pudding. We had a bath parade in the morning at the splendid showers baths at **Houchin**[293] and then a 20 minute bon respirator drill on our return. In the afternoon we marched ¾ hour away for open warfare attack. I had eggs and coffee in the evening and it has been a fine and bright day. There is a rumour that we are going on the railway construction job again.

April 22 Sunday

Breakfast: bacon. Dinner: Roast mutton with baked beans and steamed bully. Tea: jam and marg. We had a Church parade in the morning and then had the afternoon off. It was a fine and bright day and I got some violets to send to Doll.

---

[292] **Lieutenant C. W. Pimm** - Served with 12th Y&L from 15th April 1917. He was killed in action on 18th May 1917 and is buried in Bailleul Road Military Cemetery.

[293] **Houchin** - The **town** of Houchin is located in the department of Pas-de-Calais of the French region Nord-Pas-de-Calais.

I had coffee and eggs in the evening and the latest rumour is that Austria have chucked it.

April 23 Monday
Breakfast: cold bacon. Dinner: roast mutton and fig pudding. Tea: jam and marg. The bombardment which we have heard almost incessantly since coming here reached its intensest last night apparently all day along the front. We had an easy morning and then went to the bombing trenches and messed about and a lecture with No.23 Milner Rifle grenade and I was a spectator only of a bombing and grenade attack. In the afternoon we had a bit of a rifle drill then a short march along the road with outposts and we were not back until 5pm though. I had coffee and eggs in the evening again and then wrote to Doll and Mother. It has been a beautifully bright day.

April 24 Tuesday
Breakfast: bacon. Dinner and Tea together: cold roast mutton, boiled chestnuts, marmalade and marg.
We paraded at 8.30am and returned at 5pm which consisted of a field day ¾ hour march away. We had an extended order to attack on the trenches and we did it four times. I was touched in the last one and was made a casualty and was sent off. I lunched off of bacon saved from breakfast with bread, biscuits, marg and cheese. I gave in a green envelope containing the letters written yesterday. It has been a beautifully bright day again. I had coffee and a short spell of 'bru anglais' mopping in the evening and I was paid 10 francs.

April 25 Wednesday
Breakfast: Maconochies. Dinner: roast mutton and veg stew. Tea: marmalade and marg. In the morning from 9am – 11.30am we were firing in respirators and had open fighting. In the afternoon we had races and games from 2pm to 4pm and in the evening we had an open air concert and a band. The weather is fine but it was a cold day.

April 26 Thursday
Breakfast: Maconochies boiled. Dinner and Tea together, roast mutton, mashed desiccated eggs and pork and beans, biscuit pudding and marmalade and marg. We had more bread later than I can get through. We paraded at 8.15am for a field day and we were back at 4pm. We had manoeuvres four miles away beyond Magnicourt, where we had to attack twice and General Wanless O'Gowan declared us defeated by the enemy at the first attempt. I received letters from Doll of April 17th, Teddy of 23rd April and a 'Passing Show' from Maud dated 21st April. I hoped to settle down for a restful evening but instead was I was at it till long after lights out, preparing for a marching order inspection by the Brigadier. It was a fine day.

April 27 Friday
Breakfast: rissoles. Dinner: roast mutton, boiled chestnuts and turnips. Tea: marmalade and marg. C Company who were detailed for an inspection paraded

and were quite smart as regards cleanliness but not at all so in their parade drill. The Officers also got a wigging. The result was that we were in disgrace and had ½ hour close Company drill this evening on a ground a mile away. I don't think anyone will dare ask Captain Leaman which platoon has won 50 cigs per man for the smartest turned out. I had a bath again at Houchin and received a letter from Mother dated April 24ᵗʰ. The general idea is that we are going in the line in few days time. I had beer, fried eggs and coffee for the rest of the evening. It has been a fine and warm day.

April 28 Saturday
Breakfast: bacon. Dinner: stew and rice pudding. Tea: marmalade, cheese and marg. From 9am till 12 noon we had various drills and we were hard at it. From 1pm till 6pm we had ¾ hour march, a Battalion drill and an outpost scheme and then marched back again – it was a heavy day. I sent an FPC to Doll and had eggs and coffee in the evening. It has been a fine and warm day.

April 29 Sunday
Breakfast: cold bacon, very meagre. Dinner: stew, pork and beans, tea. Tea: rice pudding, marmalade. Instead of parading at 11am for a six kilometre march as announced last night, we fall in at 9.20am and do 16 kilometres. We pass through Mont St Eloi to Bray which is adjoining Ecoivres, arriving at 2.45pm, very hot and rather weary. Many fell out and the road was especially strewn with the East Lancs. It looks as if we should be over the top in a few days. I got a pass in the evening for Ecoivres and shared a bottle of vin rouge with Carter for four francs. I could have got fried eggs but there was no bread so I went without. It was a perfect day. Why do they always pinch our next Sunday for marching? We are billeted in bow huts. We were told at first that we should move at 4am in the morning but we are given late orders and parade instead for Maroeuil at 9.45am.

April 30 Monday
Breakfast: cold mutton chops. Dinner: sea pie. Tea: jam and marg. We marched off at 9.50am for Maroeuil which is only four kilometres away but we did the usual circle or rather invented a question mark of doing a good eight kilometres. We were billeted in bow huts again and were not allowed out of the camp. The weather is a long hot summer day. 114 German prisoners looking well and content, straight from the line pass our camp. Two of my platoon, for eating their iron ration biscuits, are given 28 days **field punishment.**[294] I received a parcel from Mother which contained a cake, pork pie, mince pies, apples, Kampfire, magazine. I sent an FPC to Mother and to F.E.P. Edwards and wrote to Maud.

---

[294] **Field Punishment** - Field Punishment No. 1 comprised of a British Army punishment imposed for minor offences such as drunkenness, and was often applied during the First World War. It was a most humiliating form of punishment which continued into the late 1920s, Field Punishment No.1 saw the soldier in question attached standing full-length to a fixed object - either a post or a gun wheel - for up to two hours a day (often one hour in the morning and another in the afternoon) for a maximum of 21 days.

May 1 Tuesday

Breakfast: rissoles. Dinner: stew and rice pudding. Tea: bread and marg. We fell in at 9.30am and moved off at 10am. I saw a German aeroplane fired down while waiting and the occupants are captured alive. Our destination started to be St Katherine, a suburb of Arras only five kilometres away but we marched right through it and occupy the late German 4th line, the whole neighbourhood is marked with shell holes. We have no shelter or blankets now, so we dig a shelter in the side of the trench. There are plenty of souvenirs still knocking about; helmets, ammunition, coats etc and a few corpses. I'm Corporal of the platoon guard. It has been a fine and bright day again and cool in the evening.

9
Oppy Wood and the Cadorna Raid

May 2 Wednesday

I have been resting in the trench during the day and wrote to Mother and Doll in a green envelope and am I awaiting the chance to get it posted, goodness knows when. We are the carrying party to the trenches at night as part of our Division are going over the top. We are late in arriving and come in for part of the strafe and many fellows are knocked out around me. I collect six of my platoon and make our way out as ordered. We lose our way and eventually find the Battalion at about 5.30am the next morning, who have moved since we last left. I received a letter from Doll dated April 29th. It has been perfect weather today.

May 3 Thursday

The news that the Germans are counter attacking comes at about 6.30am, we then parade at 7am for the support trench, to which we march in artillery formation straight away and we are heavily shelled all day. Captain Leaman is continually moving 11 Platoon just as soon as we'd dug in at one place to another. We had **one killed** [295] and about six wounded in the Company. The line in front of us has a rotten time and are often driven out of their trenches into the open by shell fire. We don't even know who holds **Oppy Wood**[296] in front of us till the evening when the German lights decide it. *I rather enjoy this excitement and my only worry is about dear Doll and Mother if anything happens to me.* Personally life seems so cheap now that even one's own doesn't seem of much importance. It has been fine weather.

---

[295] **31587 Private Percy Robinson Deville** - was killed in action and is buried in Bailleul Road Military Cemetery.
[296] **Oppy Wood** – and the village of Oppy are situated in a mining area in the north of France, close to Arras and is more akin to the four City Battalions from Hull who fought there, with the loss of many men.

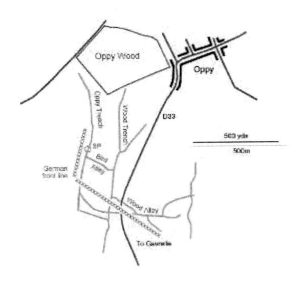

Map showing Oppy Wood and the trench system

May 4 Friday

I get decently dug in at last in a cushy spot, then of course we are moved to another part in the evening. It was very shallow and we had to start all over again. We were at it all night and I was very thirsty and had less than half a pint of water issued since we came in and we had no time to fill our bottles. Even when we started off, mine was only half full but we are well off for grub. It has been perfect weather till the evening then there was much thunder and a few spots of rain.

May 5 Saturday

We still have no water this morning. **Corporal Stimson**[297] and six men go out for six hours during the night looking for water and failed. I take two men at dinner time and a 1½ hours walk brings us to a water supply and we bring back two petrol cans each. We evacuated the trench soon after my return, in fact before I got the water going for some tea. Some of the precious water that I brought was wasted as we were saving it in the can and had no time to dish it out. We were very heavily shelled before we left and so occupy the trenches further back. It is perfect weather and we dig holes to sleep in.

May 6 Sunday

I received a letter from Mother dated April 29th and from Arthur dated May 1st. We were shelled this morning almost as much as in the front, and we had **one killed**[298] and one wounded in the Company. We were shelled in the evening

---

[297] **12/790 Corporal A. Stimpson** - a member of C Company who took part in the attack on 1st July 1916.

[298] **31626 Private William Hooton** was killed in action as is buried in Bailleul Road Military Cemetery.

186

with many casualties among passing units and artillery transport. We are the carrying party this evening and have some casualties in the Company from shell fire. The German lines that we pass through are filled with our dead, they must have been taken at a heavy cost. It has been perfect weather.

May 7 Monday

We hear that the Barnsleys have taken Oppy Wood this morning but this is as yet unconfirmed. A party is going to the army rest camp this morning so I have given in a green envelope and letters to Doll and Mother which were written on 2nd May with added postscripts up to date. They are taken to the orderly room to be carried by hand to the transport line and there posted. It is stated that we are going in the front line tonight. Later I am detailed with two men presumably as an advance party. I am pleasantly surprised to find it is to take over trenches further back still and then send out guides to same. **Major Allen**[299] passes round a bottle of whiskey and Moka Egyptian cigs which are a great treat. Rain threatens but I decide to sleep in the open in preference to the dugout or shelter. I am sorry afterwards as the rain steadily sets in and it later pours.

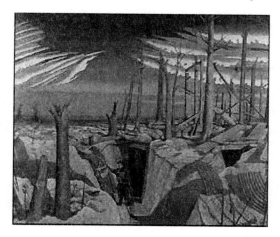

"Oppy Wood, 1917" by Paul Nash. Reproduced by permission of the Imperial War Museum, London.

May 8 Tuesday

Breakfast: boiled bacon. Dinner: bully. Tea: jam and orange. It has been pouring with rain all night. I am awakened at about 4am lying in pools of it. I am sent out with two men to look for **Corporal Hall's**[300] party and guide them home. It

---

[299] **Major D. C. Allen** – also served with the Tank Corps.

[300] **12/664 Private Herbert Hall** - was a sniper and Lewis gunner. He took part in the attack on 1st July 1916 and was later commissioned to Kings Own Yorkshire Light Infantry. In the book, Sheffield City Battalion by Ralph Gibson and Paul Oldfield he is quoted as saying: 'the food at first left a lot to be desired, after all the cooks were learning and it was 'Hobson's Choice' if it was edible or not. There was a chap in our hut at Redmires who seemed to be continuously hungry, always asking if you had any spare

is pouring all of the time and they turned up at about 7am but I missed breakfast tea. There is a rumour of a successful German counter attack. We are paraded to go up in line at once and then the order is changed to stand to. A little later on I am sent for and told that I am going with five men on a Division job. I have to go to the transport lines to draw the equipment and am given a blanket and two days rations. The result is that I am three hours late at the rendezvous and there are no signs of habitation there. I finally report to the Company at 8.30pm and am told to stop, awaiting further orders. I have been sitting about all day with a full pack etc. The job is one to do with the trenches. Blasted are visions of Boulogne and the railway jobs again and I miss the working party, which is one consolation. After a supper of salmon, cold bacon, dates, tea etc, I then enjoy a very cosy night with a blanket. I receive a letter from Doll dated May 4th given to me at transport. The weather in the afternoon turned out nice and fine.

May 9 Wednesday
Breakfast: bacon. Dinner: bully. Tea: marmalade and marg. I was awakened about 8am with a rum ration as we have had every day lately. It is a bright hot day and I get cleaned up, washed and shaved and fry rashers of bacon again. Preparations are being made to go in the front line tonight and I am awaiting instructions about my Division job. I should know by about 4pm and was ordered to report to Divisional HQ at 8pm. I met **Mr Mitchell,**[301] the Area 1 Commandant on the way, a Scotsman who impressed me very favourably as a decent sort. We live with him in a German dugout in the trenches. I have to go out and make a list with particulars of all the dugouts, shelters, tents etc in the area. I superintend the same with ten men with us, regarding sanitary conditions, maintenance and the arrival and departure of units. Our dugout is just out of shell fire on a scale but the front of our area gets it very hot.

May 10 Thursday
Breakfast: bacon. Dinner: steak. Tea: jam and marg, cheese. I was out all morning with Mr Mitchell taking dugouts etc in **Stellung**[302] he gets very tired and fed up, so leaves me to it and I don't get back till 4pm. It was a very hot day. I was appointed by one of the men as cook who looks after me very well. I sent an FPC to Doll and Mother. The 12th Yorks and Lancs went into the front line last night on a very hot sector which cost us about **50 men,**[303] so I'm well out of it. Mr Mitchell is rather pessimistic and gives this job a week but I think it will last while the Division holds this front. It's up to us to manage it properly but Mr Mitchell doesn't show much energy and takes things too easily. I shall

---

food, he must have had hollow legs. Even when in the trenches he was a fearless scrounger, always on the lookout for food. His name was 12/729 Francis Meakin'.

[301] **Captain G. Mitchell** – with the Battalion from December 1915.

[302] **Stellung** – is the German word for position. In the aftermath of the carnage of the 1916 Battle of the Somme, the German Army began to execute a skilful retirement to the prepared positions of the "Siegfried Stellung" or Hindenburg Line in late February 1917.

[303] **16166 Private Joseph Boocock , 37936 Private Wray Crabtree and 27794 Private Lewis Harrison** were among those killed. **31965 Private Alfred Beaumont** died the following day. They are all commemorated on the Arras Memorial.

have to do most of the work myself. The men are mostly duds and no use as assistants. I shall just use them at present for cleaning up around the dugout, carrying rations, water etc.

May 11 Friday
Breakfast: steak and bacon. Dinner: stew and beans, little potatoes and onions. Tea: marmalade and marg. I go out with two men in the morning but they are only a nuisance and do the middle sector of our area. Mr Mitchell also goes out with two men to do the far area. I get back about 2.30pm and find that he has returned two hours before. When we come to tabulate our results in the evening I find that he has got his mixed up and the map references are wrong, so I shall have to go and do it again tomorrow. The day is very hot again and I at work till dark going over the lists with Mr Mitchell. I draw a rum ration tonight.

May 12 Saturday
Breakfast: bacon. Dinner: cold beef and potatoes, rice pudding. Tea: marmalade, marg and cheese. I take three men with me just to get them used to the ground. There is plenty of shrapnel about the railway cutting and **Lieutenant Berry**[304] and **2 men**[305] are killed at BHQ and two are wounded just before I get there. I do all of the dugouts very thoroughly and get back at 3.30pm and then am working with the lists with Mr Mitchell until 7pm. I send letters to Doll, Mother and Orderly Corporal Dale. I hear that our Battalion has lost **48 men**[306] in the first 24 hours and that the ration party of 30 were practically wiped out. It has been a hot day again with thunderstorms in the evening. I received letters from Doll and Mother dated May 6th. Jim Wood turned up tonight with Legs 11 who is the burial officer.

May 13 Sunday
Breakfast: bacon. Dinner: steak, potatoes, baked beans. Tea: marmalade, marg, cheese and orange. I am out from 9am till 1pm listing dugouts and shelters again and tabulating the same with Mr Mitchell in the afternoon. I go down to see Jim Wood in the evening and partake of milk and rum punch with him and swap reminiscences with him till nearly 10pm. I lose myself on returning because the sky is as dark as a bag and it is drizzling after a fine close day. I retrace my steps and set off again, this time successfully, getting in at 12.30 midnight. We are living like Lords with an abundance of rations.

---

[304] **Lieutenant R. D. Berry** – killed in action 12th May 1917, he is buried in Albuera Military Cemetery, Bailleul.

[305] **43898 Private Howard Hern** who is buried at Albuera Military Cemetery and **31618 Private Henry Hooton** who is buried in Ballieul Road Military Cemetery were both killed in action on 12th May 1917.

[306] **4845 Private A. Bullivant, 12/1052 Private John William Fell, 32002 Private James Septimus Johnson, 38046 Private William Smith, 12/262 Private P. M. West** and **12/413 Private John Humphrey, 39042 Private Wilfred Handley** Were among those killed were all of whom are commemorated on the Arras Memorial.

May 14 Monday

Breakfast: bacon. Dinner: roast mutton, potatoes and beans. Tea: jam, cheese and marg. Supper: boiled ham. 1 am out all morning attempting to find various army FA brigades and only discover half but Mr Mitchell comes with results nil. It is a fine morning but very wet in the afternoon so we abandon the idea of going out in further search of the present. I spend the rest of the time reading down in the dugout which is cold and dark. Mr Mitchell gives me part of a tin of apricots for supper.

May 15 Tuesday

Breakfast: bacon. Dinner: steak, very tender, potatoes, baked beans and boiled chestnuts. Tea: jam, cheese and marg. I take an easy stroll around in the morning looking at the units of the siege Battalions close to hand, then tabulating the same with Mr Mitchell in the afternoon. The weather is misty in the early morning and then a fine bright and fresh day and chilly in the evening.

May 16 Wednesday

Breakfast: bacon. Dinner: mutton chops, potatoes, boiled chestnuts and rice pudding. Tea: as usual. In the morning I patrolled the Northern limit of our area and partly explored Bailleul and discovered more dugouts and was fortunate to hit on a quiet spell while there. I was not back till 3pm so dinner was cold and rather spoilt again. I stopped in the dugout reading for the rest of the afternoon and evening, the weather being wet. I received a letter from Doll dated May 9th.

May 17 Thursday

Breakfast: bacon. Dinner: steak, onions, potatoes and baked beans. Tea: as usual. I spent the morning in Bailleul and find a lot more dugouts. The Bosche only start to shell the place ten minutes after we leave. It has been a damp and hazy morning, turning rather wet.

May 18 Friday

Breakfast: bacon. Dinner: roast fillet of mutton, potatoes and baked beans. Tea: as usual. I went out with Mr Mitchell to the BHQ in the morning, he gets the considerable **wind up**[307] on account of the shelling around there and we return double quick. We then walk aimlessly around the tent accommodation in the afternoon. I receive a letter from Doll dated May 12th and go and chat with Jim Wood in the evening. It has been a fine and bright day.

May 19 Saturday

Breakfast: bacon. Dinner: roast fillet of mutton, potatoes, baked beans, onions, rice and raisin pudding. Tea: as usual. In our orders, 63rd relieves our Division tomorrow and we are to hand over and probably join the Battalion between then and the 22nd May. I spend the morning and afternoon checking a few points and am always in danger from shells. I receive a letter from Doll dated May 14th and

---

[307] **Wind up** – Fear, not to be confused with 'cold feet' which means to back out of duty. To have the 'wind up' was no disgrace and could be mentioned in conversation, although usually in the past tense.

write to Doll and Mother and I then went down to see Jim Wood again and borrowed 'New Worlds for Old' from him. The weather is a fine and it has been a warm day.

May 20 Sunday
Breakfast: bacon. Dinner: roast shoulder of mutton, potatoes, boiled onions and baked beans. Tea: as usual. The **HAC**[308] 63rd Division came and took over in the morning and we did not go out and are to remain here till 22nd May. I went to Arras in the afternoon to look round and get a bath and change on the way. Much of Arras is smashed up beyond repair. The Cathedral is a sad mess but many of the main thoroughfares only need resurfacing and glazing, of course all the walls are pitted with shrapnel and a building here and there is blown in. The place was fearfully crowded with troops and the estaminets were too full to get near. Mr Mitchell lent me 5 francs and I met Matthews hurrying off on leave and saw several of 113 REs in town. I received a letter from Doll dated May 17th

May 21 Monday
Breakfast: bacon. Dinner: beef fillets (roasted and tough) potatoes, baked beans. Tea: as usual. I was up at 5am to show the relief around. I should have started at 6am but the Corporal was late, so I had to wait for him till 7am and was back at 9.30am for breakfast. I did nothing for the rest of the day. We are to clear out first thing in the morning. I wrote to Doll telling her to warn Mrs B in case I get my leave.

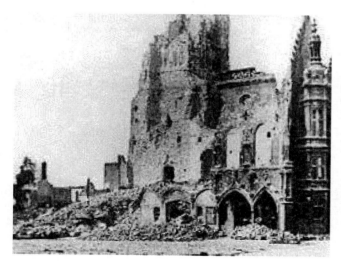

Arras Cathedral in 1917

---

[308] **H.A.C. - The Honorable Artillery Company** was incorporated by Royal Charter in 1537 by King Henry VIII. Today it is a Registered Charity whose purpose is to attend to the "better defence of the realm". This purpose is primarily achieved by the support of the HAC Regiment and a detachment of Special Constabulary to the City of London Police.

May 22 Tuesday

We had bacon as usual for breakfast but it has been raining all night and I cannot keep the fire in to boil or cook so I have a breakfast of bully beef, bread and marg. We wait in the dugout afterwards to see if the weather clears before we set out. We start off about 1am, the weather having cleared. We make a beeline for Marceuil, which was very heavy going through mud and I was fearful as I have lots of crocks with me which was a rotten job getting them along. We arrive at the Battalion at about 4pm to find them billeted in a mill in the village. I was shocked to hear that **Ellis**[309] had been killed and several others including **Mr Pimm**.[310] The beds in the billets are in threes and I get a middle one. I buy some eggs and cook part of the bacon that I brought with me for supper.

May 23 Wednesday

Breakfast: bacon. Dinner: stew (very good) and rice pudding. Tea: marmalade. We parade with the rifle grenadiers under Westby, very easy days and walk to the parade grounds about ½ mile away. We then sat down for a lecture in both the morning and the afternoon lasting about one hour each, I also go to have a bath in the morning. I receive a 'Passing Show' from Maud and was paid 30 francs. I go to the Archies concert in the evening, thinking it was the cinema, it was passable. I then made eggs and bacon for supper.

May 24 Thursday

Early morning tea. Breakfast: bacon. Dinner: rissoles, potatoes, baked beans, mutton, broth and bread. Tea: as usual. We paraded at from 7.30am till 8.45am, cleaning up beforehand for the same. We parade again at 9.30am for new CO's inspection, who turns out to be Major Allen after all and we were back at 1pm. We had no parade in the afternoon. I then wash my socks, go to sleep and go to the cinema after tea to see 'Blind Justice' which was very good. I received a letter from Mother dated May 14th. **Sergeant Gould**[311] tells me there are many promotions in C Company but Leaman won't entertain me, so I shall see other fellows put over me again. As long as he regards me as a dud and sends me off for jobs, I am content. I spend the evening writing to Doll and it is another fine day but cooler.

May 25 Friday

Early morning tea. Breakfast: bacon. Dinner: boiled mutton, onions and potatoes. Tea: dates. We had parades as yesterday but were firing on the range in the morning. We are given five rounds to deliver, I scored 19 out of 20 but at a

---

[309] **21891 Corporal Henry Cecil Ellis** was killed in action on 18th May 1917 and is commemorated on the Arras Memorial.

[310] **2nd Lieutenant C. W. Pimm** was killed in action on 18th May 1917 and is buried in Bailleul Road Military Cemetery, Blangy. He was commissioned on 1st March 1917 and served with 12th Y&L from 15th April 1917.

[311] **12/656 Sergeant Joseph William Gould**, was a teacher who served with 12th Y&L during the attack on 1st July 1916. He was killed in action on 13th October 1918 whilst serving with 5th Y&L and is buried in York Military Cemetery, Haspres.

rapid rate I only scored 9. Captain Leaman reads out the promotions for all sorts and conditions of men but as expected, pas mois. The day is fine and warm again. The Bosche drop two shells our way on the early morning parade which was very unexpected. I write to Mother and enclose a green envelope to Doll and give in. I visited **14th Yorks and Lancs**[312] and saw Mr Mitchell to pay him the 5 francs that he lent me. He took details of my Company and Battalion and said that he would ask for me, if he got another Commandant job. There is a rumour that we are likely to go back to the support trenches soon for digging, also Lestrem is not dead. Leaves look like they are getting along pretty fast again. I received letters from Mother dated May 20th, Auntie Annie dated May 21st and a 'Passing Show' from Maud.

May 26 Saturday
Breakfast: rissoles. Dinner: Maconochies stew, boiled mutton and rice pudding. Tea: as usual. We had an early morning parade as usual from 9.30am till 1pm which was a musketry and platoon drill. I am warned for Battalion orderly soon at the early morning parade, my first idea is leave but no. Then another outside job seems possible for some time. I then get an uneasy feeling that Leaman has been getting me reduced which proves correct. I'm reduced to my permanent rank of Lieutenant Corporal. No doubt Leaman wishes he could have deprived me of the lot. I told them Captain Cousins was under no misapprehension as to my parade abilities when he promoted me. Leaman's retort is that the trenches are not everything. I spent the rest of the day washing and reading.

May 27 Sunday
Breakfast: bacon. Dinner: Maconochies stew. Tea: as usual. We fell in at 8.20am to go back to the support trenches as a working party and make the usual long detour and arrive at about 11am. We are put in tents and bivouacs as far as our accommodation will allow. I rest all day and am to turn out at 8pm for digging several trenches. We work from 10pm till 2am and will have an extra hour if not enough is done by battle order. There is a well stocked canteen nearby, so I replenish my cigs, matches and biscuits. I have finished 'New Worlds for Old'. H.G. Wells's interest in socialism has revived my thinking. It took 1¼ hours to march to our job with everyone taking turns with the machine gun panniers. There is some pretty lively shelling going on around the job and we work for four hours and get back at about 3.20am and have breakfast at once. It has been a hot and bright day.

May 28 Monday
Breakfast: bacon. Dinner: bully stew mixed with potatoes and rice. Tea: as usual. I slept till midday and a parade was announced for 1.45pm, so I shaved and washed and then had a drill order. We messed about as usual with various counter orders. I dodge parade after all by going to the cobblers to get my boots repaired. It was a hot and bright day. Jeremy (Jim) Wood has given in his stripes and has gone to Transport. We are off digging in the trenches as last

---

[312] **14th York and Lancaster – 2nd** Barnsley Pals Battalion.

night and had some lively shelling again. We are given the task to work and go when we've finished which was about 1am and we were back before three and had breakfast immediately.

May 29 Tuesday
Breakfast: bacon. Dinner: bully and Maconochies stew and rice pudding. Tea: as usual. It rained a little in the night and is much cooler. I slept till 11.45am and I am told that my leave will start on 31st May, so I wrote to Doll, Mother and Arthur accordingly. We had one hour's Company drill and musketry drill in the afternoon on rotten rough ground ½ mile away. It was a bit too thick considering that we have a ten mile march battle order and four hours work each night. I have an easy night's work again and get finished by midnight and have two good rests on the way back again, returning to the camp soon after 2am but am still very tired all the same. It has been a fine day.

May 30 Wednesday
Breakfast: bacon. Dinner: rissole and potatoes. Tea: as usual. We paraded in the afternoon in our shirt sleeves but soon it began to rain so we are returned to camp afterwards and they were very heavy showers. I am told about 6pm that my leave was postponed by two days. That is all right so long as it's no longer. There is no working tomorrow, thank goodness. I went to the trenches again at night but some are full of water and tracking across the plain is dreadfully heavy going and I am done in before I arrive. Most of C Company are taken back almost immediately but the remainder of us stop till midnight doing practically nothing. We got back at 2am and were very weary and had breakfast as usual about 2.30am.

May 31 Thursday
Breakfast: bacon. Dinner: rissoles, potatoes, baked beans. Tea: as usual and I buy tea and pineapple. I slept until midday again and had an afternoon parade as usual. There is no working party tonight but there is a Brigade concert in the evening at which 20% are compelled to attend. The next leave batch is being warned for June 4th and I suppose that I shall go with them and have written to Doll and Mother accordingly. We see a fine daring lot of work by a Bosche aeroplane. Flying low, he comes over us at a remarkable speed, firing a machine gun at our observation posts, which apparently he does not hit. But four occupants of two of the same tumble out in remarkable haste in parachutes, which drift a long way towards the German lines and one looks like landing in them. The Bosche safely returns, absolutely out-distancing our shells. It has been a fine and warm day and I received a letter from Doll dated May 27th. We had a new change of clothing today and had to hand in all of our pants.

June 1 Friday
Breakfast: bacon. Dinner: rissoles, potatoes, baked beans. Tea: stewed dates and marg. I slept well at the beginning of the night but there was much enemy aeroplane activity at dawn and we continued with our anti aircraft guns and machine guns rattling away. We paraded at 12.30pm and then I dozed for part

of the afternoon. They send for me from the orderly room to ask the date when I returned from my last leave. I am getting uneasy and feel they will do me in if they can. The first draft who came to France late in April, complain that they should have their leave first. We don't parade for the working party till 8.30pm tonight. I received a letter from Mother dated May 28th. Today is a fine and bright day and it is no longer oppressive. **Major Hood**[313] has taken over our command again and we have to parade in strict battle order, with rations, ground sheet, billy can etc. We take a short cut over the trenches and it takes us ½ hour longer than usual. We work till 2am instead of the task and less work is done. A full marching order inspection is announced for 3pm tomorrow.

June 2 Saturday
Breakfast: bacon, just tea at lunch. Tea: as usual. Dinner: rissoles, potatoes, pickled onion, rice pudding. I was up at 11.45am and immediately commence operations for inspection. At 1.30pm this changed to a kit inspection at 2pm. Then a 2.15pm we get deemed for a parade and inspected to be clean as if for the 3 o'clock inspection as originally announced. We are kept at musketry and bayonet drill till 4.15pm and we do not have a minute's rest till 7.30pm after dinner. I have never been so fed up. I received a letter from Doll of May 29th. Meals are now breakfast at 4am, lunch just tea at 4.30pm and dinner at 7pm. We are parading for work at 8.20pm and deepening an old communication trench. We could have done the task in 1½ hours but we were kept till 1.30am. It has been a fine and bright day with a slight shower in the evening but then it cleared again. A German aeroplane came over while we were at work and dropped many bombs but they were some distance away.

June 3 Sunday
Breakfast: bacon – just tea at lunch. Tea: as usual. Dinner: roast mutton, potatoes, baked beans, rice pudding. We parade in full marching order for the CO's inspection. We fall in at 2pm and the inspection is most rigorous. A fellow was caught with dirty billies, making no time as his excuse and was told that they had had more time than they had ever had before. We are not parading till 1pm and only for two hours, which is pretty good considering the eight hours we do at night. I am happy again as I am down for leave tomorrow. The CSM refuses to entertain the idea of excusing us on the working party but **Sergeant Briggs**[314] sees all the officers and we are excused just as we are ready to march off, it feels quite a reprieve. It has been a fine, bright and fresh day. There is a Bosche aeroplane raid over the camp and they drop many bombs quite close at about 11.30pm. The working party has a similar experience and D Company has **three hit**[315] and one has his arm blown off.

---

[313] **Major (Lieutenant Colonel) F. J. C. Hood** – commanded the Battalion from 1st June 1917 until 28 February 1918 having transferred from 13th York and Lancaster.

[314] **23155 Sergeant G. Briggs**, he also served with 2nd Y&L and deserted on 13th October 1917.

[315] **22258 Private Thomas Chapman** died the following day on 4th June 1917 and is commemorated on the Arras Memorial and **29082 Private Harry Jones** died three days later on 6th June 1917 however CWGC have no record of his burial.

June 4 Monday

I only secure a tin of bully and a few biscuits for two days rations. I report to the orderly room at 10am and I am to be at Ecurie Station, which is half an hour's walk, at 11am. I find that the train is not due till 2pm and it actually leaves at 3.15pm. I get chocolates and biscuits at the canteen. It is a perfect day. We do not stop at Ecroives, so I cannot get further pay as per my arrangement. I arrive at Ligny at 6.25pm and we are due out at 7.40pm. I had some rotten beer and could have obtained some eggs but there was no bread. I try to send a telegram but with no success. I arrive in Boulogne at 12.45am and proceed to the billets near to the station. There is a fearful crush for the canteen for tea and biscuits. No cigarettes are available other than Woodbines and I enjoy the luxury of bed boards for a short sleep.

June 5 Tuesday

Lunch: cheese, bread, marg, jam and tea. Dinner: boiled cold beef, sauce and bread. I was up early and had a good wash and expect the boat to go at 9am. I had to buy breakfast at the canteen, duty work. We parade at 9.45am but we are marched to the next camp at the top of the hill, a horrid sweat. We are to get our passes extended and expect to sail in the morning. I get some tinned rabbit given to me by fellows at both lunch and dinner and there was a great fight for food at the canteen. It has been a hot day and was cool in the afternoon, of which I spent most of it dozing in the afternoon.

June 6 Wednesday

Breakfast: cold bacon, orange, jam. We had a reveille at 3.30am and breakfast at 4am and I obtain enough fat bacon etc for lunch on board. We parade at 6am and have our passes extended and then march off about 7am. We are on board at 8.30am and sail at 9.30am. Previously fellows with souvenirs were frightened into giving them up but no examination followed. It was a choppy passage but I saw nobody being ill. We land at 11.30am and I was in the first bout out and the last in but secure a 1st class carriage seat in the Officer's train. We leave Folkestone at 12.15pm and arrive in Victoria at 2.30pm. I go straight to the Army Pay Office and ask for £10 as I have a £12 balance. The clerk says I have nothing like it and only gives me £3. I let him have my unrestrained opinion and tell him that he ought to be at the front instead of doing incompetent work there. I send a wire to Doll and Mother about 3pm. I have a meal of two sausages, fried eggs, bread and butter, coffee and tea for 1/-. The Buckingham Palace Hotel now seems like the Church Army. I catch the 4.15pm train from St Pancras.

June 7 Thursday – June 15 Friday On leave

June 16 Saturday

I reported to the RTO at 12.40pm and was given a slip to catch the 7.20am train the next morning.

196

June 17 Sunday

No trains, buses or trams are running and I fail to get a taxi, so walk from the Norfolk Hotel in Surrey Street near the Strand to Victoria and do it in thirty five minutes. Several trains with plenty of room leave and I bid a last farewell to Doll at 8am. I arrive at Folkestone at 10.20am and go straight on board and leave at 12.30pm. I arrive in Boulogne about 2pm and am marched to the top of the hill to R Camp. We are sorted out and are to leave at 9pm tonight. We are given tea at 4pm and are to draw haversack rations at 5pm. No matches and cigs are available and the YMCA is the only place where cigs are available. It is the hottest day yet. I am given tea and haversack rations and parade for departure at 9pm. I get a comfortable stretch in the Guard's van and leave Boulogne at 11pm. We have a very quick journey and I arrive at St Eloi at 5.30am and we are met by motor buses. We arrive at transport at St Katherine's at 7am. I get bacon and tea, a wash and a shower and then sleep for the rest of the morning. SM Baines and Sergeant Lockalie arrive with me, although Briggs has not turned up yet. I send an FPC to Doll from Boulogne.

June 18 Monday

I borrow 'The Green Ray' from Jim Wood and read it all afternoon and evening. I go down to the swimming ponds in the evening and have a fine bathe. There are thunderstorms in the afternoon but otherwise it is very hot. I live on what I can get from the field kitchen and send an FPC to Mother. The Battalion are on the line and we need not join them till they come out tomorrow night. I go to sleep down at the band's billet.

June 19 Tuesday

Breakfast: bacon. Dinner: stew. Tea: marmalade and marg. I dodge the parade in the morning and then pick up a respirator from salvage. We had thunderstorms during the night and this morning. We leave on transport from Wakefield Camp at 2pm and then move to huts at Roclincourt Camp which are to be occupied by C Company alone. I have tea and bread and butter for supper and get to sleep before C Company arrives. The weather is getting cooler.

June 20 Wednesday

Breakfast: bacon. Dinner: rissoles, potatoes and lime juice. Tea: blackberry and apple jam and marg. C Company arrives at 3am and I have my breakfast right away. I sleep till about 10.30am and then clean up and we have various inspections at 3pm. It is a fine and bright day but heavy thunder and rain commences at about 7pm. I went for a swim in the bathing pools by Arras after tea and handed in letters to Mother and Doll.

June 21 Thursday

Breakfast: bacon and porridge. Dinner: rissoles, potatoes and desiccated vegs. Tea: bread only. We have an area commandant fatigue which is a cushy job and the weather is wet again in the evening and getting cold.

197

June 22 Friday ✦
Breakfast: rissoles. Dinner: stew and rice pudding. Tea: stewed dates and marg. We paraded at 8.20am to practice an attack, which is 1½ hours march away. We were back at 2.10pm and were free for the rest of the day. The weather is showery. Cigs are very difficult to obtain and matches are worse still. I receive a parcel and a letter from Mother of June 16th and finish reading 'The New Machiavelli' by H. G. Wells. There is no news from Doll yet, a phrase from the above particularly strikes me 'give me a line, the world aches for want for you'.

June 23 Saturday
Breakfast: rissoles and porridge. Dinner: stew. Tea: marmalade and marg. We paraded at 7.30am to rehearse the attack again and were back at 12.45pm. There was a compulsory parade for a concert in the afternoon, no wonder we take our pleasures badly. The concert was given by the Brecon Boys from the 5th Division who are going over with us. They were not so bad but I have seen better. I was paid 30 francs in the evening and then lost 1 franc at Solo.

June 24 Sunday
Breakfast: bacon. Dinner: stew and lime juice. Tea: marmalade and marg. We paraded at 8.30am and were rehearsing the attack again and were back at 1.45pm. I have just been out in Category B, so shall not be in the attack after all, thanks to Sergeant Gould who stands a good friend. I felt no satisfaction at first but publicity to the affair rather points to a repetition of the July 1st bluff, so on mature consideration, I will not refuse the exemption as at first I felt inclined. I was on camping parties from tonight in consequence and paraded at 7.30pm. I walked about 18 kilos (kilometres) altogether and carry three loads of barbed wire over one mile on each journey. I finish at 1.30am and am back from returning party for a short cat (nap) and arrive at the camp at 2.45am half an hour before the rest. I received a letter from Doll dated June 21st.

June 25 Monday
Breakfast: rissoles and porridge. Dinner: stew. Tea: jam and marg. I slept till midday and just parade in the afternoon to see the flare lit and how prisoners should be treated. I received a 'Passing Show' from Maud and wrote to Doll in a green envelope and also to Mother and Auntie Annie. I found a canteen where I could buy matches, cigs, dates, biscuits and oranges. I went to the cinema show at the Division after tea which was very good and refreshing after the rotten Blighty show. I was for the working party again tonight so paraded at 7.45pm and then started off at 8.15pm where I was carrying two **boxer bombs**.[316] It started to rain soon after we set out and it was wretched going over the place in the trenches. I made a beeline back on my own from Baillieul. There were heavy storms till I got back and I walked about fifteen miles altogether and arrived back at 4am.

---

[316] **Boxer bombs** - British bombs that contained a time fuse.

June 26 Tuesday

Breakfast: bacon and porridge. Dinner: fresh meat stew. Tea: jam and sponge. Supper: rissoles, porridge and tea. There was no parade at all today. The Battalion starts for the trenches at 10pm and Category B (me) are to go to the transport line where we are billeted in tents. It is a fine day and I play Solo in the evening and lost 3 francs and owe Ward 50 centimes.

June 27 Wednesday

Breakfast: bacon. Dinner: cold beef. Tea: marmalade. We parade for a rifle inspection at 9am and we are then on a carrying party for the trenches and fall in again at 8.15pm. We go round by St Catherine and St Nicholas carrying water from the transport dump to the trenches. It rains a bit on the way but it is not enough to make the going muddy. The Bosche shell a lot while we are in the trenches and some are killed and wounded at the water dump just before we get there. We are taken back through the communication trenches all the way and I must have walked about eighteen miles although I have only been carrying for about ¾ mile in actual distance. I arrive back at 4am just in time to escape a deluge. I hear that C Company have lost badly, **Sergeant Dale**[317] and **Milton**[318] are wounded and several have **been killed.**[319] I won one franc at Solo but receive for same a Belfast note (Irish note) introduced by **Gillatt**[320] who refuses to take it back.

June 28 Thursday

Breakfast: bacon. Dinner: boiled beef and veg stew. Tea: jam. I slept till 8am then had breakfast, slept till 12 and then had rifle inspection at 2pm. **Sergeant Gould**[321] turns up and has been sent back from the trenches for a commission. We hear that Leaman suffered heavy casualties and that three bottles of whiskey were smashed. The strafe (**Cadorna Raid**)[322] opens at 7.10pm and then the rain starts with thunderstorms lasting for most of the night, pouring in torrents. At about 9pm I manage the aeroplane observation. All our objectives were taken bar one small bit by the windmill (Gavrelle Windmill) which is the Barnsley's portion and we are said to be bombing the same. Later all the objectives were taken by the 5th and 31st Divisions. We had a small ration party for rum carrying out at 12.30 midnight but I managed to escape. These return about 7.30am with news that the Battalion got over without any casualties and dug in six foot and

---

[317] **12/631 Sergeant A. Dale** took part in the attack on 1st July 1916 and suffered from shellshock as a consequence.

[318] **12/733 Corporal H. Milton** took part in the attack on 1st July 1916 and was wounded on 27 June 1917.

[319] **31981 Private Windross Fletcher, 12/1059 Private W. Gilberthorpe** and **24497 Corporal Frank Johnson** were all killed in action on 27th June 1917. They are all commemorated on The Arras Memorial.

[320] **12/1809 Private F. Gillatt** who also served with the Cyclist Corps and 13th Y&L.

[321] **12/656 Sergeant Joseph William Gould**, was a teacher who served with 12th Y&L during the attack on 1st July 1916. He was killed in action on 13th October 1918 whilst serving with 5th Y&L and is buried in York Military Cemetery, Haspres.

[322] **Cadorna Raid** – the raid took part within a section of the German front line called Cadorna Trench.

are now back in the support trench, evidently being relieved. It is also reported that the Battalion has taken about 50 prisoners.

June 29 Friday
Breakfast: bully and baked beans. Dinner: ditto. Tea: jam and marg. We paraded at 9am for a rifle and communication inspection. The official message is that the whole objective was taken consolidating slight casualties. I rested all day except for about ½ hour in the evening fetching empty petrol cans from the salvage dump. It was a bright and hot day, cool in the evening with an extremely wet night. We reached our destination at midnight. We are at the **Red Line**[323] which was a very muddy and sticky march but generally fine. There is an available dugout reserved for D Company coming from the front line. We get down in the trench with light shivers during the night and I am disturbed by the cramped position and lice. The rum ration was brought up and I am looking forward to the same in the morning. I sent FPC to Doll and Mother.

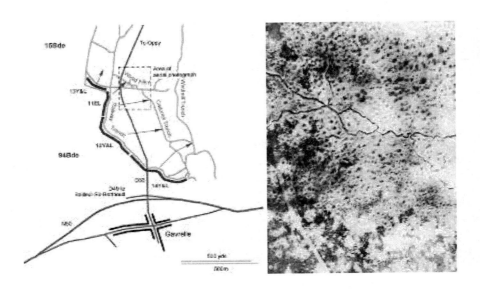

Map showing the position of 12th Y&L during the Cadorna Raid on 28th June 1917

July 1 Sunday
Breakfast: cold bacon. Dinner: cold beef. Tea: jam and marg. I find it is 11 o'clock before I finally rouse from my dozing, so I must have slept fairly well. After breakfasting nothing is seen of our officers up to midday, the usual neglect of men. There is a good rumour that we are going out tonight. The fellows tell us how the Bosche against us put up no fight at all and that they were coming out

---

[323] **Red Line** - Brigades held a portion of the line with Battalions being disposed as follows: Front line six days; **Red line** (close support) six days Brown Line (support), Roberts Camp or Springvale Camp or Cubit Camp (reserve) six days.

to meet them with their hands up and kneeling down crying 'Mercy Komrade.' They were also seen running away out of the next line which we were not even attacking. The Bosche strafe us too closely to be pleasant. I'm told to take over as Orderly Corporal on my return tonight. The day was dull, cold and threatening but there was no rain to bother. At about 10pm B and C Company were sent down to the line and the Bosche thought that there was about to be a counter attack. It remained thus for a few hours till we were relieved by the East Yorks. We got to Roclincourt Camp at about 6am and I received a 'Passing Show' from Maud.

10
Vimy Ridge

July 2 Monday
Breakfast: rissole. Dinner: stew. Tea: jam and marg, boiled bacon and pickles.
We had breakfast as soon as we arrived, then slept until 10.30am. I am not an
Orderly Corporal after all. Quarters have fixed it up with Lance Corporal Molds
and we pack up to move after dinner. The weather is fine and bright. We start
off at 3pm with a full pack and arrive at Bray at about 5.30pm. We are billeted
in a long corrugated iron shed which is fitted up for horse stalls and situated by
the side of the road near the **River Scarpe**[324] which is very convenient for
washing.

July 3 Tuesday
Breakfast: bacon. Dinner: stew. Tea: marmalade. We are still getting between a
third and a half of a loaf a day. We had a kit inspection in the morning and then
an address by General Wanless O'Gowan on the fine success of the 94th
Brigade's stint. He says that we are out for a fortnight and we are to make the
most of the training. I bathed and did some washing in the afternoon. I received
a letter from Doll and then played Solo in the evening and won 3.5 francs.

July 4 Wednesday ✎
Breakfast: rissole. Dinner: stew. Tea: jam and sponge. We paraded from 9am till
12 noon which was musketry, physical and bayonet fighting. In the afternoon we
had a reorganisation. D Company has been divided among the three other
Companies. No. 11 Platoon has been divided among the two remaining platoons
of the Company. I'm now in No. 3 section (bombers) in No. 9 Platoon. I was
paid 15 francs. An extract from the German wireless: *'The army group of*
Crown Prince Ruppreicht.[325] *Heavy fighting took place yesterday between the*
Bassee Canal and the Scarpe. Between Frenay and Garville the enemy at the
beginning suffered heavily from our fire and continued to send over fresh
troops. After bitter hand to hand fighting the English established themselves in
out front line between Oppy and the Garville Windmill. Our troops fought
brilliantly, the enemy suffered bloody loses by our magnificent defence and in a
man to man struggle'. Actually they came out to meet our Battalion with their
hands up and our losses were very slight indeed, C Company included. The

---

[324] **River Scarpe** – is located in the Nord-Pas-de-Calais in France. It is approximately 100 miles long, of
which two thirds has been turned into canals. It flows through the cities of Arras and Douai and the river
and its valley were important battlegrounds in the First World War.

[325] **Crown Prince Ruppreicht** - (1869-1955), heir to the throne of Bavaria, was born in 1869. On the
outbreak of the First World War Rupprecht was given command of the German Sixth Army.

Bosche were seen flying from the next line under our barrage without being attacked at all. The weather is fine with showers in the afternoon and I lost 2 francs at Solo in the evening.

July 5 Thursday
Breakfast: bacon, porridge. Dinner: stew. Tea: jam. We paraded at 8.45am as a Battalion and commenced by falling in to the beat of a drum – now we shall win. We had an address by the Colonel on smartening up and that we would be back in the trenches in twenty four days. We had a short parade and then baths in the afternoon. I received a letter from Doll dated July 1st and then sent a letter to her in a green envelope. I went to the pictures in Marceuil in the evening and only saw one film which was long but very good. I lost 25 centimes at Solo.

July 6 Friday
Breakfast: bacon. Dinner: rissole. Tea: sardines and jam. We paraded from 8.45am to 12.30pm as yesterday and from 2am to 3.45am on a bomber's parade under **Mr Jackson**,[326] where we sit down and do nothing. I went to the pictures in the evening which was not so good as yesterday and then afterwards saw the second half of the Battalion concert which was not up to much. It has been a fine and bright day.

July 7 Saturday
Breakfast: rissoles. Dinner: stew. Tea: sardines, jam and marg. We had a morning parade as usual and in the afternoon we were grouping on the range, I only got 12" and one wide. The weather has been fine and hot with thunderstorms in the night. I received a 'Passing Show' from Maud.

July 8 Sunday
Breakfast: rissole. Dinner: rissole hash. Tea: jam. We had a voluntary Church parade and then played chess all morning and **Whipple**[327] beat me twice. I received a letter from Mother dated July 3rd. It has been a wet morning and a fine afternoon. I reported after tea to BHQ for a scouting course. **Mr Ward** [328] said that the NCOs did not require instruction at an elementary level and that I should learn nothing but anyway we report tomorrow at 2.15pm. There was no morning instruction and the King is expected to be passing the servicing Battalion of the **RND.**[329] I had a big feed of wine, biscuits, chocolate and dates and went to the pictures, which was the same as Friday with the exception of a war film.

---

[326] **Lieutenant C. A. Jackson** –Commissioned on 28th May 1915, was a Brigade Pioneer Officer from 29th July 1917 and was a Corporal with B Company. He died on 5th November 1917 whilst serving with the Royal Flying Corps.

[327] **12/1411 Corporal H. D. Whipple** took part in the attack on 1st July 1916 and was commissioned on 23rd August 1918.

[328] **Captain T. L. Ward** – Commissioned on 1st November 1914 and also served at the Headquarters of 94th Brigade.

[329] **RND** – Royal Naval Division.

July 9 Monday
Breakfast: rissole and porridge. Dinner: rissole mash and new potatoes. Tea: sardines, jam and marg.
I was excused the parade in the morning as I would normally be on the Brigade course now. We prepared for the King's visit but the same was then postponed. I played Whipple two games of chess and won both. The subject of the Brigade class in the afternoon was the use of a primitive compass. I received a letter from Doll, July 5th and won 3 francs at Solo in the evening. It has been a fine but cool day.

July 10 Tuesday
Breakfast: rissole. Dinner: stewed mutton, new potatoes and baked beans. Tea: sardines, marmalade and marg. I had brigade at 9.30am which was map reading and setting, I also had my dinner down at the Brigade. In the afternoon I went to a tavern in Mont St Eloi for observation. We had a Company dinner and concert in the evening, which was the biggest feed since I came to France with unlimited servings; soup (mushroom), roast beef, sausage, new potatoes, baked beans, jam roll and sauce, cheese and biscuits, orange, cherries, chocolate, cigs, beer and lime juice and a very good professional comic imported from 13th Yorks and Lancs. Our new Captain was introduced, as Leaman goes on a month's course to Boulogne. **The King**[330] is coming tomorrow, so there was no parade at the Brigade this morning.

July 11 Wednesday
Breakfast: bacon far more than I could manage. Dinner: rissole, new potatoes and lime juice. Tea: sardines, jam and marg. They had us up at 6am for a 6.30am breakfast to parade to see the King at 7.30am. Breakfast was then postponed till 7.30am and only 11 Platoon were taken without breakfast, I should not have gone anyway as I have the morning off and prefer to seize the opportunity to write to Doll, bless her. This course is a snip. I know it all, so can just sit and rest all of the time. We hear that we are moving to Neuville St Vaast this afternoon so the Brigade class was cancelled and anyway I had the morning off. We set off at 4pm and arrive at the trenches for billeting at 6pm and have tea. We hear that we have been lent to the Canadians for a few days. I sent a green envelope to Doll with an enclosure for Mother. I also send a FPC to Trevor and Mrs Headland. I was then reading 'His Father's Son' and was beating Whipple at chess till 2am. It has been a fine and bright day. I share a small dugout with Whipple and have the most comfortable night that I have had for some time.

July 12 Thursday
Breakfast: bacon and bully. Dinner: stew and new potatoes. Tea: herring in tomato, currants, jam and marg. Supper: porridge. I was left alone entirely all day, with the exception of 1½ hours going to the Canadian Brigade HQ to guide the Company there in the evening. I finished my book and beat Whipple for the sixth consecutive game and he begins to get annoyed. We set off for the trenches

---

[330] **The King** – King George V.

204

at 9am and arrive at the front bombing outpost at 12.30pm. Everyone is to keep on alert all night. There is no shelling on our line or on any very near. There are lights up in front so the Bosche are probably digging an advance trench. The Canadians might be rather windy by the precautions that they display. I saw one of our balloons brought down by our anti-aircraft fire. It came right over the edge of the ridge through Frenay Wood which is very steep on this side. I am put in charge of the advanced bombing post.

July 13 Friday

Breakfast: cold bacon. Dinner: bully and beans. Tea: herring and tomato and jam. It was too cold to sleep properly early in the morning but I make up for it later. The weather then turns out very hot and bright. The Bosche appear to be shelling the support trenches but leave us alone. It was a quiet night except for our own shells bursting short and Whipple asking for trouble and getting bombs thrown at him. I have to do the guard myself practically all night through shortage of men.

July 14 Saturday

Breakfast: bully and pickles. Dinner: Maconochies. Tea: 1/6 tin of herring and tomato and jam. The rations are very poor for the trenches, 1/3 loaf and the bread is very stale and is made up with biscuits and we make our own tea. I finish reading 'The Unofficial Honeymoon' by Dolf Wyllarde which was a very good tale and commenced it yesterday afternoon, Doll must read it. We had thunder and rain in the morning but then it brightened up again. Captain Leaman and **Sergeant Boot**[331] went off on a course last night. Whipple wants me to co-operate in one of his hair brained patrols. I tell him to go to blazes and wouldn't on any account go out with him, besides after the treatment that I've had from the Army, I only do now what I must. It was showery in the afternoon and it sets in for the whole of the night pouring with rain with very heavy thunderstorms. The lower part of my body is drenched through and the trenches are up to our knees in places. There is a bombing raid by **KOSB**[332] on Frenay Wood just to our right at 3am, I was then standing to all night. I sent FPCs to Doll and Mother.

July 15 Sunday

Breakfast: a very small portion of boiled ham. Dinner: bully and beans. Tea: Honey, tomatoes and jam. We get our rations at about 6am and it has become fine again. I boil some good tea at breakfast and tea with a candle wrapped in sacking. We have only about 1½ pints of water per man, so we use muddy rain water out of the shell-hole and milk tin rations, so it is very good. It is a fine and bright morning, with showers again in the afternoon. I get a good wash and shave. Whipple and the Sergeant Major didn't return till 4pm, they were coming in about 12.30pm but were fired on by our chaps, so they thought that they were

---

[331] **12/304 Sergeant W. H. Boot** served with 12 Y&L on 1st July 1916.

[332] **KOSB** - King's Own Scottish Borderers.

approaching the Bosche line, they then got quite lost. Captain Davis[333] warns me for the patrol at midnight, to ascertain the distance to the Bosche wire and patrol about 200 yards of it and to report on the nature and condition of all trenches and discover whether they are occupied and if so in what strength and to return at 2am. I only take two of 11 platoon; **Ballinger**[334] and **Johnson**[335] I have kept fairly clear so far but I am in for it now. We took two bombs apiece, a binder rifle and bayonet. We walked out about 80 yards when a shot was fired from the trench, so we go over to investigate and proceed to crawl, when the rifles, owing to the mud soon become useless and are only an impediment

July 16 Monday
Breakfast: rissole. Dinner: Maconochies. Tea: herring and tomato jam. On the extreme right of our objective I heard a rifle bolt being worked, so finding a weak spot in the wire about 30 yards to the left got through there, leaving my men outside. I had crawled within a few yards of the trench when I heard a Bosche cough, so stopped almost immediately and two shots were fired in my direction. Being in a shell hole, I laid low for about ten minutes, then crawled back as quickly as caution would permit. It was an anxious minute getting through that wire again, wondering what a shot up the bum felt like. We then crawled all along their wire noting its condition and where the gaps were. About 100 yards along, I was crawling through a gap with the idea of having another shot at the trench when I heard a rustling in front of me and saw two prone forms. They evidently also had the wind up for did not advance, neither did I but carefully crawled away. We then made a small detour and back to Bosche wire once again. On the extreme left of my patrol everything was very quiet and I thought that there couldn't be anyone there when suddenly a bomb was chucked at us. That being the end of my journey, I made for our lines again as quickly as we could crawl. The ground was mostly thistles but they were scarcely noticed in the excitement. We got back again at 2.45am I reported to the Captain and he asked for a written report, this with a sketch I prepared for him. He said it would do very well and was worth sending in. Later he asked for me to tell me that the CO had told him to tell me that he was exceedingly pleased with my report. It took three hours to clean my rifle, then I mostly slept till about 7pm. I was sick and could eat no tea. I was detailed to find a good overland route to the lone tree at night and to lead the Company out tomorrow. We started about 10pm and got back at 2am. The weather has been slight showers all through the day and very dark at night. I received a letter from Doll, dated July 10th.

July 17 Tuesday
Breakfast: cold boiled bacon. Dinner: bully and beans. Tea: herrings, tomatoes and jam. I slept through most of the stand to and woke up in time to put my equipment on for a stand down. I consider that I have had a very easy time in the trenches this time. I then continued to sleep till 3pm. Tommies Cookies were

---

[333] **Captain K. R. Davies** – served with 12th Y&L C Company, from 8 July – 27 September 1917.

[334] **17821 Private H. Ballinger** – also served with 2nd, 7th and 10th Y&L.

[335] **31631 Private T Johnson** – also served with North Staffs and 13th Y&L.

sent with our rations for the first time since we came in and I make some decent tea. I received a 'Passing Show' from Maud. I have to go out to the lone tree which is about three miles away to guide in the Barnsleys at night and am there at 10pm. I take the Barnsleys in and then have to wait the last of all to bring the Captain and his servant in. We miss the way and have to return about 200 yards, wet and pitch dark from chalk dugouts and made an absolute beeline to the lone tree although I've never been that way before. Captain Davis is very unstable and was continually stumbling and falling and blamed me. He said he'd put me under close arrest if I didn't go more slowly and at his last fall near our destination, said if I wanted to I'd better b... well run and I'm no b... good as a guide. We arrived at the top of Vimy Ridge in our own reserve trench at 3.30am and breakfast was waiting.

July 18 Wednesday
First breakfast: rissole and new potatoes. Second breakfast: bacon. Dinner: bully, tea and new potatoes. Tea: herring and tomato and jam. **Crawford**[336] also congratulates me on what seems to have delivered the goods. I slept till the second breakfast at 10am and then till about 2pm and then cleaned up a bit. I was then on the working party going right back to the trenches at 9.30pm. I was detailed to go with a party of NCOs to recount the **Brown Line**[337] at the last moment. I just glanced at it, then went on to A Company's HQ where we spent 1½ hours in the dugout. I got to the lone tree at 1.30am and was not with the working party as directed so waited for them there. The day was very cold and wet. They had not turned up by 3.45am and as it was getting very light to cross the Ridge, so we returned without them. They arrived very shortly after at 5am. I received a letter from Doll dated July 12th.

July 19 Thursday
Breakfast: bacon. Dinner: beef, potatoes and beans. Tea: sardines, jam and marg. We had breakfast at 5am on our arrival from the working party. I slept till dinner at 1.30pm and was damp and cold so did not sleep soundly. I received a letter from Mother of July 13th who said that Arthur had just been home on leave. I wrote to Doll and Mother in a green envelope and handed them in. We had a rifle and ammunition inspection in the afternoon and then I won 1.10 francs in the evening at Solo. The weather has been slight showers with a cold wind.

July 20 Friday
Breakfast: bacon. Dinner: beef and potatoes. Tea: stewed figs and marg. We have half a loaf a day now which is more than we can manage. I went to the baths in the morning at Neuville St Vaast which was very good and had a clean change. I walked to the Canadian canteen in the afternoon and spent about 5 francs on sweets, biscuits, cigs etc. and the tea was supplied for nothing. I saw

---

[336] **Captain S. Crawford** – was commissioned on 26 September 1916 served with 12th Y&L from 25th November 1916. He also served with 7th Y&L.

[337] **Brown Line** – Brigades held a portion of the line with Battalions being disposed as follows: Front line six days; Red line (close support) six days Brown Line (support), Roberts Camp or Springvale Camp or Cubit Camp (reserve) six days.

one of our balloons brought down in the evening, the occupant of which descended by parachute. I won 2.35 francs at Solo. I was in the working party in the evening and set off at 9.30pm which was heavy all the way for about five miles without a rest which was a battle order. We do about two hours work, trench digging behind our front line. We get a machine gun turned on us with heavy fire but have no casualties. We arrive at the camp again about 3.30am and have breakfast right away. It has been a fine day but cool. **Jukes**[338] owes me 1.45 francs.

July 21 Saturday
Breakfast: bacon, ample. Dinner: beef and new potatoes. Tea: sardines and marmalade. I slept till dinner and we then moved back to Neuville St Vaast after tea for about six days rest. We are in a camp with the most splendid sand bags and corrugated iron huts and tier beds. Four of us touch for RSMs hut and we have more tea on arrival at about 6pm. The weather has been fine and bright all day. The Bosche drop one shell near the road we are billeted on, then later as the last platoon of 16th West Yorks (1st Brigade) who are taking our place were parading to march off, another shell about 40 yards from my shack fell among them with 36 wounded and 8 dead. The occupant of a balloon nearby was also compelled to descend in a parachute as his balloon was hit. I had a very comfortable night.

July 22 Sunday
Breakfast: bacon. Dinner: stew rabbit (ample). Tea: marmalade. We had a kit inspection in the morning followed by a cleanup. We were then turned out of the shacks on the road into others behind us on the plain and somebody got the wind up with yesterday's business. The weather today was perfect. I sent FPCs to Doll and Mother and I won .75 francs in the evening at Solo. I have a very comfortable bed which is warmer than the other place.

July 23 Monday
Breakfast: bacon. Dinner: stew meat, rabbit, potatoes and beans. Tea: sardines, marg and cheese. We had the pretence at a parade in the morning at 9.20am for an examination of our gas helmets and a few minutes of musketry. We then paraded in the afternoon at 2pm and then were dismissed for pay at 2.30pm and I was paid 20 francs. An aeroplane comes over firing their gun and sets a balloon on fire close by. It comes down burnt to nothing but apparently there was no observer inside. Our anti aircraft men seem asleep. Today was fine and hot and I received a letter from Doll dated July 18th and lost 2.95 francs at Solo.

July 24 Tuesday
Breakfast: Maconochies. Dinner: stewed rabbit and potatoes, with plenty left for supper. Tea: sardines and marmalade. We paraded at 8.45am till 12.30pm drills etc. and I get my hair cut during the same. In the afternoon from 1.55pm till 3.30pm we are on a wiring party. It has been a very hot day. I am on a small

---

[338] **12/1254 Private A. Jukes** – took part in the attack on 1st July 1916.

working party tonight and we are all to go tomorrow. I won .75 francs at Solo and received a 'Passing Show' from Maud.

July 25 Wednesday
Breakfast: rissole and beans. Dinner: rissole mince, potatoes and onions. Tea: cold ham and marg. There were heavy thunderstorms so we did not parade till 9.30am. I took the wiring down which took about ¼ hour followed by physical and then there was a storm again, so we finished at 11.15am. I lost 2.1 francs at Solo in the afternoon and paraded for the carrying party to the trenches at 8.20pm. It was heavy going in the rain and we walked about fifteen miles carrying wire about ¾ mile twice. I was back at 4.30am and was not so tired as I expected to be.

July 26 Thursday
Breakfast: porridge and rissoles. Dinner: rissoles, potatoes and beans. Tea: stewed figs. I slept till about 2pm after breakfast which we had immediately on our return and then slept again till 3.30pm. I gave in my name for draughtsman but think it is a mechanic that is required. The Platoon was practising for a wiring competition at 5.15pm and I'm not in it. Tea was not till 7pm so I make it up with biscuits, chocolate and ginger etc from the canteen. We parade for the working party at 8.20pm as last night but the weather was fine and we made two journeys as before and a second piquet of six each and we were back at 2.45am. We came under a heavy bout of machine gun fire at the dump. One bullet entered the ground under my foot while many plunked around.

July 27 Friday
Breakfast: bacon. Dinner: roast beef, potatoes and beans. Tea: jam. I had to wait for about one hour for breakfast after we got back and I then slept till dinner at 2pm. We then had to form a wiring party for the competition, we were second and beaten by A Company. Westby gave us 20 francs as a consolation which was 1½ francs each. I bought an early tea as yesterday and the weather was a very hot day. I received a letter from Mother dated July 19th and I am getting very tired. I am off again carrying tonight, same time and place, only one journey this time. **One man**[339] gets two bullets in the side from a machine gun and dies. I got back about 2.15am had a good rest and tea at a canteen on the road.

July 28 Saturday
Breakfast: rissole. Dinner: Maconochies, warmed. Tea: jam and marg. I slept after breakfast till dinner and then read in the afternoon and evening. I was left entirely alone and appreciate the rest. I received a letter from Auntie Annie of July 23rd.

---

[339] **3/2486 Lance Corporal Jethrew Bamford** died from wounds on 28 July 1917 and is buried in Aubigny Community Cemetery.

July 29 Sunday

Breakfast: rissole. Dinner: cooked Maconochies, cabbage and potatoes. Tea: jam. Supper: porridge, loaf and tea. We had a rifle inspection in the morning and in the afternoon take our valise to transport line as we are going up to the trenches tonight. The weather is very wet. I received a letter from Doll of July 24th and write to Doll in a green envelope with enclosures to Mother and Auntie Annie. We have supper about 7pm and start for the trenches at 9.30pm and descend Vimy Ridge by a new trench. We are billeted in a trench near to the ration dump. It is 1am before we are settled down and then have to go in the carrying party right away. Some of the men are getting the wind up over the machine gun fire. I am carrying a bundle of 12 medium **screw piquets**[340] which is too much strain altogether but it is only for one journey though.

July 30 Monday

Breakfast: boiled bacon and bully. Dinner: bully and beans. Tea: jam and marg and have brought an abundance of bread and cheese. We had breakfast on our return at about 4am and then sleep till 1pm. I make tea with dinner and tea and parade at 9.40am for the working party which is carrying spoils from the dugout in sandbags in **Winnipeg Trench**.[341] We get back about 2.30am and have a rum ration. The weather has been an unsettled and a dull day but fine at night. The Bosche machine guns have been very active with several narrow shaves.

July 31 Tuesday

Breakfast: boiled bacon. Dinner: bully and lime juice. Tea: jam and butter, scanty rations. I received a 'Passing Show' from Maud, slept, read and beat Whipple in one game of chess. I was a cloudy but fine day which set in wet in the evening. We are carrying spoils from the dugout in **Vancouver Road**[342] during the night, which was only about two hours work really but we spread it out till about 1am and then paraded at 9.30pm. We had a good rum ration on our return.

August 1 Wednesday

Breakfast: boiled bacon. Dinner: bully and beans. Tea: jam, rations more scanty. It has been a dull and wet day, during which I slept for most of the time and then had a wash and shave. We stopped in our trench in the evening and spent from 9.30pm to 1.30am improving the same followed by a rum ration.

August 2 Thursday

Breakfast: boiled bacon. Dinner: bully and beans. Tea: dates. A dull and wet day again and I slept till noon. I played Whipple a game of chess and beat him. We then were carrying sandbags of chalk from the dugout again which was the hardest evening that we have had. We paraded at 9.30am, started carrying at 9.30pm and finished at 1.20am. We handled 900 bags, lifting them up four steps

---

[340] **Screw piquet** – a stake used to secure barbed wire defence lines.

[341] **Winnipeg Trench** – A communication trench.

[342] **Vancouver Road** - A communication trench.

and then throwing them 5 feet which represented about 15 tons in weight. The night was fine and very bright, although there were heavy clouds. We were back in for 2am for a good rum ration and breakfast.

August 3 Friday
Breakfast: boiled bacon. Dinner: bully and pickles. Tea: jam, marg, cheese 1/3 loaf, rations more than ample. I slept till noon and then had a wash and shave. The day was wet and dull again. We are to go into the support trench tonight. I beat Whipple at another game of chess. We are carrying timber baulks and concrete slabs to the trenches before we go in and are finished at 2am. Whipple and I scrounge a hole together in the support line which was very tight. We had a rum ration and I sent FPCs to Doll and Mother. We have been told that we mustn't be seen outside in daytime as we are under observation.

August 4 Saturday
Breakfast: boiled bacon and rissole. Dinner: cold beef, bully and beans. Tea: jam. We had breakfast at 4am and I then slept till 12.30pm and then had wire carrying to the front line till 2.30pm. The weather is improving and is warm and cloudy but with a little rain. I beat Whipple at three games of chess again. We carried wire from Winnipeg to A Company's front line then return from the dump to Area Head Quarters then wire again from Peggy (Winnipeg) to Battalion Head Quarters. We are at it continuously from 9.30pm to 3am. **2ⁿᵈ Lieutenant Browning**[343] is an absolute dream but very anxious to stand well with the men and goes to the 12ᵗʰ Platoon after only being two days with us. That was as Booth returns to No. 9 Platoon and immediately makes himself objectionable again, he is very commonly bred. We also hear that the Colonel is back. Tonight there was no rum ration and we have much increased work, is there any connection? The sunken road has been shelled during the day.

August 5 Sunday
Breakfast: boiled bacon rissole. Dinner: cold beef. Tea: jam, marg and cheese. We had breakfast at about 5am and I received a letter from Doll dated July 31ˢᵗ and a 'Passing Show' from Maud. We turned out at 10.30am and were on a wire carrying party to Company HQ. I was put in charge of the bombers, cleaning bombs from 9pm till 10.30pm then clearing the debris of disinterred Germans over the parapet, by which we lodge rations and are finished after the journey. I was just getting down for a sleep when the Bosche commence heavy strafing principally directed on our sunken road but only one or two drop in with the exception of some shrapnel. There were only five of us left in the road however, so there was no damage. We had 23 gas casualties nearer the front line. We had a stand to at 3.30am and then had a clean-up and washed our feet. The day has been warm and dry.

---

[343] **Lieutenant D. O. Browning** - was commissioned on 30ᵗʰ May 1917 and served with 12ᵗʰ Y&L from 3 July 1917. He was gassed on 10ᵗʰ Sept 1917.

August 6 Monday

Breakfast: boiled bacon and veal loaf. Dinner: cold beef and beans. Tea: jam. We had breakfast at 4am and then slept till 10.45pm when we are turned out to carry more wire from Lewis Dump to B Dump. Lewis Dump is on top and in the open but in spite of precautions it was impressed on us these go to blazes lest we should have an idle morning. It was another bright and warm day. At stand to we are suddenly ordered to take everything to the front line. C Company are split between A and B Companies to reinforce same as casualties now amount to 40 owing chiefly to gas. There is slight drizzle during the night as we are putting out the wire and it was very quiet. There is very little accommodation for sleeping in the day but I manage to secure a good **scrounge hole**[344] myself.

August 7 Tuesday

Breakfast: boiled ham rissole. Dinner: Maconochies and loaf. Tea: jam. I rested all day and it was quiet except for a little shelling in the afternoon over us. The day turns fine and is warmer. Two of our signallers who went out to map out a wire route to our front line over the top **have mysteriously disappeared.**[345] **Lieutenant Wilson**[346] who I saw carried out yesterday gassed but looking very well is now dead. The result is that many more who tasted slight doses are now going out. Rideout has a good parcel and as I have been letting him have the tea that I prepare, generously shares with me. Just as I am about to go wiring, I am put in charge of the B Company observation post. I was very fortunate, for shortly, Bosche commence sweeping with heavy machine gunfire and attack with rifle grenades and bombs, killing one man on the working party of the 14th Yorks and Lancs. There were further attacks during the night. The stretcher bearers are turned out of our cosy little dugout for our benefit against our wishes. The **Saxons**[347] are reported to have been relieved on our front, evidently they have the wind up.

August 8 Wednesday

Breakfast: boiled bacon and rissole. Dinner: cold beef. Tea: jam. All made out very nicely by Rideout's parcel. I got little sleep as I was attending to the observation job but I find it very interesting. It was a hazy morning and a fine and hot day, followed by a heavy thunderstorm at 6pm which lasted about two hours and renders the trenches wretched again and water pours into our dugout. I sent FPCs to Doll and Mother. 90 men have been evacuated from the trenches to date, mostly due to the gas the night before last. We strafe with our trench mortars and artillery during the night. I did not get much sleep again.

---

[344] **Scrounge hole** – another name for a small dugout.

[345] **2nd Lieutenant J. Thompson** is the most like candidate for one of those missing. He was a Sheffield University Student and also served with 10th Y&L and the Machine Gun Corps.

[346] **Lieutenant F. B. Wilson** was a Sheffield University Student commissioned on 7th July 1915. He served with 1th Y&L from 7th July 1915 and died 'from wounds' i.e. he was gassed on 7th August 1917. He is buried in Aubigny Communal Cemetery.

[347] **The 'Saxons'** – The 18th West Yorks.

August 9 Thursday
Breakfast: boiled bacon rissole. Dinner: bully and beans. Tea: dates and banana from Rideout's parcel. I had cafe au lait at breakfast – long and strong and received a letter from Doll, August 3 enclosing a bandana. It was a bright and fresh morning with slight showers in the afternoon and I get some good sleep. There has been some great enemy aerial activity over us and there is a rumour that Lens has fallen. The weather is very clear and we can see men in the road in front of Douai. We were relieved at 9.30 by 14th (Yorks and Lancs) Barnsleys and billeted in **Canada Trench**[348] right to the right of the lone tree for the night. Whipple and I get a good shelter but have **Mole**[349] thrust on us also, his feet are at the least objectionable but I have a good night nevertheless. There is a tremendous pounding of big guns going on, apparently directed at Lens which must be an inferno. It was a wet evening which turns to a fine and dark night.

August 10 Friday
Breakfast: boiled bacon. Dinner: cold beef (ample). Tea: veal loaf, jam and marg. Supper: rissoles and tea. We are given an extra cig ration of 11 Navy Cut. It was a bright and showery day and I get a wash and clean up and make good tea at each meal, although water is scarce. There is great aerial activity. We are moved to a fine German dugout near Vimy Station at night where we had rum rations then rissoles and tea. We had fine wire beds and I slept splendidly.

August 11 Saturday
Breakfast: fried bacon. Dinner: stew. Tea: jam and cheese. I went to the baths at Neuville St Vaast in the morning while others went by the trench. I made a beeline over the top of the ridge and I got a magnificent view of Lens and district, a regular panorama. I laid in a stock of candles, cigs, matches and biscuits at the canteen. Coming back I discovered the most luscious blackberries and filled myself to the full, without scarcely moving. There were two varieties; one as we grow in our gardens and the other, very big and fat and as large as grapes, with the bloom of the same. I got very wet only two minutes from the dugout when it poured in torrents after a very fine morning. I wrote to Doll in a green envelope and enclosed a birthday letter to Mother with 10/-. I was on a digging party on the trenches at night and fell in at 9pm. There were showers on the way and it was fearfully muddy but it cleared up later. The trench was swept by machine gun fire once but we all got down in time and we finished at 1.30am and were back at about 3.30am and had breakfast on our return.

August 12 Sunday
Breakfast: fried bacon. Dinner: stew. Tea: marmalade, marg and cheese. I slept till dinner and was then making a barbed wire concertina in the afternoon. Five aeroplanes fight about 50 yards overhead, our plane maintains its position just above and over the enemy. He is forced to land and he appears likely to make a good job of it but then smashes in a shell hole on his nose and turns head over

---

[348] **Canada Trench** – One of the series of trenches between Garvelle and Oppy.
[349] **27585 Corporal J. Mole** – also served with 2nd and 7th Y&L.

heels. The pilot is badly shaken and had been wounded beforehand in his arm. It has been a fine and bright day but with threatening clod. I received a 'Passing Show' from Maud. I was digging in **Triumph Trench**[350] at night and go about ¾ hour out of our way, to get to it all along the front line. We only work for 1½ hours and are back at 3am when we have a rum ration and breakfast. The weather remained fine during the night.

August 13 Monday
Breakfast: fried bacon. Dinner: stew. Tea: jam and veal loaf. Supper: porridge. I slept till 1pm and then had dinner. Afterwards most of the others turned out to clear the dugout for A Company who are coming down here. We have had some rain and it was a fine night. We parade at 9.15pm for a digging party in the trenches again. We started work at 11.30pm and finished at 1.30am. We have a very meagre breakfast on our return, made out as yesterday with salvaged bully.

August 14 Tuesday
Breakfast: fried bacon. Dinner: stew. Tea: jam and veal loaf. Supper: porridge and marg. We had rifle inspection but the AOC Sergeant didn't turn up for it, I expect the exceptional gun fire just over the embankment had put the wind up him. I received a letter from Doll August 8 and a letter from Mother dated August 3rd with a Harrison pomade. It has been a threatening evening.

August 15 Wednesday
Breakfast: fried bacon. Dinner: stew. Tea: jam and cheese. Supper: porridge. I slept till dinner then pretend at cleaning out dugouts and rifle inspection. We were warned for a bombing course after tea. We set out at 9pm to report at BHQ from thence we were sent to the transport lines. I was a wet day and so very muddy and I was thankful to miss the last working party. We were picked up just after crossing the Lens/Arras road by **RFA limber**[351] and get a lift almost to the camp, great jolting and we go at a good pace. We stop at the canteen for tea, chocolate and biscuits. We arrive at 1am and I get a comfortable sleep in a forage shed. Jimmy Wood brings a mug of tea which was very good and also some bread. I receive a postcard from Doll dated August 9th.

August 16 Thursday
Breakfast: scrap of bacon. Dinner: rabbit stew. Tea: nothing – but draw next day's bread and figs. I cannot get anything from our quarters although rations had not yet arrived for us to bring when I left the Company. I find the bombing school is here in Neuville St Vaast which is hard lines as I shall be at it all the time that the Battalion is resting and enjoying are and the entertainment that has been prepared for them. I spent the day clearing up and went to the Divisional cinema in the evening which was very good indeed but a short programme,

---

[350] **Triumph Trench** - One of the series of trenches between Garvelle and Oppy.

[351] **RFA limber** – Royal Field Artillery limber. The limber is drawn by a team of six horses with a driver on one side of each pair and would have been pulling a gun, most probably an 18 – pounder field gun.

where I indulge in further biscuits and chocolate. I sent FPCs to Doll and Mother. It has been a fine day.

August 17 Friday ,
Breakfast: ¼ tin marmalade. Dinner: fried beef, potatoes and onions. Tea: Nothing for tea as I had five figs yesterday so are not out. We paraded at 9.30am till 12.30pm, inspected, lectures, practices and physical. At 2pm we were sent to Mont St Eloi for trench fighting and finished at 4.15 and get tea and cake at dismissal. I went on to Winnipeg Camp to see Battalion and get paid 40 francs. I laid in a stock of eatable at the YMCA and eggs and ham at the shop, eggs 3½ francs each. I get back in time for the cinema at 7.30pm which was very good again, Charlie Chaplin in 'Charlie's Elopement Court de Hatta' I had coffee with Jim Wood and John Bull (magazine). I went to sleep at about 11.15pm. It was a fine, hot and breezy day and I received a letter from Doll, August 12th.

August 18 Saturday
Breakfast: fried bacon. Dinner: bully, potatoes, pickles and tea. Tea: dates and ¼ loaf. We paraded as yesterday and it came on to rain just as we finished our bombing attack which was NCOs versus the officers at Mont St Eloi. We then caught a motor lorry home. I shared a tin of peas for tea for 3 francs and then went to the cinema afterwards. Received 'Lady Betty from across the Water' from Auntie Annie and read last Sunday's papers till late. The weather cleared up at night.

August 19 Sunday
Breakfast: fried bacon. Dinner: stew, potatoes and fried onions. Tea: jam and 1/3 loaf. I did not wake till 8.45 and my tea and bacon had gone cold for breakfast but fried eggs I warmed up. I then cleaned up a bit and read 'Lady Betty' absolutely all day and finished it. I intended writing to Doll but left it too late and feel very guilty and neglectful. It was a beautiful fine day.

August 20 Monday
Breakfast: veal and loaf ½ tin. Dinner: bully, boiled onions and beans. Tea: raspberry jam and marg. I was up at 6.45 and had fried eggs with my breakfast. We paraded at 9am then went straight away to Mont St Eloi for a day's trench fighting. I had tea, cake, biscuits and chocolate at the divisional canteen for 1.70 francs and then got a proper motor ride home. We had dinner and tea together and then went to the cinema. Somebody has won my tea hat and P.H. helmet, so I went to the dump afterwards and replaced them. It was 9.30 pm before I finally settled down to continue my letter to Doll which I sat up and finished and enclosed a green envelope with one to Mother and to Auntie Annie to send off tomorrow morning. It has been another fine day again.

August 21 Tuesday
Breakfast: veal and loaf ½ tin. Dinner: fried steak and potatoes. Tea: raspberry jam and marg. We set out at 8.20am for St Eloi. A team of us was selected to

take on the Barnsleys but I was not included, so had a very easy time all morning. I made a meal of the same as yesterday at the canteen and bought some more eggs. We were throwing line bombs in the afternoon. We got a motor lorry coming and going back and was in the camp again at 4.30pm so had dinner and tea combined and went to the pictures in the evening. I received a letter from Doll dated August 16th and a 'Passing Show' from Maud. It has been a lovely day again.

August 22 Wednesday
Breakfast: bully. Dinner: fried beef and beans. Tea: jam. We had a full day in the camp which was mostly lectures. I boiled two eggs for breakfast which were stale and went to the pictures in the evening which was rotten. I finished 'Wither the Law' which I commenced at about 11pm last night. There are rumours of a stint on for us when we go back to the line. It has been another fine and warm day.

August 23 Thursday
Breakfast: fried bacon. Dinner: bully and beans. Tea: jam and marg. I had a fried egg with my breakfast and then we all paraded at the camp. I got none in the throwing trials. We had two slight showers in the evening and went to the pictures, which was poor. Later we were chucked out of our shelter and put in a tent. I was up till 2am reading 'Butane the Smith' by Farnol.

August 24 Friday
Breakfast: fried bacon. We paraded at 9am and were sent to Mont St Eloi for the day and got a motor lorry there and had trench fighting in the morning. Our Battalion goes in the line today and we go with rations tomorrow. C Company start that night, so we may miss it. I got lunch at the canteen which was ½ tin of peaches, cake and tea for 2.20 francs. We then had rifle grenades and throwing bombs in the afternoon and then got a Motor lorry back at 4.30pm. I received a letter and handkerchief from Doll, August 19 and went to the pictures after tea. The Corps Commander is to attend so we were delayed by ½ hour till he arrived. He apparently hadn't seen 'The Sort of Girl who comes from Heaven' which we had had before, this was substituted for another being very good, 'Charlie in the Bank' which was also very amusing. The windows were opened between every section for ventilation, so it didn't finish till 7.45pm. We were shifted out of our tents again to brigade huts and I was up till 1am reading 'Butane the Smith'.

August 26 Saturday
Breakfast: fried bacon. Dinner: stew. Tea: jam. We had an examination all day which finished at 3.30pm.I did very well in detailing and knowledge of bombs etc. The incapacity of officers in this diction was well nigh incredible. It was exceedingly amusing to hear them mixing German and British and mixing the parts together. I devoted all my spare time to finishing my book and managed it with about two minutes to spare. We left the camp with about transport at 7.45pm. I laid in a stock of cigs, toffee, biscuits and chocolate and put my packs

on some limbers. We went a long way round by Farbes village and got to CHQ at 11pm where I was put in charge of No. 3 post. It was a very quiet night. One of the eggs that I fried this morning was practically bad, 3½ francs each – the French robbers. It has been a fine, bright and breezy day.

August 27 Sunday

Breakfast: cold boiled ham. Dinner: 1/3rd tin of Maconochies. Tea: jam, margarine and cheese. I stood down about 4.30am then boiled billy for tea and breakfast and afterwards slept till 1pm. I was supposed to be working 1pm till 10pm with one hour off for tea. It was a bright and fine day. Bourne who left as acting sergeant is to take a commission has returned to us as a Private. Wood comes to ask me to take charge of the covering party on stint in place of Stimpson who is away on a course. I thought that I might object as I was away when we practised and he wants to be as fair as possible. I tell him not to bother about that point of view as I've been in the Army quite long enough to realise there's no such thing as fairness in it. He then further asks if I would like to go on patrol tonight. I tell him after my treatment, that I now volunteer for nothing but if ordered, I will do my best. So he says that he wishes me to go. He asks what my grievance is and I tell him. I go out 2am till 4am and find a new line of wire and trenches newly made but unoccupied as yet. It poured earlier from 8.30pm till 9.30pm then quietly rained till about midnight with further occasional showers, so I got fairly wet. I was writing to Doll but was interrupted by Wood. **Rushby**[352] and Rideout went with me. Wood and **Sergeant Jarvis**[353] were fairing back as our covering party. Rushby turned tail, so we two went on alone. Wood and James also desert us.

August 27 Monday

Breakfast: boiled bacon. Dinner: cold beef and beans. Tea: jam. Rations were rather late so did not finish until about 8.30am. It was a fine and bright morning. I slept until 2pm to find it raining again which kept on all day, so proceeded to doze on till evening. I took charge of the post again at 8.30 and was sent for at 10.30pm. The Colonel specially detailed me to get particulars of the occupied post I discovered last time in, a ticklish job, and I am only to take one man too. **Crossland**[354] was waiting for me and Wood gives me some whiskey before setting out. I arrived with a revolver and two bombs. We had only gone about 40 to 50 paces outside of our wire with Crossland following behind, when I was suddenly challenged 6 yards on my right by a German. Getting no reply he called again and immediately fired at me, followed by two others as hard as they could go. I slipped into a shell-hole which was fortunately just on my left. One German advanced, thinking that he had hit me, apparently. I fired point blank at 3 yards; he collapsed with souam and groan. The two others continued to fire. I returned to another shell-hole further on the left. They saw me and followed with their fire. I eventually dodged and got back through our wire only

---

[352] **12/1558 Private L. Rushby** - served with C Company.

[353] **18582 Sergeant R. A. Jarvis** – was wounded in the attack on 1st July 1916.

[354] **12/1411 Private J. Crossland** also served with 2nd and 13th Y&L.

losing the seat of my trousers and part of my tunic. The night was dark and stormy and as dark as a bag. I could not have got my direction without the aid of a magnetic compass. It was a most exhilarating sensation, shooting Germans in self defence.

August 28 Tuesday (Mother's Birthday)

Breakfast: bacon and rissole. Dinner: Maconochies. Tea: gooseberry and strawberry jam, cheese, marg. Rum issue. I got in from the disastrous patrol about 1am. I was on my way to report at Company HQ, telling the tale in one of the bays, when a new draught man suddenly holds me up with a levelled rifle bayonet, saying you are not Corporal Meakin. It took me about ten minutes cursing and blaspheming to convince him that I was not a German spy, he had even started to march me off with my hands up. It was the **other Meakin**[355] that he knew.

After reporting, I went back to our wire and called to Crossland but there was no result. After making my report and cleaning my rifle, it was 10am before I got down for a rest. I was fetched out again at 12 noon to don camouflage and go out to the scene of affray to see if I could discover anything but there was nothing but Bosche footmarks and trampled grass. Wood afterwards discussed the big fighting patrol that he is taking out and I have to lead, he seems to have great confidence in my judgement. No more sleep for me, then I was writing to Doll for rest of evening. The patrol assembles at 8.30pm, it is raining again but clears later. We are out till 1am and consider we might have had one German except for the hindrance of flank men and an officer to whom the word was passed up 'Man 4 yards away' and allowed him to get away again. Crossland has not come in and is certainly captured now. **Sergeant Footit**[356] who saw us out to the wire and when I saw walk back along the parapet and disappear at big burst of machine gun fire, is also missing. I was soaked through again and we got rum in return, which was very acceptable. This makes four patrols in three days for me.

August 29 Wednesday

Breakfast: rissole. Dinner: cold beef, beans and marmalade. Tea: blackberry jam. The front line has been evacuated but for machine gun posts as we are strafing the enemy with gas shells at 2am. To save walking out, I go the machine gun post and stand to with my gas helmet on, so my rest had been delayed again. I return to my scrounge hole and am awakened at 7am by the Sergeant and told that I must make a shelter nearer the sentry post and to clear out by 2pm. I receive letters from Mother August dated 23rd, Arthur dated August 25th and a 'Passing Show' from Maud. I talk to the Sergeant again who lets me give the order to move. It has been showery all day. There is still no

---

[355] **24055 Corporal A. Meakin** was the 'other' Meakin. He also served with 7th and 10th Y&L.

[356] **19187 Sergeant P Footit** also served with 2nd and 9th Y&L. As stated, Frank saw him disappear in a burst of machine gun fire and for several nights, search parties looked for him. He was never found. On 21st November 1917 Frank spoke with the brother of **12/1411 Pte J. Crossland** who confirmed that his Mother had heard that both his Brother and Sergeant Footit had both been taken prisoner that night and were in good health.

news of Footit yet, although we have searched for him. I lead out a fighting patrol again at 9pm and we are back at 10.30pm as we are to strafe again with gas. I am out long enough though to get wet through again. I wrote to Arthur, Doll and Mother.

August 30 Thursday

Breakfast: boiled bacon and rissole. Dinner: bully and beans. Tea: jam. I got down at 2am till 7am but did not get much sleep as my feet were too painful. We had a rum issue in the morning and I made a hot billy of cocoa for breakfast done out nicely. I got Wood to censor Arthur's letter and he took it and gave it to Divisional quarters. **Taylor**[357] placed deuce with me for not having moved from my scrounge hole. I had my first wash and shave since I first came to the trenches. I then finished my letter to Mother. It is not worthwhile moving now but I had better not sleep again. I was relieved at 10pm and there is a fighting patrol to go out for one hour but I'm let off this time. There is a constant search made for Footit but no result, this is a mysterious front. The Barnsleys captured a German Scoutmaster a few days ago, he and two others nearly succeeded in grabbing a man out of their trench and that this would have made his 9th capture. He told them that their patrol had captured Corporal Roberts and another signaller who had mysteriously disappeared the last time we were in No Man's Land. The weather has been slight showers on and off and I received a parcel from Mother.

August 31 Friday

Breakfast: boiled bacon. Dinner: cold beef. Tea: jam. We came to Canada Trench last midnight and I washed my feet and changed my socks. Whipple is back and he has bagged a fine cubby hole, a **Baby elephant,**[358] very cosy. I opened Mother's parcel, the plums had caused damage to all eatables but one, very luscious cakes not much the worse. I slept till 10am then breakfast and cleaned myself up a bit. The Chaplin gave me a tin of **Goldflake**[359] between two. I handed in my green envelope to Doll with an enclosure to Mother. I also posted acknowledging cigs from the pupils of St Lambeth, Church Street Infants School and am feeling quite cheerful again. We paraded at 8.30pm for the working party and had to fetch picks and shovels and take them back there afterwards from Vancouver Dump, although the pile by our trenches is a mile extra walk. We then were digging in Triumph Trench which was quiet. It was sad that we had to work till 3am but the RE corporal said no one stopped after 1.30am, so we cleared off then. Stimpson is in charge of No. 9 Platoon and is very easy going and doesn't insist on much work and lets us smoke in the bottom of the trench. I got breakfast on our return about 3am. It had been a fine

---

[357] **Lieutenant A. L. Taylor**, commissioned to 4th Y&L on 25th October 1916 and served with 12th Y&L from 8th January 1917.

[358] **Baby elephant** - An 'elephant' was a large corrugated iron shelter developed in late 1916. A baby elephant was a small shelter.

[359] **Gold Flake Cigarette** Sun Cured Virginia tobacco available in tins (which are most probably the tins that Frank kept his diaries in as they are the perfect size ...)

and bright day except for slight drizzle once or twice. It was a cold and clear night.

• *September 1 Saturday*
Breakfast: boiled bacon. Dinner: rissole and beans. Tea: jam. I fried my bacon for breakfast and slept till 2pm to find a dull cloudy day turning to rain. I washed my socks. Our front line seems to be getting strafed pretty heavily. Just before the working party turns out I am told that they've detailed me for a course. I am to report to transport tomorrow for dugout construction with the 170th tunnellers from **CRE**.[360] The SM says it is only for two or three days which means that I will be back again when we go in the front line, my usual luck. I'm to go out with transport tonight. I stay for letters to be sorted so the transport goes without me and I miss the ride but it is worth it as get a cracking letter from Doll, August 27. I go straight over the ridge and arrive only ½ hour after the transport. I get some tea and fry the boiled bacon that I've bought and make a good supper. I get down at about 1am in the forage shed next to a goat and wake up at 4am itching all over, so no more sleep. Today has been a dull and wet day at first and a fine evening.

September 2 Sunday
Breakfast: bacon. Dinner: boiled beef and desiccated veg. Tea: jam. I got a bath and a change of clothing in the morning with B Company. I was refitted with a new tunic, trousers and boots, the latter being 7's (the only size obtainable) they seem to fit although I've been wearing 9s. I go to the cinema in the afternoon which was good and I get an order for 50 francs pay. I do some cleaning up and then have coffee with Jim Wood at night. I get down extremely comfortable on chaff bags in the forage shed and slept soundly all night. I received papers and 'The Shumable' from Auntie Annie. It was a bright day with occasional brief showers. I sent FPCs to Doll and Mother and received a letter from Arthur.

September 3 Monday
Breakfast: bacon. Dinner: bully. Tea: jam and cheese. I met the lorry at La Targette at 7.15am and didn't wake till 6.15. We went right round by Roclincourt and go to Ecoivres and I drew 50 francs. We got to Nolux les Mines at 12 o'clock but I don't start till tomorrow. I am in a frame hut with electric lights and canvas frame beds. I have some very good beer at the camp canteen and have four ½ pint glasses. I go out and buy tomatoes for 7½ **livre**[361] and some fine peas for 5 livres and sauces to go with bully for dinner. I then have a nap till tea. I go to the French cinema, had started the 6.30pm pictures which was moderate and came out at 8.30pm in the midst of a pseudo Chaplin film which was rotten. We were shelled a bit in the afternoon and an aeroplane drops bombs about 9.15pm. We passed some Chinese and Portuguese working parties on the way.

---

[360] **CRE** – Commander of the Royal Engineers.

[361] **Livre** – a unit of Belgian currency.

September 4 Tuesday
Breakfast: bacon. Dinner: stew. Tea: jam and butter. We paraded at 7.30am and I was put in charge of a section and we are set to continue with a dugout on our own. I chucked it for dinner at 12.30pm and was at it again from 1.30pm till 4.30pm it was go as you please but the fellows worked very well. I went exploring the town in the evening and got peaches for 1.50 francs per livre and four for .75 francs. I dropped in for supper of two eggs and chips, bread, butter and coffee for 1.80 francs. I wrote to Mrs Crossland and also to Doll. It has been a perfect day, although cool down in the dugout.

September 5 Wednesday
Breakfast: bacon. Dinner: beef, pickles and cocoa. Tea: jam and cheese. I was in the working party as before and do a good morning's work and start putting in timbers in the afternoon. A few shells were put over us after tea. I stopped in as my new boots were too painful to walk out, so I read all evening. I was full up with fruit, biscuits, chocolate and canteen tea. I wrote to Arthur enclosing a Nolux les Mines frame note to give him the tip. It was a very hot day. I received a 'Passing Show' from Maud.

September 6 Thursday
Breakfast: tin of sardines. Dinner: stew. Tea: Jam and butter. I get in a set of timbers and excavate half way for fresh set. I went to the concert at the YMCA in the evening, 99th Labour Company, which was fairly good but my boots spoiled my evening. I am eating beaucoup of fruit. We had a thunderstorm in the evening.

September 7 Friday
Breakfast: bacon. Dinner: loaf, pickles and cocoa. Tea: jam and cheese. I move to deep dugout in HQ yard which has a shaft, corridor and a chamber 12 feet wide and **RSJ**[362] beams, otherwise treated the same as a corridor. They have fine William pears in the market for .35 francs and I was charged .75 in the evening for plums. I went to a French cinema which was exceptionally good, Charlie Chaplin 'En Famille' and also 'Syd Chaplin' I left my socks off altogether and had some comfort at last. I was a fine day.

September 8 Saturday
Breakfast: bacon. Dinner: Maconochies. Tea: jam and butter. We were working as before. A drunken sapper goes down well with us to put up the set. We warn him that the roof should not be touched any more till it is set under the end but he insists on the piles being raised with fresh wedges under the end. Levering up the same standing at the face, he brought the lot down. It was a large pocket about 10' x 6' x 6' which came down with poles and the last set including a 57.3' RSJ on top of him. I thought that he must have been killed for certain. I put the accident down to the leaning post to which I had drawn to the attention of the R.E. when starting the job. While the others sent for assistance he called

---

[362] **RSJ** – Rolled Steel Joists.

out quite cheerfully for help. I crawled over the top and uncovered him to his waist before the R.E.s arrived. He was cut about the head and thought that his leg was broken with the RSJ. His mates worked like Trojans while there were further little showers coming down from time to time. He was got out with nothing more than cuts and bruises. There was no more work after 3.30pm when I got a bath and a change of clothing. My cap was buried so I got a new one from the Quarter Master's Stores and then went to the cinema in the evening which was good again. I consumed some grapes, chocolate and biscuits and peaches in the morning. I was a fine and warm day.

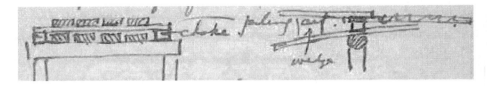

Sketch of the dugout

September 9 Sunday
Breakfast: bacon. Dinner: stew and rice pudding. I worked from 7.30am to 12 in the evening clearing out the fallen in dugout and I recovered my cap. I got a pass for Bethune and got a lift in a motor lorry and arrived at 3pm. I had a fine ice cream at a patisserie for .50 francs and coffee and cakes for 1.90 francs and had a tin of toffee de-luxe at the **E.F.C.**,[363] which has gone up to 1.60 francs. I couldn't find a place for a decent dinner, everywhere was likely for officers only. I intended to get a photo taken, the only likely place was 12 francs for six, the others were ghastly for 4.50 francs for six, the thieves. I walked back and had two eggs, bread and butter and coffee for 1.30 francs on my return. A find and warm day and my boots are getting easier.

September 10 Monday
Breakfast: bacon and porridge. Dinner: Maconochies and cocoa. Tea: raspberry jam and marg

I was making the staircase up from the inside of the dugout and put in one set. I went up to see the 'Fancies' in the evening but they don't perform till Thursday so afterwards I went to a concert of Durham Light Infantry at the YMCA which was good variety. I had eggs and coffee for supper. It has been a fine day but I have a cough and cold developing.

---

[363] **E.F.C.** – Expeditionary Force Canteen – a canteen set up behind the lines for the sale of foodstuff and liquid refreshments.

11
Return to Blighty

September 11 Tuesday
Breakfast: cold bacon. Dinner: stew and raisin pudding. Tea: jam and cheese. I was working as yesterday putting another set of stairs in. I felt too ill to rouse myself to work in the afternoon, so dozed on the steps. I am losing my appetite. I lay down all evening. It was a fine day and the Bosche were shelling during the night.

September 12 Wednesday
Breakfast: bacon. Dinner: bully, pickle and rice pudding. Tea: raspberry jam. I felt like nothing at all today. I hid myself and lay down in the morning after getting quinine tablets from the MOs orderly. I slept in the hut in the afternoon, my appetite has completely gone, I have a headache and a swimming feeling in my head. My cough is shaking up my inside. There is free beer and a concert the canteen with biscuits and cigs tonight but I don't feel equal to it. I got down again in the evening. Today has been a fine day and cooler.

September 13 Thursday
Meals are of no interest – I can't eat any. I have been dodging work and have been dozing all day except for a lecture in the afternoon. I received a 'Passing Show' from Maud. I am getting very concerned about Doll, not a line from her since I came here. It has been a fine day and rather gusty. I must see the 'Fancies'[364] as I realise it may be my only chance before I really layup. I quite enjoy them in spite of my condition, so they must be good and are probably quite equal to anything that I've seen. I got a bottle of real Bass at the interval but it made me terribly thirsty. I was up urinating and drinking all night. There were slight showers in the night.

September 14 Friday
Meals: ditto. I reported sick and was ordered to transfer to the cabins at the Regimental Aid Post. My temperature is 99. No further notice was taken of me all day, I fear that I shall die of weakness through lack of nourishment as I have only been eating fruit lately. I get an old lady and her daughter to beat me one egg in milk twice during the day. They are very decent and charge only a bare cost. It is a long time since I came across anything French at all disinterested. I

---

[364] **The Fancies** – The 6th Divisional Concert Troupe which gave regular concerts. The troupe consisted of nine artistes and two girls known as 'Glycerine' and 'Vaseline'. One was a refugee from Lille and the other was the daughter of an estaminet keeper at Armentieres. The most priceless turn in the show was the singing of 'I'm Gilbert the Filbert' by one of the two girls who could not speak English.

lie down all day and I can neither read nor write. The fellow sharing the cabin with me has swollen glands and can swallow nothing. I felt very lightheaded all day. All the time I seem to dealing with 1000s upon 1000s of sandbags and miles and miles of piles and never seem to allow myself to rest. *(At this point Frank seems to be hallucinating)*

September 15 Saturday
Meals: ditto. I am still providing for myself and get peaches and grapes also. My temperature in the morning is 100.6. The Doctor orders another man for hospital and he's only just returned from leave. He says that he will come to see me again today and get some nice medicine about mid-day but see no more Doctor. I write to Mother and give to our hut orderly to post. There is no news of Doll yet, this brain that won't keep quiet conjures up all sorts of horrible things. The Germans are dropping shells very frequently during the last three days and are very close. I just had a cup of coffee brought to me from the house, the best I've struck out here. I managed to shave this morning and do some reading. Hospital may be the soldier's paradise but the Regimental Aid Post is certainly purgatory. I get bread and milk from the house for supper.

September 16 Sunday
Breakfast: sardines. Dinner: bully and rice pudding. Tea: jam and marg. I managed some sardines and pudding out of the above today and I had poached eggs at dinner. My temperature is down to 98 this morning, so I expect getting sent back to the unit tomorrow. My limbs are black with the dye out of the blankets which are simply passed on to men coming here for detention, I should get something catching out of all that's in them. I went to the camp this morning to see my kit, my tin hat has gone, so I brought the rest with me. I sent a letter to Doll. There is a board across my bed to prevent sagging which caused me to dream mostly a sort of comic drama story where I was usually the bottom man and woke up protesting against the destruction of Government property. Some weird solution for the existence of the board but I shall forget it. *(At this point Frank seems to be hallucinating again)*

September 17 Monday
Breakfast: porridge, bread and marg. Dinner: beef and pickles, rice pudding and cocoa. My temperature is only 97.6 and the Medical Officer does not come in to see me but marks me discharged. I pack up and buy some splendid black grapes and peaches. I make further enquiries about my letters and we are told that the last five were returned to the Battalion yesterday. The motor lorries start off at 1.30pm and we arrive at Ecoivres at about 3pm and find that the Battalion are still at Silverdale Camp, where I report and am told that we are going in support tomorrow. I go down to the Divisional cinema after tea which was very good. I see the postman and get letters from Doll August 30th and September 4th and 8th and from Arthur September 5th, 8th, 13th which prove delicious entertainment for the rest of the evening. It has been a fine day. Arthur writes to say that he is coming over tomorrow. Carter tells me that he has put me down for Boulogne next on 21st September.

September 18 Tuesday

Breakfast: bacon. I awakened at 6am and was told that packs had to be in at 7am as we are moving to the trenches. I go sick hoping to be left behind then I can see Arthur. I just report that I have come straight from the Regimental Aid Post but my temperature is now only 98.9 and I am told by the Medical Officer to report at 6pm to the trench. I receive letters from Mother and Mrs Crossland both September 10th. I fall in at 9.30am for the trenches and am rather done in carrying my kit. We are turned out of the decent baby elephant that I find to make room for stretcher bearers and only get open ones after. Arthur turns up about 2pm with a friend of his who cooks very well and it puts me in good spirits to see him. He consults me about him getting a commission and I advise not while he is as cushy as at present. Carter comes along and advises that he has put my name down for a commission in the Cyclists' Corps. Arthur leaves at 6pm and says that he will come over again as soon as we are out resting. I gave him 5 francs. I report to the Medical Officer and my temperature is 100, Carter is also taken bad, his temperature is 102.6 and both of us are sent into dock which looks like blowing my rest. We landed at 94th **F.A.**[365] in Roclincourt. My temperature is 101 and I get a pill, some hot milk and a very comfortable nights' rest on stretchers and plenty of blankets. It has been a fine and breezy day.

September 19 Wednesday

Breakfast: bacon, brad and marg. Dinner: stew and cabbage. Tea: jam, veal beef and marg. Supper: cocoa and jam. I was sent to 95th F.A. as a stretcher case in the morning and was carried out on a stretcher for the motor ambulances and carefully unloaded at the other end. My temperature is 98, so I am an ordinary case to go to 94th Corps Rest Camp F.A. and go in a horse wagon, taking my own equipment. I arrive at Ecoivres where my temperature is taken and I have time for tea. I am allotted to Ward D, I have had better billets in the trenches. I have been trying to get returned to the Battalion all day but each insists in forwarding me on. I understand that now I cannot possible get away till about 2pm on 21st which will be too late for my rest, so will have to stick out as long as possible. There was a concert in the canteen after tea which was rather good. It was a beautiful day with rain in the night.

September 20 Thursday

Breakfast: cold bacon and porridge. Dinner: beef, beans, veg and rice pudding. Tea: jam, sardines and marg. Supper: soup. My temperature is 97 to 98, so lest I get back too quickly, I decide to tell the Medical Officer of my diabetes. He seemed a very decent sort and the inspection wasn't till 2pm. I was ordered a test for sugar in my urine and then spent the day reading and writing to Doll. I had my breakfast at 7am, dinner at 12 Midday and tea at 4pm, 5pm and 7pm and am getting a tonic pill. I am in wire beds in tiers similar to the big billets. The weather has been fine.

---

[365] - **F. A.** – Field Ambulance.

September 21 Friday

Breakfast: Porridge, herring in tomato. Dinner: stew and rice pudding. Tea: sardines, jam, cheese and marg. There is evidently plenty of sugar in my urine and the Medical Officer marks me for the **CCS**.[366] I go tomorrow morning and I expect to get to base now for dieting. I send a green envelope to Doll with an enclosure for Mother and Auntie Annie, I also write to Mrs Crossland. The weather is fine. I should get very fed up with this place, although the food is decently cooked.

September 22 Saturday

Breakfast: porridge, bully, pickles and marg. Dinner: stew. Tea: 2 eggs, ½ slice of bread and butter. Supper: cocoa, bread and butter. I left the CCS about 10.30 and had a nice drive in the driver's seat of an F.A. Car to Aubingy, where I enter 42nd CCS which seems to be very full. I did not get accommodated with a bed till the afternoon and there was no rice pudding when I had dinner. It was a pleasant surprise to find Carter here; his temperature is down but he feels rotten. I'm put in D ward where he was and he's turned out to K ward to make room for more serious cases. He says this is a rotten hole. I'm feeling as fit as usual and I'm made to get to bed and am placed on a diet right away. I have a special mug of tea made without sugar and am only allowed ½ slice of bread and butter but get two boiled eggs and am the only one in the ward to get jam. The bed feels very cosy but the sheets are not very clean. I get a lovely hot shower bath before getting down. The weather has been beautiful. I had ½ slice of bread and butter with cocoa for supper which was said to be against orders and the man next to me gave me his as well.

September 23 Sunday

Breakfast: porridge ½ slice of bread and butter. Dinner: mince, potatoes and rice pudding. Tea: jam, marg and cheese. Supper: cocoa. I was turned out of D Ward to K Ward, which was a marquee with stretchers on trestles. I saw the Doctor and was then sent to J Ward where there were stretchers on the floor where I did not see a Doctor. I was aroused at 5pm to wash in warm water and after a starvation breakfast, I was left to get the rest of my meals in the mess room, so did better and had no dieting. The weather has been fine. I was then reading all day with plenty of magazines about. I saw **Captain Simpson**[367] who had a bullet in his arm going out to investigate for an A Company.

September 24 Monday

Breakfast: porridge and bacon. Dinner: mutton and potatoes. Tea: jam and bread and butter. Supper: cocoa and cheese. I was marked for evacuation sitting without seeing the doctor. I had attack of faintness and feeling sick whilst awaiting dinner. I embarked on the hospital train in the afternoon about 3.30pm and left about 4.30pm. I was in very comfortable sitting accommodation with

---

[366] **C.C.S.** Casulty Clearing Station.

[367] **Captain Vivian Simpson M.C.** – also served with 13th Y&L and was killed in action on 13th April 1918. He is buried in Outtersteene Communal Cemetery.

tea and supper served in the train. The seats let down in three tiers for sleeping at night. Tossing up I had to share one tier but had quite a comfortable night's sleep though. I arrived in Rouen about 4am and was taken in a motor to 12th General Hospital, where they were all American.

September 25 Tuesday

Breakfast: porridge with beautifully made bread and butter. Dinner: meat loaf and gravy and sago pudding. Tea: bread and butter. Supper: cocoa. I get a wash and shave then have to go to bed and am provided with a blue suit. The beds are nice with white sheets and a counterpane in a marquee which is all open at one side. The doctor sees me about 9.30am and seems very decent and says that there will be no movement for three days. The medicine came around in style, in neat little glasses by nurses. I was reading and writing all day and wrote to Doll and the Post Corporal of 12th Yorks and Lancs. My temperature is over 100 due to stoppage I expect and my urine has been taken for a test. The beautiful weather continues. My cards are taken away in the evening. *I am told my condition means a Blighty which is incredulous.* I have a restless night thinking about it.

September 26 Wednesday

Breakfast: porridge, bread and butter. Dinner: stew and semolina pudding. Tea: bread, butter and cheese. Supper: cocoa. I am told by the sister first thing this morning that I'm for Blighty. My diabetes is *severe* on the card, I **smile,**[368] it is also marked E. Pacecoadial Systalic. I am given clothes but again they are not my own. The stretcher bearers come for me at 10am but I insist on walking. I just started off when I remembered that I'd left my false teeth in a bowl in the wash house. I start walk to look for same much to the consternation of the stretcher bearers who insist that I must be carried from the dispatch tent to the motor ambulance and from thence on board have the arm of the attendant put carefully around me to guide me to my bed in the **Aberdonian.**[369] I leave Rouen about midday and whiskey is brought round to most patients after dinner but there is none for me. I get up and go on the deck in the afternoon where I saw splendid scenery that rather reminds me of the lakeside end of Windermere. Later the sunset effect at the lower reaches of the Seine with a low shore, then fringe of bushy topped trees and a glorious red and orange behind, only wanted a camel to complete the picture. I had very nice comfortable berths but the food is very plain and the orderlies were very obliging. I sent my letter to the Post Corporal of 12th Yorks and Lancs. It has been a fine day and rather cloudy. I had a slight movement in the morning.

---

[368] **I smile** – the significance of this smile is that Frank had known he was diabetic when he signed up in 1915 and did not declare it, as he would not have been able to join the Sheffield City Battalion. He managed to hide the fact for over two years by making sure that he ate on a regular basis, hence his obsession with food.

[369] **S. S. Aberdonian** - was in service as a hospital ship from 16th October 1915 until 16th June 1919, and was one of the smaller hospital ships with accommodation for 245 wounded.

September 27 Thursday

Breakfast: hard boiled eggs and bread and butter. Dinner: stewed beef and beef tea. Tea: diabetic biscuits. Supper: boiled milk. I slept well during the night, the boat rolls a bit and some were sick. We arrive off Southampton about 7am. This is the last ambulance boat across for 10 days on account of the moon. We do not sail as a hospital ship but the markings are painted out and we carry guns. The ship can only do 11 knots. I had a slight movement this morning. We unboarded at 10am and were taken off in sections ascending to home. No.3 is for Leicester, Nottingham, Derby, Sheffield etc but the Embarkation Officer who is to fill up the trains, shoves us in anywhere and the result is that I arrive in the Cheltenham train. They insist on making a stretcher case of me and I could have run rings around them. I sent letters to Doll, Mother and Arthur. I was taken to the Racecourse Hospital and the rule was to have a milk diet till the doctor comes around the next day but get given solids on the sly. I had a fine, hot bath and part with all my clothes. As far as I can make out, I am likely to remain here. It has been a fine day.

September 28 Friday

Breakfast: milk. Dinner: mutton, cabbage and junket. Tea: buttered toast. Supper: milk, toast and butter. I am allowed to get up and am supplied with a blue suit and take a walk around the grounds. There is a billiard table which is horribly cut up. I write to Doll, Mother, Auntie Annie and C Company Quarters. I shall be very lonely till I can get Doll down here. I see my gravity is only 1.025, I should have considered myself cured before the war at that.

September 29 Saturday

Breakfast: toast and butter. Dinner: mutton, cabbage, toast and custard. Supper: buttered toast and milk. I went out after breakfast and filled my pockets with a sort of sweet red crab apple, which are very good. I receive a telegram from Doll already and I am delightfully excited that she is coming to stay with the **Kerrs**[370] here. I get a pass out in the afternoon and send a telegram and letter to Doll and then went to the pictures at the Palace followed by tea at George's where I had filleted sole, anchovy sauce, buttered toast, tea for 2/1d. We rode down and back in a taxi, six of us at 4d each. They have funny ideas of a diet, I have plenty of milk and plenty of bread if it's only just browned over as toast and I am not allowed any sausage meat, minced salmon or porridge. It has been a beautiful day and my gravity is a bit higher, I hear.

September 30 Sunday

Breakfast: fried egg, toast and butter. Dinner: roast mutton, beetroot, apple and blackberry out of pie and custard pudding. Tea: toast and butter. Supper: ditto and milk. I received a letter from Doll and Mother, September 29th and wrote to Doll and Mother. I did not go out and gave voluntary aid with the washing up. I had some apples and nuts in the afternoon and am getting 5 cigs per day. It has been a beautiful day, which I have spent mostly reading.

---

[370] **Kerrs** – relatives of Doll's older sister Maud, who married Malcolm Colin Kerr.

1 October Monday
Breakfast: bacon. Dinner: fish and cabbage with no sauce. Tea: custard pudding. Supper: buttered toast and I got plenty of sausage meat surreptitiously. I received a letter from Doll, September 30th and then went out for the afternoon and started looking up digs for Doll. I walked to Prestbury then got a car into town. I found the Kerr's address in the directory at the Town Hall. I then had tea; 2 poached eggs on toast and a bun and china tea for 1/2d. I just had time to go down to the Kerrs who were very kind and pleasant and were pleased to have Doll and I laid stress on paying. I got back in time to finish my letter to Doll telling her the good news. I am feeling very pleased tonight.

2 October Tuesday
I received a postcard from Mother who is coming over for the day. I get an early pass for 10.30am and meet her at 12 midday. Bring her up to the hospital. It is a beautiful day and she returns at 5.50pm.

3 October Wednesday
I received a letter from Doll, she is coming today and I meet the midday train again. She misses it but arrives by 1.10pm looking exquisite. I bring her up to the hospital, feeling very proud. I just have time to take her to the Kerrs, have a little tea and then go back again. Sister says that I'm five minutes late - her watch is that fast. I hear that special diabetic bread has been ordered for me. Doll brings me a beautiful basket of fruit and eggs and some cakes the latter of which I distribute. I note that my gravity latest is 1.025 as when I came in and my water only averages about 70.3. I had a shower at 6am and after was pulled again by the nurse for being four minutes late by her fast watch. It has been a fine day.

4 October Thursday &
I received a letter from Auntie Annie and a confirmation telegram from Doll saying that she was coming by the next train. It poured all morning and then cleared through for me to start out to meet Doll at 1.45pm. Mrs Kerr brought her up. Doll and I went to **Clara Butt's**[371] concert, a lady pianist and probably the best in town. They get special bread for me now. I had my first **spoon**[372] all afternoon.

5 October Friday
I received a letter from Maud and then write to Maud and Mother. I meet Doll near the hospital and walk to Lover's Lane, intending to take the tram up to Clive Hill and walk to the top. We went to the pictures at the Winter Gardens

---

[371] **Dame Clara Ellen Butt DBE** (1 February 1872 – 23 January 1936), sometimes called Clara Butt-Rumford after her marriage, was an English contralto a remarkably imposing voice and a surprisingly agile singing technique. Her main career was as a recitalist and concert singer.

[372] **To spoon** - A form of affection between a couple.

which was rotten. I arrived back too late for tea but make it up with plenty of tea and butter for supper and beaucoup fruit.

6 October Saturday
I received a letter from Mother, October 5th and she wants one to fire up the digs for a week, bringing Tony. I meet Doll but the shops are closed in town and the pictures are off, so we go straight to the Kerrs. They are very considerate and leave us alone a good bit, we had a fine time. Mrs Kerr lends Doll a lovely fur lined coat and had intimated that she is willing to sell it. I insist that Doll is to clear for anything up to £5. I am getting more venturesome, after giving in my pass, I go out for a good spoon on the stand till 7pm.

7 October Sunday
I get out at 9.50 with an early pass and find that there are no trams running so have to walk to Lickhampton. It is raining heavily with thunderstorms which cleared in the afternoon but we stopped at the Kerrs all the time. Doll and I are left alone pretty well, so I enjoy myself – you bet! Elsie is coming, which means that I must look out digs for Doll and have her nearer at any rate. Mrs Kerr is exceedingly nice. Doll comes up with me again and stops till just gone 7pm, the Sister was out. Some egg custard was saved for me from dinner and feel that my appetite has been satisfied for once. My temperature is 99.8 and my pulse 100 and I am sent to bed early by the nurse.

8 October Monday
My temperature was right down in the morning but I was curtly told by the Sister that I must get into bed for a day or two. I didn't agree to a word! It was a dreadfully wet afternoon but Doll turns up when I had begun to give her up. I am feeling absolutely fit and my temperature is normal at night as is my pulse.

9 October Tuesday
My temperature and pulse are all OK again and the Sister says that I can get up if the Doctor says so but the way that she puts the question leads him to say 'Just as well these are wet, damp day' so I am done again. It was pouring at the time. Doll comes in the afternoon and brings the sunshine with her. I expect her to fire up digs on her way back. I notice that the sweeping is not done so well as when I take it in hand.

10 October Wednesday
I was kept in bed all day and Doll has tea with me. My temperature is 99.4, so it is hopeless for tomorrow.

11 October Thursday
I am kept in bed all day but can sit up in the afternoon. They forget to take my temperature, so I ask the night nurse to. It is normal but she forgets to put it down, so I don't get the credit.

12 October Friday
I am allowed to sit up in the afternoon and Doll came to tea with me. My temperature was 99 at night. I asked the Sister to ask the Doctor if I can go out. She puts it quite fairly but says it is better not to as a chill might be serious. I rather misjudged the Sister, she is being nicer to me.

13 October Saturday
Dr Charles, Military Inspector comes at mid day and rushes through like a whirlwind, marking men for duty etc. He arrives at me our sister ensuring him that I really have diabetes says 'I would like to get him home, wouldn't you' of course 'Yes!' He then marks me recommend for discharge.
I am allowed to get up in the afternoon around the Ward. Doll is incredulous when the ward forestalls me with the news. My temperature is normal at night. There is a splendid concert in the Recreation Room at night and I enjoyed it more than Clara Butt. Doll came with me. The weather has been fine.

14 October Sunday
I am allowed up in the morning and out in the afternoon, when I go to Doll's digs. I push a fellow in a bath chair on my return. My temperature is 99 which is uneasy for the morrow. I wrote to Mother. The weather has been fine.

15 October Monday
The Sister lets me off this time and I sit out in the grounds with Doll in the morning. The Doctor on his rounds fills in my papers for the next Board. I go to the pictures in the afternoon and get some food for a good tea but there is no time for same. There is a concert and temperature check in the evening and Doll goes with me. I try the cold water dodge with my temperature and overdo it and not holding the thermometer properly have no temperature. Fortunately it is only the nurse, so she tries again and it is normal.

16 October Tuesday
Doll called in the morning and we spent the afternoon at her digs. I sent letters to F.E.P. Edwards and Frank Twinn. I drank three mug fulls of water and then my temperature wasn't taken. It was a wet morning and then fine.

17 October Wednesday
Weather was fine in the morning and then Doll came up. We went to the pictures early in the afternoon and then went to Doll's digs. My temperature was only 97.8 at night. I had bacon and tomatoes for tea.

18 October Thursday
I went with Doll to the pictures to see Chaplin the 'The Curse' one of his best. I had a tripe tea with Doll which was fine. I received letters from F.E.P. Edwards and Mother, October 17 and a 'Passing Show' from Maud.

19 October Friday
I take my early pass and have dinner with Doll; chicken and three veg and delicious apple dumplings. We went to the top of Cleeve Hill with the most intensive views of the Severn Valley, the Malvern Hills and the Welsh Mountains. I received a PC from Frank Twinn.

20 October Saturday
Doll came in the morning and we went to the pictures in the afternoon. I wrote to Mother and it was a fine day. My gravity is only 1.020 and sugar is reduced to 10 grain per Oz and I weighed in at 10st 3lbs, a gain of 10lbs in three weeks. Thank goodness that the Board meets on Tuesday or I shall be entirely cured before it meets. I had cold chicken for tea.

21 October Sunday
Doll came up in the morning and we went to the Kerrs for tea, a good feed. I promised to go again before I leave. Another convoy arrives at the hospital and I hear that the Board are not likely to meet till next week after all.

22 October Monday – 29 October Monday
Frank remains in hospital, going out shopping and to the pictures with Doll and regularly taking his temperature.

30 October Tuesday
Medical Board I was the last man that the Doctor saw. He was in a desperate hurry to catch his train so asked me no questions at all except about my teeth and cracked plate and could I do my own work. He marked me down C3 right away, to be on the safe side I suppose. I am given to understand from the RAMC Sergeant that I should go back to my civilian employment.

31 October Wednesday – 10 November Saturday
Frank gets into a routine of meeting Doll each day and going shopping, going to the pictures and concerts and attempts to gets his teeth mended, which involves having a cast taken of them in wax.

11 November Sunday – 18 November Sunday
On leave

19 November Monday
I returned to the depot and was sent to Hending Road Schools in Sunderland. I arrived in Sunderland at 7.20pm. There was a good canteen and soup provided for supper. A fellow has heard that the Battalion are in Italy.

20 November Tuesday
I had a good breakfast of liver and bacon and was sent to Fulwell Schools which is five minutes from the sea and I have a seaview. Dinner was not bad but badly served, we had the same plate for dinner and pudding. Tea was a scramble for margarine and the last one got none, it was the same with the treacle. I went to

the Roker Palace at night and afterwards had supper at **BWTA**[373] which was the best place that I've ever struck, good meat pies at 1½d, coffee and tea for ½d and teacake and marg for 1d. I drew equipment but there is no small kit yet, so I have to manage meals with a jack and a pen knife. I then wrote to Doll and Mother.

21 November Wednesday
I reported sick for my teeth and went to Harfield Schools. I saw there, Crossland's brother who said that his mother had heard from him (12/1411 Pte J. Crossland) several times and he had said that he was alright as a prisoner and that Sergeant Footit was with him too. I keep seeing old Battalion fellows. One has heard that the Battalion is now wiped out. In the afternoon, I go down to Grangetown dentist at the Military Hospital. He won't tackle the metalwork but will prepare casts of my mouth for one to send to John. I go to the Empire in the evening and have supper as before at BWTA and then write to John.

22 November Thursday
Breakfast: Quaker oats, bacon, bread and sausage. Dinner; stew, potatoes and turnips. Tea: ham, bread and marg. I went down to the town fetching my clothing this morning. In the afternoon I was on the Quarter Master's fatigue, moving equipment. The licking soup experience was carried out with great difficulty, drinking soup out of a soup plate. I spent the evening at the BWTA and had supper as usual.

23 November Friday
Breakfast: Quaker Oats, kipper, bread and marg. Dinner: stewed beef, potatoes, turnips and rice pudding. Tea: beetroot, bread and marg. I replaced a man reporting sick as L/C of guard till 3pm. I received a letter from Doll, November 22nd and was paid 5/-. I then went to the pictures and had supper as usual.

24 November Saturday
Breakfast: sausage, dripping and bread. I went to the dentists in the morning, he would have made me a new set if I had not been **B111**.[374] I left the price with casts and a letter to be sent to John Edwards. I had a bath on the way back and then wrote to Doll. I had tea at the Wesleyan Chapel in Roker Road. It was very nice with meat pies only 1d each. I had supper at BWTA as usual.

25 November Sunday
We had a Church Parade in the morning and then tea at the Wesleyan Chapel in Roker Road; brown bread and butter, various cakes and buttered tea cake ad lib, collection only 2d understood. I then had supper at BWTA as above with tea and collection only 1d understood.

---

[373] **BWTA** – The British Women's Temperance Association.
[374] **Form B111** – documentation completed for a 'short service'.

26 November Monday
I spent the morning fetching stencils from Chester Road Schools and noticed **Ingold**[375] there and got my specs mended on the way for 1/-. I went to the Roker Palace in the evening and had supper as usual. I received a letter from Mother.

27 November Tuesday
I went to Whitburn in the morning for a gas experiment in a gas chamber. I received a letter from Arthur and applied for leave to go and see him but was refused on the grounds that I have not been here long enough, so I write to Arthur. I hear that I am down for MOs inspection on Friday.

28 November Wednesday
I am put out on parade. I find that they persist in putting me down as 'Private'. I tell the Doctor that I have diabetes, he says that I ought to have been discharged and sends me to Bede Towers. There is a motor waiting so that I cannot return to Fulwell Schools. The Captain at the hospital orders a test and says that I ought to be marked B&W and will take me before the Major. We stop for dinner and tea and I do not see the Major but am told that they are sending me to hospital for discharge. I arrive in the evening and have broth for supper.

I then wrote to Doll as follows:

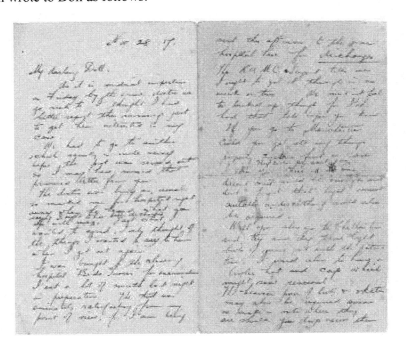

---

[375] **Lieutenant G. J. H. Ingold** - a Sheffield University student who was wounded during the attack on 1st July 1916. He was commissioned on 18th September 1914.

My Darling Doll,

As it is the medical inspection on Friday by the same Doctor we go sick to, I thought that I had better report this morning just to get him interested in my case.

We had to go to another school nearly a mile away before the post was served out so I may have missed that promised letter from you.

The Doctor was very busy as usual, so marked me for hospital right away when he heard what was up with me, saying that I ought to have been discharged, which is just what I wanted to avoid. I only thought of the things that I wanted to say to him when I got out again.

I was brought to the clearing hospital 'Bede Towers' for examination. I ate a lot of sweets last night in preparation. The test was eminently successful from my point of view for I am sent this afternoon to the war hospital here for **discharge**. The RAMC Sergeant tells me I ought to get it through in a week or two. We mustn't feel too bucked up though for I've had that tale before you know.

If you go to Manchester could you get all my things properly together first in case I join you there. One decent suit would be enough and don't forget that light overcoat and suitable underclothing would be required.

Will you also go to Cheltenham and try and dig those light boots of mine out with the patent toes. I used to also have a bowler hat and cap which might save renewal.

The heavier pair of boots and skates may also be required soon, so make a note where they are should you drop across them.

Won't it be fine lovely, if we are together after all for Xmas. I do long for you now.

I tried to get off yesterday to see Arthur but no go as I'd been here such a short time. I will drop you a card as soon as I know my definite address again.

Yours ever xx

Frank

29 November Thursday
I stay in the ward all morning for the Doctor who does not see me. I am put down for the Empire at night and go up to Fulwell after dinner (they let me have two helpings of rice pudding after steak and greens). I get a letter from Doll, November 27th and John Edwards, November 26th. I hand in my equipment etc. my towel, a pair of socks and cardigan are already missing. I hear that I was down for prequit last night as on my papers I'm classed as 'private'. The trams are free also the pictures which I attend in the afternoon, 'Gertie Gitana' at the Empire. I write a PC to Doll and a letter to John Edwards. They only give me sweet snacks for tea and allowed me no butter or marg, so I protest and ask if they have my complaint right. I get coffee and plenty of brown bread and butter

8 December Saturday
I asked the Sister how my discharge was getting on. She knew nothing about it. She says that Campbell will be coming this week. I am expecting the usual re my dates for discharge i.e. Board, Form B3 etc.

Frank continued to write his diary and his entries became very brief and continued to revolve around food, his letters, the repair of his teeth and his day to day existence in hospital.

25 December Tuesday (Christmas Day)
Breakfast: bacon. Dinner: turkey, sausage, ham, Brussels sprouts, plum pudding, mince pie, chocolates, apples, grapes, packet of cigs, cigar and lemonade. The merriest, if not the happiest Xmas Day I've ever spent, if only Doll could have shared it. I woke to find a stocking filled with a razor strop, 45 cigs and matches, two lots of milk chocolate, tobacco and a new penny. It must have cost about 7/6 altogether. We had a dance and a concert at night. I surprised everyone by letting myself go and danced to everything. Cigs, sweets, crystallized fruit, cigars, apples etc were passed around during the evening. I received a present from the hospital of 30 cigs, some matches and a handkerchief.

1918

1 January Tuesday (New Year's Day)
Spoke to Doctor Modlin about my discharge, he said that I should get it and when I mentioned a voucher for Doll he said it wasn't worth while her coming now.

10 January Thursday
O C from A Company 3rd Yorks and Lance sends to ask the date of my embarkation and return. I give him December 21st 1915 for the former and mention that the pay book opens on December 20th. I then went to the Empire in the evening and wrote to Mother

11 January Friday
I went to a whist drive and then wrote the following letter to Doll:

Jeffrey Hall Hospital
Monk Street
Sunderland
January 11. 18

My Darling Doll

I got your dear letter late last night on return from the Empire pantomime. It was a poor show but word of you again made me forget all else. I read your letters over and over again till I know them by heart.

You know very well dearest, you can get whatever you want, so when you want something badly and see it at bargain, snap it before you lose it. Get the coat by all means.

I won't forget a card for Lucy's birthday but in the meantime spend £1 on her from me will you please.

Various indications suggest my Board coming along presently. I had a note from my depot yesterday wanting to know _immediately_ the dates and duration of my service overseas. So I should think they are filling forms in too. The Colonel from *the War Hospital was also around on Wednesday seeing every man but he passed me without any enquiries as to my condition as though my case was quite cut and dried. No Doctor here yet has put any questions to me as regards my complaint.*

I quite expect I shall have had my Board before you have had a fortnight in Manchester. I rather think love from the interest that you are taking now in the sticking of our future home, you really have an idea this time I'm going to get that discharge.

I got a surprise outing on Wednesday night. The St John's Ambulance were giving their annual whist drive and dance and being short of gentlemen sent for a few men who could dance from Jeffrey Hall. I was the first selected having established quite a reputation in that line.

The whist drive took place first. I was nowhere as usual. Dancing commenced about 10pm after supper. The Doctor here had said we could stop till 11pm but it was after 12 o'clock when we reluctantly left and the dance was to continue till 2am. All my partners were nurses from this hospital and I only had one dance with each. I acted more decorously, even than though you had been there pet, for in that case I should only have wanted one partner all the time.

We have a whist drive here tonight. Have you had any skating at all yet, there's nothing doing here. The frost is very severe at times but never lasts more than two nights. Don't forget to put my clothes ready before you go to Manchester.

I never thought of Lucy as being anywhere near 21, it makes me feel very old when I can remember her at Rhyll as a kid with a spade and bucket. I little thought that 1918 would find me still ...

This letter remains unfinished as the second page is missing

13 January Sunday
I stopped in all day and expect that the Board to make a decision in a few days as I was sent for into the office for my particulars.

16 January Wednesday
The Board ring up for me without any notice and I get my discharge quite easily. With view to particular details, I tell them that it is an old complaint.

17 January Thursday
I went to the pictures in the afternoon and a whist drive in the evening and scored 142 over twenty games but missed a prize. I received a letter from Doll and wrote to Mother and then wrote the following letter to Doll:

January 17. 18

My Darling Doll

Another dear letter to feed my longing. I know that you don't really think I shall feel life flat when I leave here. I am looking forward to absolute intoxication. I feel those sweet lips and the kisses I'm thirsting for.

Who's offered £16 for the clock? If it's a dealer, don't sell it but I should be inclined to let it go if it is a private collector but wait a bit first to see if he increases the offer.

I share your disgust at Jack's characteristic action. Why not return him the voucher and ask him to get the Matron to alter it. I'm sure there would be no difficulty. It might postpone you visit till Monday that's all.

I don't want any underclothing sent dear, only the suit and overcoat, a decent tie if I have one and a soft collar or two. I shall have to buy a cap I expect as mine will be packed away at Cheltenham.

The concerts we get here are not as a rule up to much but would form much material for sly amusement if only you could share it with me. It was a N. E. Railway glee concert party last night and they were not an exception. They brought plenty of cigs along though to bribe us into endurance. It is another whist drive tonight.

Hasn't there really been any skating round home yet, perhaps there will be a chance after I get home after all.

I wonder if there will be another letter for me in the morning. I should like to keep the ball rolling like this.

Love and xxxxxs
Yours ever

Frank

I received a letter from Doll, wrote to F.E.P.E. and wrote the following letter to
Doll:

Jeffrey Hall Hospital
Monk Street
Sunderland

January 18. 18

My Darling Doll

*I'm so glad you share my joy at our real prospect at last of establishing that little oft
dreamed of nest together. I know we are going to make each other very happy. I feel
as if I was just going to get really married.*

*The hospital Doctor with another, came round ticking men off this morning. He
just referred to me as the 'diabetic patient' and passed on as usual. The other
Doctor seemed rather surprised and remarked there didn't seem much wrong with
me. They can say what they like now though. I certainly don't look ill but I'm getting
far too much tummy. I think it will have to be a flat with plenty of stairs so you can
set me running up and down continually for coals and exercise dear.*

*I shall be wanting to make a few purchases before I leave here, so do you think
the exchequer could stand me another pound love.*

*By your account, Gladys does seem spoilt. Just tell her she will be 21, herself all
too soon, then the parents she now envies won't compensate her for the increased
care and responsibilities age brings.*

The weather has broken up here, it's raining today.

*I nearly won a prize last night. I missed the fourth by two points. I quite thought
that I was going to win one for I got 142 tucks in the twenty games but the scores
were unusually high last night. The first gent's prize was a watch, the second a
safety razor, third a pocket watch and the fourth a shaving glass. Anyway there will
be a few more chances for me yet.*

*As soon as I get back to you dearest you will know how I have loved and wanted
you.*

Yours ever

Frank x

28 January 1918

This is the last entry that Frank made in his diary

I weighed myself on Rocket Promenade. I was 11st 8lbs, deducting 4lbs for boots leave 11st 4lbs. That is a 1 stone 11lbs gain since I came to England and 13lbs gain since I left Cheltenham.

6 February 1918

Frank was finally discharged on 6th February 1918. The Sheffield City Battalion itself, which had lasted for three and a half years, was eventually disbanded on 28th February 1918, twenty two days after Frank had been discharged. Over the duration of the lifetime of the Regiment, over 3,000 men had passed through the ranks, with over 700 being killed.

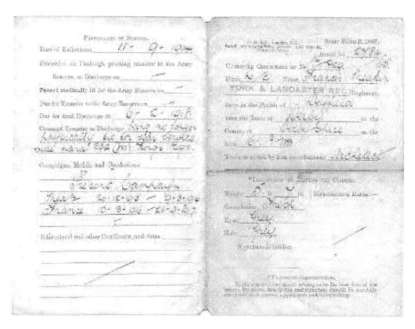

A copy of Frank's Particulars of Service

Frank received his War Badge on 17th April 1918, as did all surviving members of the Sheffield City Battalion.

There was a great deal of contention over the awarding of these, as the Battalion should have been entitled to the 1914 - 15 Star. The 1914 -15 Star was approved in 1918 for issue to the Officers and men of the British and Imperial Forces who served in any 'theatre' of the War between 5th August 1914 and 31st December 1915. Officially, the Battalion did not start their active service until they set foot in Egypt on 1st January 1916 which, if they had not been delayed by submarine activity, would have entitled them to the Decoration.

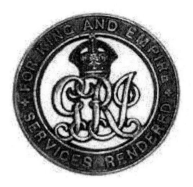

A copy of Frank's War Badge and supporting documentation

1935

Following his early discharge from the Sheffield City Battalion, Frank returned to work as an architect at the City Architect's department at the Town Hall in Sheffield, alongside Mr F. E. Pearce Edwards, the Chief Architect. He continued to study and became a full member of the Association of Architects, Surveyors and Technical Assistants on 14th June 1933. Throughout his war campaign the 'A.A.' had sent parcels to Frank no matter where he was.

The Sheffield City Battalion held Annual Reunions, Known as the '12th Club' and Frank was always a regular attendee. The Club was basically a 'Survivors Club' and consisted of members of the Battalion who had joined prior to 1st July 1916. Other members had to be elected by two other members of the 'Club'.

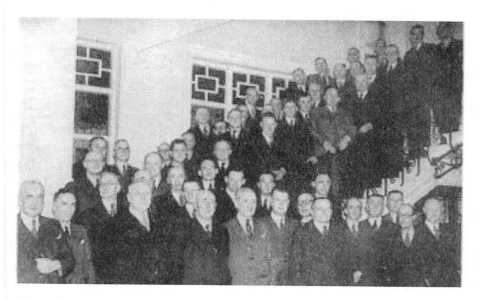

The photograph above is a Reunion of the '12th Club' in the early 1930s. Frank can be seen standing as the bottom of the stairs, the fourth person from the left.

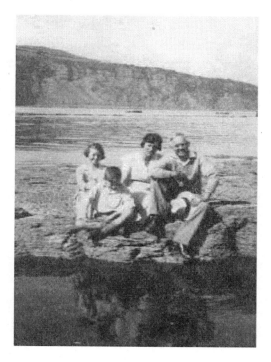

Frank, Doll with their son James and daughter Margaret on holiday in Bridlington.

243

Frank and Doll had two children, Margaret who was born on 20th August 1919 and James who was born on 29th April 1924. Life continued to revolve around working at the Town Hall and family life.

Frank and Doll had a very good lifestyle and travelled a great deal. In 1935 they were planning a cruise with P&O Cruises to Naples, which was becoming a highly fashionable new type of 'holiday'.

During the summer Frank and Doll tended to take the children on their summer holidays to the east coast of England with Bridlington being one of their favourite destinations. Holidays lasted for several weeks and during that time Frank would return to Sheffield during the week and then each weekend return to join the family.

The following letters are three letters that Frank wrote to Doll in August 1935 while she was on holiday with the children in Bridlington:

6 August 1935

City Architect's Department
Town Hall
Sheffield 1

6 August 35

My Dearest Doll

Got home very comfortably at 11.50, the journey seemed very quick. The house seemed very empty without even a dog in. I absent mindedly turned on the wireless and nearly jumped when I heard a voice.

I got the milk all right this morning and a big breakfast, there was an egg left. Think I shall buy some hams and a custard and take them home and gather some logans for dinner.

Enclose a very nice letter from Bill Parkes, expect it's the standard one concocted with his Dad before he set out. Have also forwarded another letter addressed to you.

Love to you all and best regards and thanks for many comforts to Mrs Thompson.

Yours lovingly

Frank xxx

13 August 1935

City Architect's Department
Town Hall
Sheffield 1.

13 August 35

My Dearest Doll

Had another nice ride home, just a few drops of rain on the way and was back three hours as usual. I didn't envy you at the seaside yesterday, very dull and seemed likely to freeze here. It's bright again today but still not warm.

If Mr Thompson cannot bring me on Saturday, it looks pretty convenient to come by train; Sheffield 12.33, Bridlington 3.15. Sunday return is 9pm, arrive Sheffield 11.28. There is a train at midnight. Edith has been getting on with the wash today. I spliced an extra bit on to the flea so she could get on with the ironing. I will post it when it is done. I also took home 6lbs of black currants 8d per lb, she will jam them and let you have some jars if we haven't enough. I'm running down most evenings to Mellor getting my teeth fixed. I think he prolongs the process to make it seem worth more.

They sent me the P&O shore excursion booklet this morning. The Naples excursion is 2/- less than McLacclan's, so he is dropping his and will book us all P&O. I note in his hints what to take, that plus fours are not de rigour on a cruise.

Having got some screws I looked for the leg of the sink stand but couldn't find it, did you put it safely away? I suspect Edith of swallowing it but she declares she's never seen it. The day before we left it was on the window shelf. Edith cooked me a chop with potatoes and peas today and made me pancakes afterwards. I noted there was enough batter left to make some for her kids who were there. I told her to give it to them.

If I come by train Saturday we will have another evenings dancing and start an hour earlier.

Love to all

Your loving Frank xx

P.S. Yorkshire are playing Derbyshire at Scarboro Saturday, Monday and Tuesday. If Derbyshire who are runners up for the Championship do well in their intervening matches, it will be a keen fight for the Championship. There should be cheap excursions from Brid. If you feel like going on Monday or Tuesday let me know where your Members ticket is and I will bring it.

P.P.S. I have just found out that the cricket match is tomorrow, Wednesday, Thursday and Friday. It should be well worth visiting as Derbyshire as they have just beaten Essex and whoever wins this match will almost certainly take the Championship. Here are your tickets. Edith has evidently taken the money home as clothes and the iron are missing, so expect I shall be sending them off tomorrow.

22 August 1935

City Architect's Department
Town Hall
Sheffield 1.

22 August 35

My Dearest Doll

I scarcely dared open your letter this morning, I felt it was to say that you were all returning at once. I was relieved at the note of levity with which it opened.

Edith has brought the washing back, I have packed our towels and what I suppose are Margaret's things but am not sure about a decent light pair of combies and a pink pyjama set with cream braiding but am bringing them.

I bought bilberries today to bottle, a lot dearer than usual but haven't had time to pick my own. The plums are coming in, I shall perhaps have to buy some last thing before I go.

The sales are pretty well over. Kate Down has her sale in the window and also Bradmores. There is a linen dress there with chocolate and pink spots and looks rather well, 23/11. Anyway it was payday today, so I shall not be short if you want to pick up something next week.

Give Margaret my love and best wishes for many happy returns. Of course I remembered her at parting. I hope to get over early on Saturday but shall not know what time till John has been tonight.

Love Yours affectionately

Frank xx

24 August Saturday

Frank arrived in Bridlington on Saturday 24th August and to celebrate his daughter Margaret's birthday they went dancing at the hotel where they were staying. Margaret often spoke of dancing with her Father that night...

The next day on Sunday 25th August 1935 after breakfast, Frank went swimming in the sea at Bridlington.

Whilst he was swimming he came into difficulties as a result of his diabetes. Margaret was watching the commotion on the beach from a distance, not realising the tragedy that was unfolding before her. Despite the desperate attempts of many who were forced to move him further up the beach as the tide came in, Frank died. His Death Certificate records the cause of death as 'Death by Misadventure' and states that 'He was bathing in the sea and was drowned'.

It is so very sad that having survived the horrors of the trenches and escaping death on several occasions, his fate was to drown twenty years later, whilst on holiday with his family. The shock of this was one of the reasons that both Doll and the children never read his diaries.

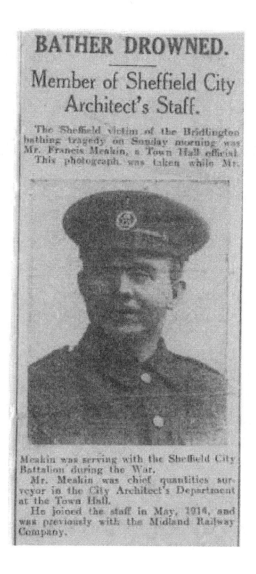

BATHER DROWNED.

Member of Sheffield City Architect's Staff.

The Sheffield victim of the Bridlington bathing tragedy on Sunday morning was Mr. Francis Meakin, a Town Hall official. This photograph was taken while Mr.

Meakin was serving with the Sheffield City Battalion during the War.

Mr. Meakin was chief quantities surveyor in the City Architect's Department at the Town Hall.

He joined the staff in May, 1914, and was previously with the Midland Railway Company.

26 August Monday

It is unimaginable what the family went through over the next few days. Frank was 54 when he died and only had a few years left until he would have been able to draw a pension from the Architect's Association. It was quite clear from the letters that Frank wrote, that they maintained a very good lifestyle. Frank was held in very high regard at Sheffield Town Hall working as the Chief Quantities Surveyor in the City Architect's Department.

Doll received many letters of condolence and in particular one from Mr F. E. Pearce Edwards.

Mr F. E. P. Edwards
F.S.A. F.R.I.B.A.
Ansley Lea
Torquay

26 August '35

Dear Mrs Meakin

I am deeply distressed to hear the news of the dreadful tragedy which has overwhelmed yourself and your children in the terribly sad and sudden loss of poor Frank and I hasten to send you at once my most heartfelt sympathy. We had many years happy association at the Town Hall, where his sturdy integrity and loyal service earned my gratitude and confidence. It is poignant to think that in a very few years he would have earned a retiring allowance for his own private pursuits and leisure. I can only hope the Corporation will be duly mindful of their obligations to his family and I think that Whittaker and the Guild can be depended upon to move urgently in the matter.

I trust you will be upheld in your deep sorrow and find some comfort in the sympathy of many friends. Believe me dear Mrs Meakin.

Yours sincerely

F. E. Pearce Edwards

Let me know if I can do anything

Frank's body was brought back by road to Sheffield a few days later and he was buried in Shire Green Cemetery in Sheffield on 30th August 1935. 12/729 Lance Corporal Francis Meakin can be found in plot number 3816 in Section D of the Cemetery.

Doll continued to live in Sheffield and received some support from the Architect's Association and her family. She died in 1977, surviving Frank by forty two years.

Frank's diaries, together with the last letters that he wrote to Doll, were carefully placed in her writing box where they lay, unread, for almost eighty years.

12
Their Legacy

The Cemeteries and Memorials

Now is your opportunity to visit these wonderful, brave young men. Uniquely, many of them are buried where they fell.

The map below shows the location of the major cemeteries, which are predominantly close to village of Serre on the D919 road from Albert to Bapume.

I would recommend that you devote at least two days to your pilgrimage and stay either in Amiens or in one of the many bed and breakfast establishments in the Somme area. The best by far is 'Les Galets', located on the British front line in Auchonvillers / Beaumont Hamel, owned by Mike and Julie Renshaw, who are guaranteed to add to your experience

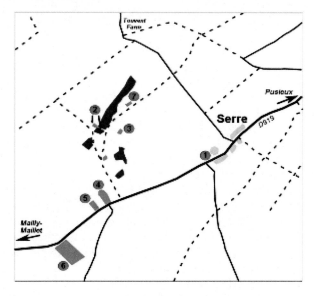

1.   12th Yorks and Lancs Memorial in Serre Village
2.   Sheffield Memorial Park and Railway Hollow Cemetery
3.   Queen's Cemetery
4.   Serre Road No. 1 Cemetery
5.   French Cemetery and Chapel
6.   Serre Road No. 2 Cemetery
7.   Luke Copse Cemetery

The 12th York and Lancaster Memorial

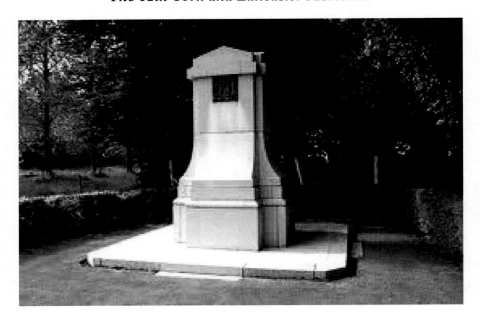

This Memorial was raised by the City of Sheffield for her Pals and is dedicated to the 12th Yorks and Lancs, Sheffield City Battalion. The Monument was designed by Mr J. S. Brown, an ex-Sheffield City Battalion solider who had studied architecture at Sheffield University before the war. Monsieur Augustin Rey was the sculptor in Paris who carried out the final work. It was unveiled on the 21st May 1923, by Lieutenant-Colonel Wedgwood, in the presence of around 150 men who had fought at Serre in 1916. Unfortunately we do not know if Frank attended the ceremony.

Prominent citizens from Sheffield were also present at the ceremony, including Gresford Jones who had been the Vicar of Sheffield during the War and who dedicated the Memorial. Newspaper reports on the 4th July 1916 stated that Serre had been taken on the morning of 1st July but then appeared to have been retaken by the Germans. This suggested even a temporary success here, which was far from the case. However some men from the Sheffield City Battalion had actually reached Serre and their bodies were found by 3rd Division troops when they briefly entered Serre during the unsuccessful attack on 13th November 1916 attack, four months later.

Serre village was 'adopted' by Sheffield after the war.

Sheffield Memorial Park

After the war, the City of Sheffield purchased the area from which the Battalion fought from on 1st July 1916 which is now known as Sheffield Memorial Park. It is situated off of the D919 road close to the village of Serre.

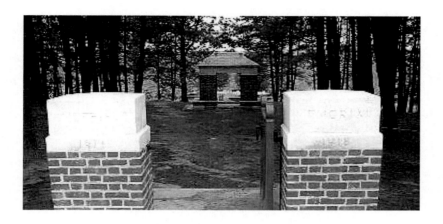

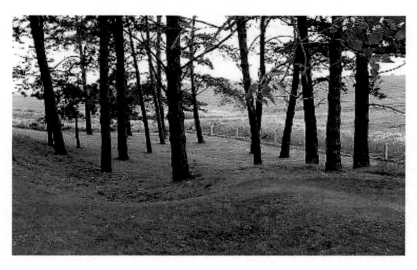

Sheffield Memorial Park is a wooded area where the original frontline trenches and the shell-holes in the ground have been preserved. It is the only piece of British Front Line that is preserved on the Somme and was opened as a Memorial Park in 1936. There is a recent information tablet placed by Sheffield City near the front of the park which has a coloured map, showing the positions of the various Battalions that fought here on July the 1st 1916, along with the

German trenches and machine-gun positions that they advanced towards. Also located here are Memorials to the Accrington, Barnsley and Chorley Pals, who also suffered huge losses on that day. Sheffield Memorial Park is also the location of the four copses, Matthew Copse, Mark Copse, Luke Copse and John Copse, however Matthew Copse, which was sited just to the south of the Memorial Park, has not grown back into a wood.

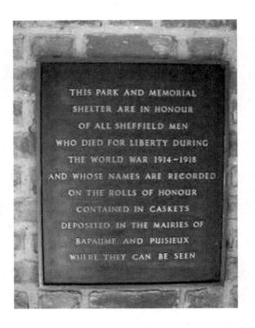

THIS PARK AND MEMORIAL
SHELTER ARE IN HONOUR
OF ALL SHEFFIELD MEN
WHO DIED FOR LIBERTY DURING
THE WORLD WAR 1914–1918
AND WHOSE NAMES ARE RECORDED
ON THE ROLLS OF HONOUR
CONTAINED IN CASKETS
DEPOSITED IN THE MAIRIES OF
BAPAUME AND PUISIEUX
WHERE THEY CAN BE SEEN

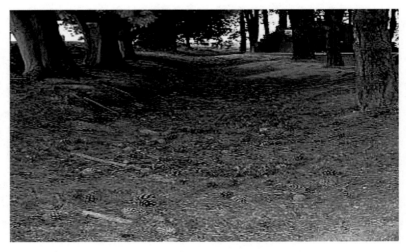

Queens Military Cemetery

This Cemetery is located in No Man's Land, which is relatively unique in terms of the Somme. It contains a large number of Sheffield City Pals who attacked from their trench in John Copse on 1st July 1916, which is now within the Sheffield Memorial Park.

In the spring of 1917 the battlefields of the Somme were cleared by V Corps and a number of new Cemeteries were made. Queens Cemetery, originally known as Queens V Corps Cemetery No 4 was designed by N. A. Rew. The graves are from 31st, 3rd and 19th Divisions who died on 1st July 1916, 13th November 1916 and in February 1917. There are 311 graves in total and 131 of them are unidentified.

Buried here from the Sheffield City Battalion and mentioned in the diaries are:

Harry Thomas Hale, John William Parker, Gordon Henry Saddler, Alfred James (Alf) Thorne and Albert (Tommy) Webster who all died on 1st July 1916.

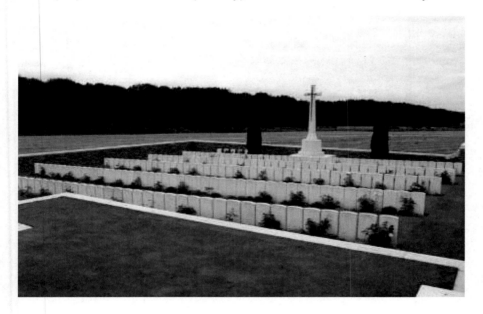

Luke Copse Military Cemetery

This cemetery, originally known as V Corps Cemetery No. 19, stands in No Man's Land and is the closest to the front line trench from where the Sheffield City Battalion fought on 1st July 1916.

It is a small cemetery with only 72 burials, 28 of whom are unidentified and contains the men of the Sheffield City Battalion who attacked here on 1st July 1916 and 13th November 1916. Many of the burials feature double headstones.

Buried here from the Sheffield City Battalion and mentioned in the diaries are:

Horace Driver, brothers Frank Gunstone buried in Grave No. 11, William Gunstone who is buried in Grave No. 21 and Arthur James Hollis who all died on 1st July 1916

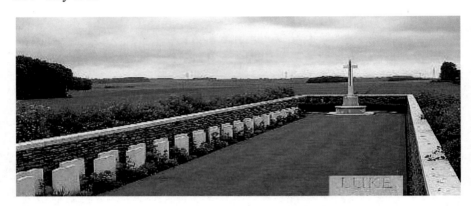

Sucrerie Cemetery

The Sucrerie Military Cemetery is situated on one of the main routes from Colincamps to the front line of 1st July 1916, Colincamps being a village 11 kilometres north of Albert. Colincamps and "Euston", a road junction a little east of the village, were within the Allied lines before the Somme offensive of July 1916. During later Somme battles mass graves were prepared for the casualties. It was started by the French on the south side of a tree lined road coming down from Colincamps. Camouflage netting hung along the edges of the road to protect troops from the German artillery.

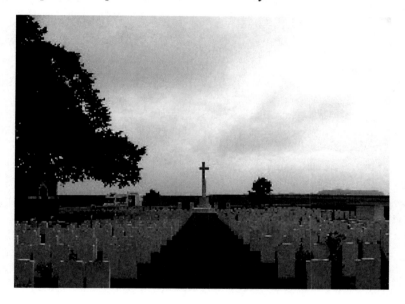

Buried here from the Sheffield City Battalion and mentioned in the diaries are:

Alexander McKenzie who died on 4th April 1916, William Arthur Emerson and Harry Handbury who both died on 8th April 1916. Arthur Douglas Frost, Stafford Hardwick, Edward Gordon Rogers, Harold Todd and Gilbert Unwin who all died on 3rd May 1916. John William Ellis and Percy Charles Richards who both died on 4th May 1916

A. E. Arrowsmith, Wilfred Barlow, Percy Burch, Gilbert George Cook, Horace Bradley Dowty, Edwin Furniss, Clement Johnson, Robert Haly Bruce Matthews, Bernard John Register, Alfred Slack, Richard Elvidge Smith, Joseph Strickland, Thomas William Stubley, Wilfred Henry Cranstone Tucker and Richard Henry Walker who all died on 16th May 1916. Frederick Walker who died on 27th May 1916

Bertrancourt Military Cemetery

This Cemetery was used by a British Field Ambulance station in 1916. Buried here are casualties from the Battalion's tour of the front line of in June 1916.

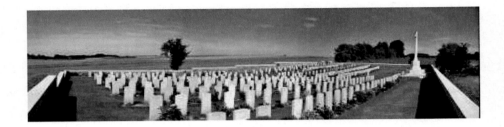

Buried here from the Sheffield City Battalion and mentioned in the diaries are:

Henry Charles Clay and Ernest Clifford Thomas who both died on 17th June 1916, Francis Gleave who died on 14th June 1916 and Cecil George Ibbotson who died on 21st June 1916

Serre Road No.2 Cemetery

There are many 'concentration' cemeteries in the Somme area where bodies were buried, often some distance from the place where they were killed. Serre Road No. 2 Cemetery located on the D919 is an example of this. This huge Cemetery was designed by Sir Edwin Lutyens and contains over 7,000 burials. This cemetery is probably a good place to visit first, to begin to understand the sheer scale of human sacrifice. This was also the site of the German stronghold known as the Quadrilateral or Heidenkopf. Remembered here from the Sheffield City Battalion is A. E. Bull who was killed in action on 1st July and has a private memorial in Sheffield Memorial Park.

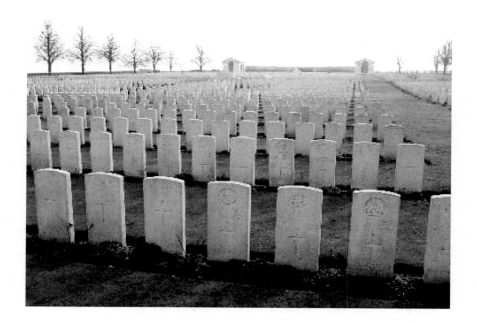

Thiepval Memorial

This structure is a Memorial to over 73,000 men who have no known grave and fell on the Somme between July 1916 and March 1918. It was designed by Sir Edwin Lutyens and stands 140 feet high, dominating the surrounding area.

It has sixteen piers on whose faces the names of the Missing are inscribed. The Missing are listed firstly with the Regiment, then ranks in order of seniority and then within each rank names in alphabetical order.

Remembered here from the Sheffield City Battalion and mentioned in the diaries are:

Company Sergeant Major William Marsden who died on 17th June 1916

Henry Cecil Crozier who died on 16th May 1916 and William H. Marsden who died on 17th June 1916

Cyril Atkinson, Arthur Carter, Arthur Clarke, George Colley, Rodney Frank Devey, Horace George Parkin, Walter Thomson, Sidney George Wardill and his brother C. H. Wardill, Nelson Waterfall and Harry Wood who all died on 1st July 1916.

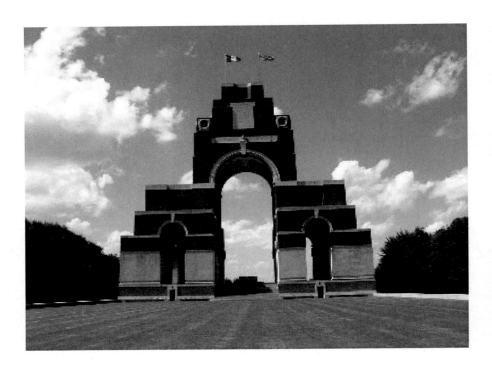

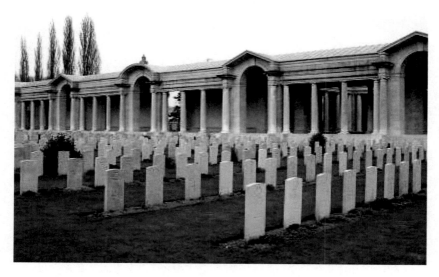

The burials that are in Arras and Bailleul Road tend to be from NCOs who joined the Battalion after the Battle of the Somme as a result of depleted numbers in the Battalion.

Arras Memorial and Cemetery

The Arras Memorial commemorates almost 35,000 servicemen from the United Kingdom, South Africa and New Zealand who were killed in the Arras sector and have no known grave.

Remembered and buried here from the Sheffield City Battalion and mentioned in the diaries are:
Joseph Boocock, Wray Crabtree and Lewis Harrison who all died on 10th May 1917. P. M. West, A. Bullivant, John William Fell, Wilfred Handley, John Humphrey, James Septimus Johnson, and William Smith who all died on 12th May 1917. Henry Cecil Ellis who died on 18th May 1917. Thomas Chapman who died on 4th June 1917. Thomas Dunne who died on 16th June 1917. Windross Fletcher, W. Gilberthorpe and Frank Johnson who all died on 27th June 1917.

Bailleul Road Military Cemetery

Bailleul Road East is a large cemetery which has a fairly irregular layout with the Cross of Sacrifice standing at the front. On one side of the cemetery are two cupolas with the Stone of Remembrance between them. During the war, belts of barbed wire were to be found around the position the cemetery now occupies. There are 1287 men buried here, with only 42% who are identified.

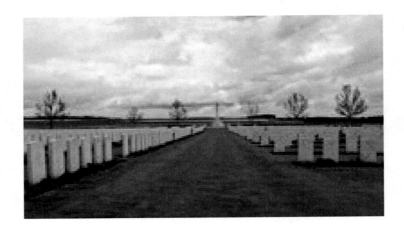

Remembered here from the Sheffield City Battalion and mentioned in the diaries are:

Percy Robinson Deville who died on 3rd May 1917, William Hooton who died on 6th May 1917, Henry Hooton who died on 12th May 1917 and C.W. Pimm who died on 18th May 1917

There are many other cemeteries both on the Somme and in the Arras and Vimy areas mentioned in the diaries where you will find members of the Sheffield City Battalion. These include:

In the Somme and surrounding area:
Couin Military Cemetery
Courcelles Military Cemetery
Euston Road Military Cemetery
Hebuterne Military Cemetery
Louvrencourt Military Cemetery - which was the site of a British Field Ambulance Hospital
Merville Community Cemetery
Sailly au Bois Military Cemetery - which was the site of a British Field Ambulance Hospital

In the Arras and Vimy areas:
Albuera Military Cemetery, Bailleul
Aubingy Community Cemetery
Awoingt Military Cemetery
Hooge Crater Military Cemetery
Le Touret Military Cemetery, Richbourg
Loos Memorial
Roclincourt Military Cemetery

Two years in the making
Ten minutes in the destroying
That was our history

(Covenant with Death by John Harris)

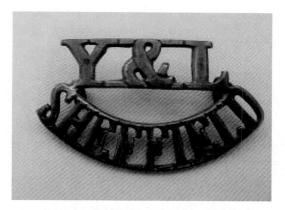

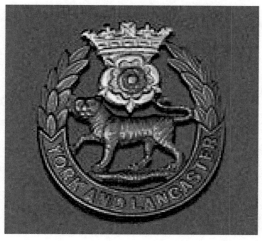

Bibliography

The following books and documents have been used for reference in the compilation of this work:

Published Sources

Gibson, R. & Oldfield, P. *Sheffield City Battalion*. Pen and Sword 1994
Special thanks are given to Ralph Gibson who wrote giving his permission to use any of his information in the production of this book

Bilton, D. *Oppy Wood*. Pen and Sword Battleground. 2005.

Brittain, V. *Testament of Youth*. Arrow/Hutchinson 1960.

Brown, M. *Wipers Times*. Little Books Limited 2006.

Cave, N. *Beaumont Hamel*. Pen and Sword Battleground. 1994.

Cave, N. *Vimy Ridge*. Pen and Sword Battleground. 2004.

Coombes, R. MBE. *Before Endeavours Fade*. After the Battle. 1983.

Gliddon, G. *The Battle of the Somme, a Topographical History*. Leo Cooper 1990.

Harris, J. *Covenant with Death* (novel). Hutchinson 1961.

Holmes, R. War *Walks from Agincourt to Normandy*. BBC Books 1996.

Holt, Major and Mrs. *Ypres, Battlefield Guide. Pen and Sword 2001.*

Holt, Major and Mrs. *Somme, Battlefield Guide*. Pen and Sword Battleground. 1996.

Horsfall, J. & Cave, N. *Serre*. Pen and Sword Battleground. 1996

McCarthy, C. *The Somme The Day by Day Account*. Brockhampton Press 1998.

MacDonald, L. *Somme*. Michael Joseph 1983.

McPhail, H. *Wilfred Owen Poet and Soldier 1893 – 1918*. Gliddon Books 1993.

Malins, G. H. *How I filmed the War.* Herbert Jenkins 1920.

Michelin Guides: *The Somme Volume One.* Michelin 1919.

Middlebrook, M. *Somme Battlefields.* Martin Middlebrook 1991.

Middlebrook, M. *The First Day of the Somme.* Allen Lane 1971.

Putkowski, J. & Sykes, J. *Shot at Dawn.* Wharncliffe Publishing 1989.

Reed, P. *Walking the Somme.* Pen and Sword Battleground. 2011.

Sheffield, G. *The Chief: Douglas Haig and the British Army.* Aurum Press 2012.

Official Sources

The National Archives

The Commonwealth War Graves Commission for records of burials and memorials

Websites
www.pals.org.uk
www.britishnewspaperarchive.co.uk
www.ww1battlefields.co.uk
Accrington Pals website
Great War Forum website

Selective Index

Neuville St Vaast, 240, 207, 208, 213, 214
New Zealand troops, 172
Nolux les Mines, 220, 221
Norfolk Barracks, 18

O

Oppy Wood, 185, 186, 187
Orange, 58

P

Parados, 65, 75, 80, 104, 107, 146
Passing Show, 56, 61, 63, 122, 149, 159, 162, 182, 192, 193, 198, 201, 203, 207,
    209, 210, 211, 214, 216, 218, 221, 223, 231

Personnel:
Allen – Major D. C, 100, 187, 192
Appleton - 40185 Lance Corporal Cyril, 168
Arrowsmith - 12/25 Private A. E. 80, 255
Askew - 12/578 Corporal Herbert, 120, 140, 143
Astill - 41080 Private A. 52
Atkinson - 12/1381 Private Cyril, 43, 45
Ballard - 12/582 Private E, 162
Ballinger - 17821 Private H, 206
Bamford - 3/2486 Lance Corporal Jethrew, 209
Barlow - 31558 Private John, 137
Barlow - 12/291 Private Wilfred, 80
Bartholomew - 12/293 Sergeant H, 30
Beaumont - 31965 Private Alfred, 188
Beley - Captain G, 42
Berry - Lieutenant R. D, 147, 189
Blacktin - 12/596 Private S. C, 110, 147
Blenkarn - 12/597 Lance Corporal William, 117
Boocock - 16166 Private Joseph, 188, 259
Boot - 12/304 Sergeant W. H, 205
Bourne - 31348 Sergeant W. K, 159
Bradshaw - 12/602 Lance Corporal J. E, 41
Bramham - 12/1668 Private George Henry, 134
Briggs - 23155 Sergeant G, 195, 197
Brookes - 12/317 Sergeant, 144
Broomhead - 12/319 Private J, 45
Browning - Lieutenant D. O, 211
Bullivant - 4845 Private A, 189, 259
Burch - 12/1267 Private Percy, 80, 255
Carter - 12/1716 Private Arthur, 38, 258
Carter - 12/1323 Private W. R. 155, 159, 160, 165, 168, 183, 225, 226
Cavill - 12/1190 Private Albert, 71
Chadwick - 38013 Lieutenant John Henry, 152, 170

Chamberlain - 12/889 Private Charles Frederick, 133
Chapman - 22258 Private Thomas, 195, 259
Charlesworth - 12/561 Sergeant F, 66, 74, 122, 151, 163
Clarke - 12/73 Private Arthur, 44, 45, 258
Clay - 12/1388 Sergeant Henry Charles, 90
Cloud - Lieutenant C.C, 80, 84, 99, 131
Clough - Major T. C, 64, 99
Coats - 12/620 Private W. 35
Coates - 40092 Private W. 120
Cook - 12/622 Private F. 33, 83, 140
Cook - 12/1469 Private Gilbert George , 255
Colley - Captain W. A, 20, 22, 28, 32, 42, 49, 51, 61, 70, 71, 83, 85, 88, 91, 96,
    100, 258
Colquhoun - Captain J. F, 23
Cousins - Captain A. N, 23, 34, 40, 49, 61, 63, 101, 113, 115, 116, 117, 118,
    120, 193
Cowen - 12/78 Private H, 46
Cowen - Captain J. C, 134, 157
Crabtree - 37936 Private Wray, 188, 259
Crawford - Captain S, 151, 160, 164, 207
Crossland - 12/1411 Private J, 217, 218, 233
Crossthwaite - Colonel J. A, 23, 99
Crozier - 12/628 Sergeant Henry Cecil, 23, 73, 74, 81, 258
Dale - 12/631 Sergeant A, 199
Davies - 39129 Lance Corporal H. G, 114
Davies - Captain K. R, 114
Davies -12/916 Private L, 168
Devey - 12/1336 Private Rodney Frank, 89, 97, 258
Deville - 31587 Private Percy Robinson, 185, 260
Dowty - 12/638 Private Horace Bradley, 16, 60, 69, 80, 255
Driver - 12/641 Private Horace, 64, 254
Dunne - 38015 Private J. E, 170
Dunne - 38016 Lance Corporal Thomas, 170, 171, 259
Ellis - 21891 Corporal Henry Cecil, 192
Ellis - 12/644 Private J. S. Ellis, 165
Ellis - 12/560 Company Sergeant Major John William, 20, 74, 75
Ellison, 12/910 Sergeant C, 115, 125, 138
Emerson - 12/358 Private William Arthur, 68, 255
Evans - 12/912 Sergeant C. C, 144
Everatt - Company Sergeant Major T, 150
Fairclough - 12/2047 Private Joseph Seamore, 121
Faker - 12/647 Acting Sergeant Major F. L, 74, 134
Fell - 12/1052 Private John William, 189
Fisher - Lieutenant Colonel H. B. 123
Fletcher - 31981 Private Windross, 199, 259
Flint - 12/1375 Private W, 86
Footit - 19187 Sergeant P, 218, 219, 233

Ford - 12/100 Private William Edgar, 137
Foxon - 12/105 Private Alan Hugh, 120
Frost - 12/1238 Private Arthur Douglas, 75, 255
Furniss - 12/651 Private Edwin, 80, 255
Gallimore, 12/1123 Sergeant R, 117
Gamble - 39135 Corporal F, 163
Garfitt - 12/652 Private L. 83
Garvey - 12/653 Private F. J, 37
Gilberthorpe - 12/1059 Private W, 199, 259
Gillatt - 12/1809 Private F, 199
Gleave - 12/1354 Private Francis, 88, 256
Gough, General, 161
Gould - 12/656 Sergeant Joseph William, 192, 198, 199
Grant - Captain D. E, 33, 36, 38, 39, 40, 41, 44, 45, 46, 47, 62, 72, 75, 77, 79, 80, 81, 121
Greaves – 12/1406 Private E. F, 42
Greaves - 12/385 Private T. A, 43, 71
Gunstone - 12/660 Lance Corporal Frank, 86, 254
Gunstone - 12/661 Private William Walter, 86, 254
Gurney - Major C. H, 105, 107, 122, 128
Hacking - 38057 Sergeant William, 159
Haddock - 7595 Private J. A, 118, 119
Haig - Field Marshal Douglas, 78, 110, 119, 263
Hale - 12/663 Private Harry Thomas, 16, 26, 28, 71, 72, 83, 89, 99, 253
Hall - 12/663 Private Herbert, 104, 147, 154, 157, 160, 187
Handbury - 12/388 Private Harry, 68, 255
Handforth - 12/133 Private Charles Haydn, 21
Handley - 39042 Private Wilfred, 189, 259
Hardwick - 12/668 Lance Corporal Stafford, 75, 255
Harrison - 27794 Private Lewis, 188, 259
Hern - 43898 Private Howard, 189
Heslington - 12/395 Private F. H. 46
Hill - 12/676 Corporal Jeremy, 72, 77
Hill - 12/677 Corporal Tommy W, 38
Hills - 12/678 Private A. J, 165
Hollis - 12/687 Private Arthur James, 81, 254
Hood – Major F. J. C, 195
Hooton - 31618 Private Henry, 189, 260
Hooton - 31626 Private William, 186, 260
Hough - 12/691 Private Ernest Hough, 105
Hughes – Colonel H, 19
Humphrey - 12/413 Private John, 189, 259
Ibbotson - 12/416 Private Cecil George, 92, 256
Ingold - Lieutenant G. J. H. 234Jackson - Lieutenant C. A, 203
Jarvis – 18582 Sergeant R. A, 217
Johnson - 24497 Corporal Frank, 117, 259
Johnson - 12/700 Private Clement, 255

Richards - 12/757 Private Percy Charles, 16, 75, 255
Rickman, Colonel of East Lancs, 84
Rideout - 12/758 Private F.O, 45, 212, 213, 217
Roberts - 12/761 Sergeant A. W, 23, 74
Roberts - 12/762 Corporal C, 23
Roberts - 12/1029 Sergeant E. W, 41
Roberts - 12/765 Lance Corporal N. W, 219
Rogers -12/767 Private Edward Gordon, 16, 75, 255
Rush - 12/770 Private B, 78
Rushby - 12/1558 Private L, 217
Saddler - 12/771 Private Gordon Henry, 16, 90, 253
Schofield - 12/1185 Private H, 42
Sharpe - Private 12/943 J. T, 108
Simpson - Captain Vivian M.C, 226
Slack - 12/516 Private Alfred, 80, 255
Smith - 12/1057 Lance Corporal Richard Elvidge, 45, 80, 255
Smith - 38046 Private William, 189, 259
Stimpson - 12/790 Corporal A, 217, 219, 186
Strickland - 12/1480 Private Joseph, 80, 255
Stubley - 12/1145 Private Thomas William, 80, 255
Tagg - 12/528 Private Reginald, 46
Taylor - 12/1997 Corporal E, 144, 219
Thomas - 12/249 Private Ernest Clifford, 90
Thompson - 11225 Sergeant A, 177
Thompson - 2nd Lieutenant J, 212
Thompson- 12/1069 Sergeant Walter, 95, 258
Thorne - 12/799 Private Alfred James (Alf), 16, 52, 57, 59, 60, 99
Todd - 12/802 Private Harold, 16, 37, 75, 255
Tucker - 12/805 Private Wilfred Henry Cranstone, 80, 255
Tyzack - 12/1846 Lance Corporal W.H, 42
Unwin - 12/807 Private Gilbert, 16, 74, 75, 255
Varley - 12/808 Corporal J. S, 47, 91
Walker - 12/1084 Lance Corporal Frederick, 84, 255
Walker - 12/1268 Private Richard Henry, 80, 255
Walton - Private G. 106
Wardill - Lieutenant C. H, 95, 96, 258
Watson - 23165 Private J, 143
Webster - Tommy Webster – 12/1165 Private Albert (Tommy), 64, 97, 253
Welsh - 12/550 Lance Corporal W. A, 46
West - 12/262 Private P. M, 76, 259
Westby - 2nd Lieutenant F. H, 94, 102, 192, 209
Weston, (Hunter) General & Corps Commander, 94, 100
Whipple - 12/1411 Corporal H. D, 203, 204, 205, 210, 211, 213, 219
Whittaker - 12/265 Private George W, 146
Wilson - Lieutenant F. B, 212
Wilson - 12/1412 Private Hector Atkinson, 117
Windle - 12/826 Private G, 46

Warnimont Wood, 136, 139

Y
Yellow Line, 146
Ypres, 170

Z
Zeppelin raid over Derby, 48